Health Sciences Collection Management for the Twenty-First Century

Medical Library Association Books

The Medical Library Association (MLA) features books that showcase the expertise of health sciences librarians for other librarians and professionals.

MLA Books are excellent resources for librarians in hospitals, medical research practice, and other settings. These volumes will provide health care professionals and patients with accurate information that can improve outcomes and save lives.

Each book in the series has been overseen editorially since conception by the Medical Library Association Books Panel, composed of MLA members with expertise spanning the breadth of health sciences librarianship.

Medical Library Association Books Panel

Lauren M. Young, AHIP, chair
Kristen L. Young, AHIP, chair designate
Michel C. Atlas
Dorothy C. Ogdon, AHIP
Karen McElfresh, AHIP
Megan Curran Rosenbloom
Tracy Shields, AHIP
JoLinda L. Thompson, AHIP
Heidi Heilemann, AHIP, board liaison

About the Medical Library Association

Founded in 1898, MLA is a 501(c)(3) nonprofit, educational organization of 3,500 individual and institutional members in the health sciences information field that provides lifelong educational opportunities, supports a knowledge base of health information research, and works with a global network of partners to promote the importance of quality information for improved health to the health care community and the public.

Books in the Series

The Medical Library Association Guide to Providing Consumer and Patient Health Information edited by Michele Spatz
Health Sciences Librarianship edited by M. Sandra Wood
Curriculum-Based Library Instruction: From Cultivating Faculty Relationships to Assessment edited by Amy Blevins and Megan Inman
Mobile Technologies for Every Library by Ann Whitney Gleason

Health Sciences Collection Management for the Twenty-First Century

Edited by
Susan K. Kendall

ROWMAN & LITTLEFIELD
Lanham • Boulder • New York • London

Published by Rowman & Littlefield
A wholly owned subsidiary of The Rowman & Littlefield Publishing Group, Inc.
4501 Forbes Boulevard, Suite 200, Lanham, Maryland 20706
www.rowman.com

Unit A, Whitacre Mews, 26-34 Stannary Street, London SE11 4AB

British Library Cataloguing in Publication Information Available

Library of Congress Cataloging-in-Publication Data Available

ISBN 9781442274211

Contents

Figures

Tables

Preface

Collection management, including collection development, as an area of health sciences librarianship does not always get the spotlight these days. Newly graduated librarians who are interested in the health sciences are often focused on the outward-facing activities of teaching, instructional design, liaison, and embedded librarian or informationist roles. Others, interested in the "back end," are absorbed in assessment, usability, creating metadata, and developing repositories. Compared to some of these areas, "collection management" can sound old-fashioned, but *Health Sciences Collection Management for the Twenty-First Century* sets out to show that collection management is anything but old-fashioned. To be sure, new roles for health sciences librarians are exciting and demonstrate our diversity of talents. But, despite a lot of talk to the contrary, collections are still at the heart of the library and are a huge part of what users are looking for when they approach their health sciences librarian and library (whether physical or online). In fact, most of the roles mentioned above are simply new ways for librarians to put users in touch with the collections. Collection management librarians are learning that their jobs are increasingly complex and that they need to consider the concerns of pedagogy, design, discovery, usability, metadata, and other related fields when they make purchasing decisions. All departments of the library are interconnected, with the collection at the center of activities. What is the purpose of discovery tools if there is no collection to discover? Alternatively, why have an excellent collection that no one can find or use well? Collection management librarians are collaborating even more than ever with librarians in other roles to create a library that is user-centric. This book was written to demonstrate the breadth of issues involved in collection management, to inspire and advise those interested in and doing collection management, and to acquaint other librarians not doing collection management with many of the ways that what they are doing in the library is informed by and informs collection matters.

Health sciences libraries have long been on the cutting edge of trends in the library world, thanks in part to the nature of the health care field, which puts an emphasis on timely access to current information, and in part to leadership from the National Library of Medicine in the United States. In the 1960s, the National Library of Medicine developed the Medical Literature Analysis and Retrieval System (MEDLARS), the first library application of computers to search for scientific literature (Dee 2007). In the early 2000s, biomedical publishers were early experimenters with open-access models, and biomedical funding agencies were some of the first to implement open-access policies. Even more recently, by necessity, health professionals have been early adopters of mobile devices for information retrieval in clinical settings, and health sciences libraries have been licensing apps to meet those needs. For two decades, health sciences librarians have been leading the way in focusing on electronic resources. A more recent outcome of that focus has been dramatic decisions by some health sciences libraries to go almost totally electronic, deaccession physical collections, move materials off-site, and re-purpose space. Just how radical are the changes occurring for collections in libraries today? The chapters and stories in this book document these changes.

This book is intended for those with any level of experience in health sciences collection management. For those new to the field, it will cover the basics and more. It won't tell new librarians what to buy, but it will give them background information and criteria that can educate their decision making. For experienced librarians, this book also goes deeper than that, exploring the bigger picture of trends in collections and how changes in the field will affect choices today and in the future. Single chapters about collection management have appeared in general books about health sciences librarianship, but this book is able to go into much more depth on each topic. Every effort has been made to be inclusive of different types of health sciences libraries, but the reality is that academic librarians spend much more time writing and speaking at conferences about their activities, and there is simply more data and more information available about them. Also, most of the authors of this book are at academic or research institutions. It certainly should be acknowledged that there can be vast differences between managing collections in a hospital versus a community college or a research health sciences library in a medical center. However, there are also many similarities in the concerns of health sciences librarians in all these institutions, and the hope is that all will find something of value in these pages.

Chapter contributors are all working in the United States, but in different regions and institutions. The varied perspectives they bring to the topics discussed demonstrate the thoughtfulness of today's health sciences collection management librarians. Interspersed between the chapters of this book, library stories illustrate the topics discussed in practical, specific, and timely detail. While whole books go into some of these subjects on their own in depth, the treatment of each topic here focuses on the unique perspective and concerns of the health sciences collection manager.

The book begins in chapter 1 with the current context of health sciences publishing. It is important for health sciences librarians, and especially collection management librarians, to understand how trends in the publishing industry affect libraries. There is a discussion of the varied types and formats of materials available to libraries and the challenges facing both publishers and libraries today with licensing, preservation, open access, Big Deals, and predatory publishing. A recommended list of sources for keeping current on scholarly publishing is included in this chapter, and a story about librarians developing a collection to support a brand-new medical school follows.

Chapter 2 is very practical. It covers all the details that librarians need to know and understand to manage a twenty-first-century health sciences collection, from collection policies to selection and deselection of monographs, journals, databases, and other types of media. The focus is naturally on electronic materials, although print materials are covered as well. Topics such as staffing, collaboration with other librarians, and licensing also comprise significant sections of this chapter. A story about a major medical center health sciences library's weeding project follows.

Chapter 3 is about budgeting and includes practical concerns such as how to develop a budget, how to allocate a budget, how to deal with price increases, and how to factor such services as interlibrary loan, pay-per-view, aggregated access, and patron-driven acquisitions models into an overall strategic purchasing scheme. The chapter also explores the effect of Big Deals and open-access publishing on health sciences collections budgets. It concludes with a sizable section on how to negotiate with vendors, with many tips for both new and experienced librarians. Following this chapter is a story of the creation of a hospital library consortium for group purchasing.

Chapter 4 introduces the concept of evidence-based librarianship and covers user-oriented assessment of collections, an area attracting growing attention in this age of demonstrating return on investment. All forms of assessment are discussed: benchmarks, usage statistics, citation analysis, surveys, and focus groups. The story following this chapter is about a large library system's cancellation of a major vendor product. Assessment of the collection and user needs was a part of that account.

Chapter 5 brings in the very timely theme of collaborative collection management. Collaboration has been a part of health sciences libraries for decades and today involves collaborative licensing, collaborative purchasing, and collaborative print repositories. An example of the success of one such repository is illustrated in the story following.

Chapter 6 covers discovery of the collection. Collection managers cannot simply be satisfied with building a collection, they must be concerned about whether users can find it. Discovery means that access is provided on multiple levels: the resource level, the title level, and the article level. It also encompasses the role of liaison librarians in publicizing and embedding the collection, and the story following this chapter demonstrates how parts of a collection were embedded in a reimagined medical school curriculum online.

Not only must users be able to find the collection, they must also be able to use it, and chapter 7 covers usability and accessibility of the collections health sciences librarians are building. Both of those topics are growing concerns for libraries, and the terms are defined and described as they relate to online library resources. Accessibility, especially, is a consideration that librarians are taking much more seriously, as it has moral and legal implications for their institutions. The chapter contains very practical tips about working with vendors to ensure the accessibility of resources that are licensed, and the story that follows illustrates putting these tips into action at a large university library.

Chapter 8 is about a new area for collection development—collecting data. Helpful considerations are included for the concerns of collecting data sets and databases as well as collecting locally created data from one's own institution. Because it is a new area, the policies of many different institutions are described and presented as potential models for libraries that have not yet written their own policies.

Chapter 9 is about special collections in the health sciences, a field not always covered in books about health sciences collection management. But collection managers have much to learn from colleagues in special collections. The collections purchased today will eventually be historical collections, a fact that raises questions about how well we are preserving today's material for the future. Considerations for collecting and preserving materials from the seventeenth century to the mid-twentieth century to the websites of today are all a part of this chapter.

Finally, chapter 10 concludes with thoughts about and a discussion of the future for health sciences collections. Thinkers of the past and present have predicted and described many different, sometimes conflicting, visions for collections for the future. The chapter considers a selection of them, along with the challenges and opportunities that optional futures present for librarians.

The hope is that librarians will find in these chapters new ideas to consider and perhaps pursue further. Librarians are grappling with tough questions: "Are collection policies still relevant in the age of Big Deals?" "What if our users don't care about finding the best information and just want the easiest to find?" "What does it mean to *own* an electronic book or journal?" "Can we preserve materials that we don't own?" and "What will researchers one hundred years from now think of some of the pragmatic decisions of today's librarians?" Collection management librarians can find themselves caught up in day-to-day realities and emergencies, in selecting and deselecting amid budget cuts or space downsizing, or in figuring out how to respond to user demands. It's easy to ignore the bigger picture. Occasionally, however, it is important to take a step back and consider the larger questions of how each of these daily decisions affects the identity and the future of health sciences libraries and possibly health care. This book aims to help facilitate that kind of reflection. It is often noted that health sciences libraries do have a unique kind of user and unique kinds of resources, but, if the past is any indication of the future, health sciences libraries will continue to be leaders among all types of libraries in thinking about the future of collection building and management.

REFERENCE

Dee, Cheryl Rae. 2007. "The Development of the Medical Literature Analysis and Retrieval System (MEDLARS)." *Journal of the Medical Library Association* 95 (4): 416–25. doi: 10.3163/1536-5050.95.4.416.

Acknowledgments

I want to acknowledge all the authors of the chapters and stories of this volume. Each one brought unique expertise and experience, and I learned so much from them throughout the revision and editing process. The final work is enriched by having different viewpoints from different places. I especially want to thank Susan Swogger for her advice and feedback and Steven Sowards, my supervisor at the Michigan State University Libraries, for his support through the book editing process.

Chapter One

The Health Sciences Publishing Environment

T. Scott Plutchak

There may have been a time when good collection management librarians didn't need to know very much about the publishing industry. They could become familiar with the materials in their subject areas and figure out what to buy based on subject priority and availability of funds. While librarians never thought that they had enough money to buy everything they ought to, a book was a book, a journal was a journal, the price was the price, and they could make good choices without knowing very much about the business, business practices, and operations of the publishers they were dealing with.

No longer. Few industries have been upended as dramatically as publishing and libraries. For several decades now there has been considerable hand-wringing among librarians about how to remain "relevant" and whether the disruption brought about by the internet will result in the end of libraries altogether. Certainly publishers feel these same anxieties as deeply, if not more so. Effectively navigating the intersection of the two requires a level of knowledge and sophistication that goes far beyond what was required in the days when print ruled.

This chapter is intended to provide an overview of the current publishing industry, with an emphasis on the scientific, technical, and medical (STM) sector and, in particular, the health sciences. It is necessarily a snapshot in time, some of it inevitably outdated by the time it is published, but it should provide some orientation to this necessarily fluid area and help to guide collection management (or "content management") librarians in the direction of increasing their own knowledge.

SCHOLARLY PUBLISHING LANDSCAPE

Librarians speak of "publishers" as if they were a single monolithic entity, but, of course, there are as many variations among publishers as there are among librarians. Here is how the *Oxford English Dictionary* (OED) defines "publisher":

> 1. A person who makes something generally known; a person who declares or proclaims something publicly. 2b. A person or company whose business is the preparation and issuing of printed or documentary material for distribution or sale, acting as the agent of an author or owner; a person or company that arranges the printing or manufacture of such items and their distribution to booksellers or the public; *(U.S.)* a newspaper proprietor. (OED Online 2017a)

"Publishing" is defined as follows:

> 1. The action of making something publicly known; official or public notification; promulgation, public announcement. 2. The action or business of preparing and issuing books, newspapers, etc., for public sale or distribution; an instance of this. (OED Online 2017b)

These ostensibly simple statements encompass a wide variety of complex activities.

Scholarly publishing involves both journals and books, but journals and books fill very different functions, particularly in the health sciences. Unlike scholarship in history, for example, where the discipline lends itself to long-form treatment, research in the sciences is an unending succession of small, concrete experiments, reported as close to when they actually happen as possible. Journal articles track the science as it is happening, and researchers are the biggest users of these. Review articles in journals or collected works, which summarize the current knowledge of a particular narrow subject, are also frequently consulted, but the practicing researcher in the biomedical sciences has relatively little need for most books. On the other hand, clinical textbooks, which summarize current practice, tend to be used by clinical professionals and students in professional programs such as medical or nursing schools. Some of this need is increasingly fulfilled by other sorts of online products, but many remain important classics.

Databases of various sorts also comprise a key component of scholarly publishing in the health and biomedical sciences. Publishers may tend to focus more on one type of publication than the others, but many publishers have offerings across all three groups. Even in these cases, however, the journal, book, and database divisions are likely to operate fairly independently.

Journal Publishing

Health sciences librarians are predominantly concerned with publishers that focus on STM materials, especially those that publish journals. According to the statistics compiled by the Association of Academic Health Sciences Libraries (AAHSL), the typical academic health sciences library in 2014–2015 spent about 72 percent of its content budget on serials (Squires 2016). There are no comparable statistics for hospital libraries, but it is reasonable to assume that the breakdown in spending is not markedly different. The most authoritative compendium of information on STM journal publishing comes from the report commissioned by the International Association of Scientific, Technical and Medical Publishers (typically referred to as the STM Association) and coauthored by Mark Ware of Mark Ware Consulting and Michael Mabe, executive director of the association.

The fourth edition of *The STM Report: An Overview of Scientific and Scholarly Journal Publishing* (March 2015) celebrates the 350th anniversary of journal publishing (Ware and Mabe 2015). It notes that in 2014 there were, according to some estimates, about 28,100 active, peer-reviewed English-language journals publishing some 2.5 million articles per year across all disciplines (27). Biomedical journals were the largest single subject area, representing about 30 percent of these. The number of journals grows at a steady rate of approximately 3.5 percent per year. This has been the case for the last three centuries aside from a slight acceleration in growth during the three decades following World War II when there was a substantial increase in research funding.

Overall, the largest STM publisher, by number of journals, is Springer. This was so even prior to its merger with Nature Publishing Group in the spring of 2015. Elsevier comes in second, followed by Wiley, Taylor & Francis, and Sage. These five accounted for 38.1 percent of STM journals (Ware and Mabe 2015, 45). The top 100 publishers (out of the approximately 650 noted in the *STM Report*) account for 67 percent of all journals. While the ranking of publishers shifts slightly when one considers only the health sciences (Elsevier publishes more health sciences journals than Springer, for example), the overall picture is of a market dominated by those same five commercial publishers, another ninety-five or so commercial and not-for-profit publishers, each with a range of journals, and then hundreds of publishers with only one or two titles each. Many of these publishers, such as scholarly and professional associations, have primary identities outside of publishing. The Medical Library Association (MLA), for example, is a significant publisher for health sciences librarians, even though its single title, the *Journal of the Medical Library Association*, is only a very small part of MLA's overall activity. The report quotes an analysis done by Elsevier of the ThomsonReuters (now Clarivate Analytics) journal citation database that suggests that 64 percent of article production comes from commercial publishers (including publishing done by these publishers for societies), 30 percent from society publishers, 4 percent from university presses, and 2 percent from "other" (Ware and Mabe 2015, 45).

Because publishers view their internal operations in the nature of trade secrets, it is notoriously difficult to determine what publishing actually costs, the totality of what publishers do, or how publishers set their prices. Although it is possible to calculate overall operating margins for some publishers (Dorsey et al. 2011), there is very little information available on what expenses are actually involved in publishing individual articles. Because of this opacity, estimates of what publishing could or should cost vary widely (Van Noorden 2013). In an effort to buck this trend, the electronic-only journal *eLife* publishes an annual financial report. The journal *eLife* is far from typical, but its example does shed some light on the kinds of costs incurred by highly selective, high-quality journals (Patterson and McLennan 2016a). The expenses for *eLife* are divided between publishing and nonpublishing costs. Nonpublishing costs include "[t]echnology and innovation: Major product innovation and development work that goes substantially beyond incremental improvements to the existing website and products." These accounted for 22 percent of total expenses in 2015. The rest of the expenses were for publishing costs: 33 percent for payments to editors, 8 percent for staff and outsourcing, 9 percent for online systems, 24 percent for article processing, 12 percent for features, and 14 percent for marketing. The journal handled 6,024 new submissions and published 833 articles in a year. Overall, *eLife*'s publishing expenditures amounted to £3,025,000 (about US$4.72 million). While the relative proportions of expenses and total costs will vary tremendously among journals, these categories are representative of the publishing costs for most major journals published by professional publishing houses (whether commercial or not-for-profit). Some journals reduce those expenses by relying solely on volunteer editors and doing relatively little marketing.

Depending on the publisher and the product, publishers rely on a number of revenue sources: subscriptions (individual and institutional, often set at different levels), advertising, reprints (typically sold in bulk to pharmaceutical companies that use them in their marketing efforts), membership dues (for some society journals), author page charges, or article processing charges (for some open-access journals or hybrid journals publishing open-access articles). Some of the more prominent open-access journals received substantial grant funding in order to launch. For example, the Public Library of Science (PLOS) journals were started with funding from the Gordon and Betty Moore Foundation and the Sandler Family Supporting Foundation. The journal *eLife* was initially supported entirely by the Howard Hughes Medical Institute, Max Planck Society, and Wellcome Trust. In July 2011, PLoS announced that it was now completely self-supporting (Jerram 2011), and, in 2017, *eLife* instituted an article processing charge (Patterson and McLennan 2016b). The *STM Report* quotes a 2008 study from the UK Research Information Network that claims that journal revenues came "primarily from academic library subscriptions (68–75% of the total revenue), followed by corporate subscriptions (15–17%), advertising (4%), membership fees and personal subscriptions (3%), and various author-side payments (3%)" (Ware and Mabe 2015, 23). Note that these are average revenues across the entire industry. The revenue mix for any individual journal may vary substantially from these numbers. Advertising, for example, primarily from pharmaceutical interests, has been a very significant source of revenue for some clinical journals, while many biomedical journals accept no advertising at all. As with all other aspects of publishing, the shift into the digital world has up-ended the revenue balance for scholarly journals. Publishers of all types have had to think creatively about ways to preserve revenues as these sources have changed.

While the health sciences publishing marketplace is dominated by a handful of large companies, there is a very large number of smaller publishers that produce important material. Size does not necessarily correlate with for-profit or not-for-profit status since there are small commercial publishers and large not-for-profit publishers. Of the top ten journal publishers (by number of journals) mentioned in the *STM Report*, however, only two are not-for-profit (Cambridge University Press and Oxford University Press) (Ware and Mabe 2015, 45). Estimates for the breakdown of commercial versus other publishers also vary widely, depending on how the universe of publishers is calculated. Because of their size, both in number of journals and number of articles produced, the business practices of the largest commercial publishers tend to dominate discussion about the present and future of scientific publishing. It is important, therefore, to keep in mind the very large number of publishers that may publish only a small number of journals or even just a single journal.

The commercial versus not-for-profit split is muddied by the fact that many societies contract with commercial publishers to produce their journals. Depending on the terms of the contract, the society may retain complete editorial control while turning over all business aspects to their publishing partner. As the economics of journal publishing continue to evolve, there appears to be increasing pressure on societies to take this route (Clarke 2015). For some societies, the journal publishing program represents their major financial activity, providing revenues that are used to support scholarships, educational activities, and other society priorities. Contracting with a commercial publisher can be an effective means of protecting this revenue stream, although it may also threaten the society's control over its publications.

Recent years have seen the emergence of academic libraries providing a variety of publishing services. These may include partnering with their institution's traditional university press, providing a number of publishing support services, or setting themselves up as full-fledged publishers for hire. The University of Pittsburgh's libraries are an example of the latter, using OJS (Online Journal Systems) as a platform to support journals across a variety of disciplines, with various business models from subscription to open access with article processing charges (ULS 2017). While relatively small within the overall context of scholarly publishing, these efforts emphasize new roles for libraries and librarians and offer a measure of competition to the legacy publishing industry. The Library Publishing Coalition has been formed to support libraries in developing sustainable publishing services (LPC 2017).

Book Publishing

The same mix of commercial and not-for-profit publishers that produce journal content also produces books. Doody's Core Titles in the Health Sciences (DCT) is the primary selection tool for books in the health sciences, tracking the roughly 3,000 new books published in health sciences disciplines each year (out of approximately 134,000 currently in print) (Doody's 2017). The 2016 edition identified 2,276 of these as "Core Titles," with 578 designated as essential purchases. These are produced by some eighty to one hundred publishers. As with journal publishing, scholarly and professional health sciences book publishing is skewed with just a few commercial publishers producing the majority of titles. Elsevier, Wolters Kluwer, Springer Nature, Taylor & Francis, and McGraw-Hill dominate. In the second tier are some twenty-five specialty publishers, including society publishers. The majority of these also publish journals and generally seek to increase their journal portfolios. The remainder of book publishers tend to be small operations producing only one or two titles per year.

Individual books account for only a small proportion of health sciences library spending, although that does not necessarily mean that these libraries are not spending on books. The major publishers have invested heavily in platforms for the distribution of the digital versions of their books. Very expensive products like ClinicalKey and McGraw-Hill's Access platforms include significant book content that used to be purchased on a per-item basis when in print. Many of these packages of electronic books from major publishers are offered to libraries only as subscriptions, essentially making book package purchases similar to serial purchases. Statistics on health sciences library book spending can be misleading when book packages are counted as "databases."

The major development affecting book publishing, however, has been the rise of point-of-care products like UpToDate and DynaMed. UpToDate, in particular, has been a marketing marvel and is in wide use in health care institutions of all sizes. The effectiveness of these tools in providing quick, authoritative answers to clinical questions has made clinical reference books much less important for the clinician in the health sciences than they were previously.

WHAT DO PUBLISHERS DO?

The dictionary definition quoted earlier indicates that "publishing" involves preparing material and making it available to the public. But what does this actually entail? Regardless of the business model, the size of the publisher, or the type of material being published, there are some general commonalities.

As noted in the 2009 version of the *STM Report*, "The journal has traditionally been seen to embody four functions: registration (establishing the author's precedence and ownership of an idea), dissemination (communicating the findings to its intended audience), certification (ensuring quality control through peer review and rewarding authors), and serving as the archival record (preserving a fixed version of the paper for future reference and citation)" (Ware and Mabe 2009, 12). How these functions are performed is the subject of much discussion. In 2008, the Scholarly Kitchen blog was established by the Society for Scholarly Publishing. The blog features daily posts from a pool of regular contributors. The "chefs," as they are called, come from diverse backgrounds, affiliated variously with society or commercial publishers, academic libraries, and independent consultants. With its often lively and sometimes disputatious comment threads, the Scholarly Kitchen has become one of the primary venues for discussions around the evolving nature of scholarly publishing. While STM journal publishing is the primary focus, issues related to book publishing and publishing in the humanities and social sciences are also covered.

In 2010, Michael Clarke published an influential post in the Scholarly Kitchen asking, "Why Hasn't Scientific Publishing Been Disrupted Already?" (Clarke 2010). Clarke, who has worked as a digital information consultant as well as an editor and publishing executive with Silverchair Information Systems, the American Medical Association, and the University of Chicago Press, reviewed the history of scholarly journals from their invention in the mid-seventeenth century. In his analysis, Clarke breaks out the functions mentioned above differently and suggests that journals were originally created to address two issues: dissemination—getting the results of scientific experiments into the hands of an interested audience; and registration—publicly claiming credit. Over time three more fundamental functions were added: validation—providing some assurance that the purported facts in an article are indeed true, which is provided through the mechanisms of peer review; filtration—mechanisms to help people figure out what is new and interesting and worth reading; and designation—providing a record of a scholar's achievements. Clarke argues that these general purposes of scientific publishing are fundamental enough to have made the transition from print to digital without causing the kinds of disruptions seen in other forms of publishing (newspapers, magazines, and the commercial book trade). They are not so dependent on the form in which the content is delivered. So, while paper has generally given way to digital publishing, and many new tools and functions have been developed, the basic structure of scholarly publishing has not been disrupted to any significant extent.

The tasks that are involved in these functions can be broken down much further. On the same blog, Kent Anderson (whose long career in publishing includes executive positions with the American Academy of Pediatrics, the *New England Journal of Medicine*, JBJS, Inc., and the American Association for the Advancement of Science) wrote a series of updated posts identifying ninety-six things that publishers do (Anderson 2016). Anderson groups his items under these headings: Editorial, Marketing, Community, Technology, and Finances and Business. The editorial task includes relatively familiar items like managing the peer-review process, which, for a publisher handling hundreds or thousands of manuscripts a year, represents a major undertaking, even if the actual reviews are written by academic volunteers. It also includes increasingly important tasks like checking for plagiarism, integrating new standards like ORCID for researcher identification and FundRef for reporting funding sources, and participating in a variety of archiving programs. These are all activities that readers and authors take for granted but that involve substantial commitments of effort and expense. Similarly, while printing and physical distribution costs have been eliminated for born-digital publications and substantially reduced for journals that still produce print versions, they have been replaced by the costs required for investing in sophisticated technology platforms. The community services that Anderson describes are perhaps the most overlooked. They include collaborating with other publishers on the array of services provided by CrossRef, developing reports, providing continuing education and continuing medical education certifications, and addressing conflicts of interest and potential violations of research ethics.

Inspired by Anderson's post, Francine O'Sullivan, an editor with Edward Elgar Publishing, created a list of "60 Things Academic Book Publishers Do" (O'Sullivan 2013). Her list is similar to Anderson's but emphasizes differences in the production and marketing aspects for books versus journals. She also highlights the differences in financial arrangements. The book publisher generally makes a much more substantive upfront financial investment, which is paid off only if the book is successful. In most cases, academic book authors also receive royalties.

As publishing technology has advanced, one of the central controversies about scholarly journal publishing has been how the many roles the publisher plays are truly essential and to what degree publishers should be compensated for them. Critics of the current system argue that journal publishing could be done much more cheaply (Van Noorden 2013). Every aspect of the journal publishing chain has been questioned. Unlike books, journal article authors are not paid royalties for journal articles, and those performing peer review are also unpaid volunteers, typically professors or researchers employed by universities who do such things as part of their service to the profession. The caricature version of journal publishing is that since authors and peer reviewers are typically uncompensated, publishers are demanding "exorbitant" subscription fees while contributing very little to the final product. Publishers' reticence to share information about costs exacerbates the problem, as does the wide variation in quality among journals. Librarians have little concrete information to use when comparing publications and are typically unable to make considered judgments about the value being delivered for the prices being paid.

Publishing has always been a service industry, and there is an increasing emphasis among publishers on the services that they perform for authors. Peer review, content editing and copy editing, checking for plagiarism, preparation of figures and charts, using editorials to provide context, assigning digital object identifiers (DOIs), and marketing through traditional means and through social media are all services provided by publishers to authors and readers. But the degree to which these services are provided varies considerably among journals, making cost comparisons very difficult. A top-tier journal like the *New England Journal of Medicine*, for example, has a large cohort of experienced professional editors and technical staff who can work with authors to validate the research and make sure it is presented in as thorough and compelling a fashion as possible. From initial submission, through possibly several rounds of revision, copy editing, proofreading (especially important to ensure that dosages, for instance, do not contain errors), typesetting, and final publication, each article passes through many hands. Such a process is obviously going to be far more costly than the per-article cost for a journal in which the volunteer editor makes the decision to accept or reject based on a single round of review, requires few, if any, revisions, does no substantive editing, and uses the author's final manuscript to generate camera-ready copy. Compounding the difficulty of comparing costs is that high-volume journals that also have low acceptance rates have to handle the submission, peer review, and decision process for the very many articles that do not make it into the journal. The revenue generated by the articles that are published, whether through subscription fees or open-access article processing charges, must cover the costs associated with the rejected articles as well.

Finally, while some journals have sufficient resources to actively court authors, for example, by attending conferences and engaging with presenters or conducting seminars and information sessions on university campuses, most journals rely on unsolicited submissions for their content, and the authors are not compensated financially. Book publishers, on the other hand, are much more likely to develop the concept for a new book or book series and actively solicit authors. Editorial staff will work closely with these authors to develop the final text, and substantial resources are devoted to design, illustrations, supplementary material, and the like. Book contracts are more likely to include royalty payments, and the authors of a successful textbook that goes through multiple editions may realize significant income over time.

TYPES AND FORMATS OF PUBLISHED MATERIALS

Print vs. Electronic Journals

Standard practices for electronic journals have reached the point where it seems reasonable to consider jettisoning the print product altogether, and some publishers have already done that. Electronic journals have achieved widespread acceptance among university students and faculty and clinical professionals, but most journals (except for those that were born digital) continue to produce a print counterpart. Some publishers argue that despite e-journals' widespread acceptance, many market segments, particularly in the developing world where internet access may be unreliable, still demand the print product.

In light of this, some publishers are experimenting with a divergence between their online offerings and the associated print product. The *BMJ*, for example, continually updates the content on their website, directed at a global audience, while selecting from that content to produce a weekly print edition directed primarily to the interests of the UK members of the British Medical Association. Similarly, many other publishers, while continuing to produce a print product, include much more content in the electronic version. New articles are frequently made available online as soon as they have passed through the copy-editing process. Where early e-journals were sometimes just a partial electronic version of the print product, now the print journal is more often just a subset of the content that is available online.

For those journals that are only published in electronic format, the designations of volume, issue, and page number are increasingly archaic, and many have abandoned them. For electronic searching and discovery, the article is the important unit rather than the journal volume, although the journals themselves remain important signifiers of quality. But a new complication has arisen with the increasing availability of multiple versions of any one article: the final published version in print (if it exists), the final published version on the journal website, and a pre- or post-print version hosted in a repository or on the author's own website. This variability led the National Information Standards Organization (NISO) to develop their recommended practices in *Journal Article Versions (JAV): Recommendations of the NISO/ALPSP JAV Technical Working Group* (NISO 2008). This document supplies standard definitions for the major versions that are most likely to be found when one is searching for a particular article. The "version of record" (VoR) is defined as "a fixed version of a journal article that has been made available by any organization that acts as a publisher by formally and exclusively declaring the article 'published.'" Most publishers now consider the online version to be the version of record.

Print vs. Electronic Books

In contrast, textbook publishers continue to struggle with developing electronic products that are functionally equivalent to print books, let alone superior, and the electronic book market is far from attaining the level of standardization that has occurred with electronic journals. Both librarians and library users can find the differences among the various e-book platforms confusing and frustrating. Some e-book platforms allow users to download the entire book as a PDF; some allow the user to "check out" the book for a certain length of time; some allow users to download PDFs of chapters individually; and others only make the material available in HTML format without the pagination of the original print book. Many have limits on the numbers of pages that users can print, and others allow no printing whatsoever. Some require downloading special software or use of software that will not display properly on some mobile devices. None have the ease of use that trade book publishers have created for their products on e-book readers. Concern over illegal posting of their electronic textbooks to websites has led many health sciences publishers to take away functionality from their electronic books, making them more difficult for readers to use.

Book publishers are also engaging in similar experiments with shrinking their printed publications. It used to be the trend for textbooks to grow larger with each new edition as more content was added. Now, some printed textbooks have become smaller as publishers move whole sections and chapters as well as supplementary material, multimedia, and supporting data to the web, accessible by means of a single-user access code. The whole second half of the student version of the classic textbook *Molecular Biology of the Cell* is now online only. An added complexity is that, while publishers typically think of libraries as the target market for journal subscriptions, they often see individuals as the primary market for books, particularly textbooks.

As a consequence, the access mechanisms for these online-only materials are usually geared toward individual readers and not usable at the library level.

People use books very differently from the way they use journals, particularly if the book is a long-form treatment or a textbook rather than a collection of individual articles. A 2015 article includes a substantial review of the literature demonstrating that students across disciplines tend to prefer print (Millar and Schrier 2015). A Hewlett-Packard survey reported in *Publishers Weekly* indicated that ease of use and note-taking ability were the primary reasons for college students preferring print textbooks, although this may be more relevant to individual purchases rather than library purchases if students are primarily interested in marking up the text (Tan 2014). Prognostications about the end of print books have largely disappeared. A recent Pew report indicates that the reading population in general continues to prefer print (Perrin 2016). It is difficult to draw too many conclusions for health sciences libraries from these studies because they tend to survey readers about *any* kind of reading and not specifically professional reading. A recent study of medical students and residents at Tulane Medical School also showed a strong preference for print textbooks over electronic among first- and third-year students. The relative preference shifted for residents, although 56 percent still indicated a preference for print (Pickett 2016). How the e-book market will play out and when (or if!) publishers develop e-book formats that people find more useful than print books, with business models that librarians view as fair and affordable, remains to be seen.

Multimedia

Publishers have been slow to embrace the possibilities of multimedia in their electronic publications, in part due to the high costs of development. The all-video journal *JoVE: The Journal of Visualized Experiments* debuted in 2006 and now exists in a number of sections. Other journals, while still primarily text based, have begun to incorporate video, animation, and simulations.

Databases and Aggregators

While journals and books have tended to occupy most of the content management librarian's time and energy, databases of various sorts demand increasing attention and, because of their frequently high prices, will consume a greater portion of the budget relative to their number. It should be noted that this division of published materials into categories is increasingly artificial and archaic. Librarians use the terms because they are the categories that they are familiar with from print, but, as digital technology advances, the products using the technology diverge in greater degree from their print antecedents. At the basic technical level, all of these online materials are databases, and, at the functional level, the distinctions between them are increasingly blurred. Books are frequently licensed in the same way as serials, and large databases of factual material share qualities of both journals and books. There are databases of abstracts, databases of book collections, databases of journal articles, databases of streaming video, databases of pharmaceutical information, databases of test preparation materials, and databases of point-of-care information.

Bibliographic abstract databases were the earliest, and they index primarily the journal literature, although many also index book chapters. MEDLINE, now usually searched through the PubMed search interface, is the oldest publicly available bibliographic abstract database and the one most central to the majority of a health sciences library's clientele. But there are many other such databases, from very narrowly tailored to very general, that the health sciences librarian must consider. Abstract databases, while remaining very important for information retrieval, almost seem old-fashioned now in an age of full-text searching of aggregated content, Google Scholar, and comprehensive publisher products like ClinicalKey. Librarians have to work harder to help people understand their usefulness.

Vendors that license content from multiple publishers and make it available in packages at prices that are considerably less expensive than would be the case if one were licensing the same content individually are called "aggregators." The tradeoff is that, in many cases, the most recent content is embargoed and the available content may be incomplete. EBSCO, ProQuest, and Ovid are the major vendors of aggregated content for health sciences.

In the health care arena, factual databases have become increasingly important. Neither journals nor books, these databases are designed to provide specific, authoritative answers to particular questions. Of particular interest to health sciences librarians is the category known as "point-of-care" tools, designed to be used in clinical situations to provide quick answers to specific clinical queries. UpToDate, initially launched in 1994 and now owned by Wolters Kluwer, is the best known of these and is very popular with medical students and residents. Competing, although quite different, products include EBSCO's DynaMed and Elsevier's ClinicalKey.

CHALLENGES OF THE ELECTRONIC PUBLISHING ENVIRONMENT FOR LIBRARIES

The "Big Deal"

By the early 2000s, many of the larger journal publishers were offering packages typically referred to as the "Big Deal." The multi-title journal bundle was first lunched by Academic Press in 1996 through their IDEAL program (Dobbins 1996). In his 2001 article "The Librarians' Dilemma: Contemplating the Costs of the 'Big Deal,'" Ken Frazier, librarian at the University of Wisconsin, popularized the term, while cautioning librarians about the inherent dangers. Frazier himself pointed out several years later that "the advice was nearly universally ignored" (Frazier 2005). As defined by Frazier, in the most common version of the Big Deal, a publisher offers access to all of the titles it produces at a price that is some supplement above the cost currently paid by a library for those titles it already licenses. The pricing is adjusted in such a way as to make the cost per individual title within the package much less than the library would pay per title outside of the package. Big Deals became very popular, particularly among larger libraries, since they enabled them to add a large number of new titles that they would not otherwise have been able to afford.

The downside for libraries was that, since these are typically multi-year deals with guaranteed price increases and tight restrictions on what titles within the package could be canceled, they locked in a significant portion of library budgets, reducing librarians' flexibility in responding to the needs of their communities. While journal bundles continue to be a major source of acquisitions, these are typically smaller than the full title list. In their 2012 survey of ARL (Association of Research Libraries) libraries, Strieb and Blixrud note that "research libraries appear to have pulled back from the 'Big Deal' substantially. Even in the 2006 data, it appears that the 'Big Deal' was not a dominant market model among the largest publishers" (Strieb and Blixrud 2014). For example, their data show that while 92 percent of ARL libraries licensed an Elsevier bundle, only 23 percent licensed the full title list (Strieb and Blixrud 2013). The figures are similar for the three other large publishers that they document (Springer, Taylor & Francis, and Wiley).

Big Deals of varying sizes continue to be important for many libraries, while their pros and cons continue to be debated, as evidenced by a series of articles published in the February 2017 issue of *Against the Grain* (Ismail 2017).

Purchasing versus Licensing

Although librarians continue to talk about "collection development" when addressing issues related to content, it can be argued that many health sciences librarians today are not developing collections in any meaningful sense of the term. Rather, they are managing content, licensing resources to provide access, without ever achieving ownership of the material itself. This is particularly true of health sciences librarians working in smaller libraries, in new born-digital libraries, and in hospital libraries, while those working in large academic health sciences libraries are often still grappling with the desire and perceived need to develop collections for posterity.

This change creates subtle shifts in how librarians think about the context of the material they are providing access to. In the traditional model of collection development that dominated practice in the age of print, librarians sought to build balanced collections that mirrored the academic and clinical programs they served. For example, librarians might try to collect virtually everything that was published in a particular area where the institution had PhD programs, while collecting more selectively in disciplines supporting master's or bachelor's degree programs. The goal was to collect material "just in case" it was needed. Interlibrary loan services were relied on to supply materials that fell in the gaps.

In the current environment, librarians tend to focus more on the immediate needs of their library users. Usage can be tracked much more granularly in the electronic environment, and librarians are under increasing pressure to ensure that material they are paying for is well used. "Cost-per-use" has become an important metric in deciding what to keep or cancel.

But the switch from owning to licensing content has resulted in some casualties, interlibrary loan being an important one in some cases. Interlibrary loan remains a challenging area for licensing negotiations as librarians argue for terms that enable them to make use of electronic materials as freely as copyright law allows for print, and publishers seek to impose restrictions that will make it more difficult for librarians to use systematic interlibrary loan as a substitute for licensing. Licensing terms for books remain even more problematic as publishers continue to experiment with models that can satisfy the needs of librarians while maintaining an acceptable revenue stream. This has proved to be very difficult, as the restrictions on multiple simultaneous access, or the prices charged for such access, are often perceived by librarians as unacceptably onerous.

Whereas librarians never needed to pay much attention to some of these concerns in the print world, becoming a knowledgeable and effective negotiator is now an essential part of the skillset of the collection management or content management librarian. More on the topic of negotiating is discussed in chapter 3 of this book.

Preservation and Archiving

The licensing versus purchasing conundrum raises concerns about long-term archiving. As was noted above, archiving has been seen as part of the publishing function in that journal articles verify the particulars of a scientific discovery in terms of what, who, where, and when. Publishers, however, were not concerned in the past with preserving this record—that was the role of libraries. The emergence of electronic versions of print products and, increasingly, "born-digital" documents that do not have a physical version has disrupted that balance. Academic librarians now routinely negotiate "perpetual access" clauses in their licenses in an attempt to ensure some level of ongoing access to licensed content for the future in the event of a license being canceled (Carr 2011). Such clauses may include continuing access at a nominal charge or the option of downloading the content to the institution's servers. But experiences with exercising such clauses have been limited, and the success that librarians have reported has been variable. Furthermore, such clauses can depend on the publisher having the technical infrastructure, the technical expertise, and the desire to preserve digital content even when it is no longer profitable. Over time, several third-party solutions to digital preservation have emerged, and both publishers and libraries now rely on agencies like LOCKSS, Portico, and PubMed Central.

The LOCKSS program (Lots of Copies Keeps Stuff Safe), based at Stanford University Libraries, operates on a distributed model, with many libraries participating in a network of servers that provide constant error correction by comparing the version of a publication stored on any single "LOCKSS box" with versions stored on other LOCKSS boxes. In the event of network failure or a publisher going out of business, access to e-books and e-journals is provided through these archived versions. LOCKSS is seen as a low-cost option that enables libraries, in partnership with participating publishers, to continue in their traditional preservation role. Portico, originally developed by JSTOR but now operated by the nonprofit Ithaka Harbors, Inc., is a centralized preservation service hosting e-journals, e-books, and other digital objects. Portico operates as a "dim" archive, providing access to its stored content only in the event that the publisher is no longer able to do so. PubMed Central (PMC), although viewed primarily as a source of open-access journal content, plays a vital role in the National Library of Medicine's preservation strategy. Unlike "dark" or "dim" archives, the PubMed Central strategy is based on the theory that continual use of the archived material is a fundamental component of the preservation strategy.

While developments such as LOCKSS, Portico, PMC, and other large-scale preservation projects have made great strides in alleviating some worries about the long-term preservation of formally published electronic books and journals, there remains considerable cause for concern. There are many publishers, particularly smaller ones, that do not participate in these services. There is an increasing profusion of digital objects that fall outside traditional publishing streams and thus are beyond the scope of some of these services. Many of these materials may be stored in local institutional repositories that do not have adequate preservation protocols in place.

A further complication is created when publishers continuously update an electronic work. Even if there is a preservation protocol in place, that does not necessarily mean that every update to an electronic database is preserved. Most academic health sciences libraries have had the experience of helping lawyers needing to find superseded editions of major textbooks in order to establish the standard of care in effect at a particular time in the past for a malpractice case. This may become more difficult as the specific online resource consulted by a physician at some point in the past is no longer available.

ISSUES IN SCHOLARLY PUBLISHING

Copyright

In the print world, copyright law governed the use of materials purchased by a library. The first sale doctrine protected the ability of a library to lend the physical items that they had purchased, and library exceptions for interlibrary loan and classroom copying were well established. Some publishers chafed under these restrictions and saw an opportunity with electronic materials to develop specific contract licenses for their use that would be more restrictive. What librarians must understand, and library users often do not understand, is that a signed license contract supersedes any allowances under copyright law. Librarians and users cannot rely on copyright law to provide guidance in how those electronic materials can be used if there is a license in place governing their use instead. While knowledge of copyright and its impact on the use of a library's materials remains a critical area of knowledge, and librarians are often viewed as the copyright experts in their institutions, the licenses that the institution signs will generally provide the definitive guidance. All the more reason for librarians to be vigilant in negotiating licenses that provide the broadest range of permissible uses by the members of their communities.

Open Access

No single issue has dominated discussion of scholarly publishing in the early part of the twenty-first century as much as open access (OA). Much of the discussion has been contentious, pitting librarians, who in general, favor easier access to content, against publishers, who, while often willing to experiment with open-access models, tend to be very conservative about implementing innovations that may threaten successful business models. A full discussion of OA, its variants, and the debates that continue to swirl around it are far beyond the scope of this chapter. While many early OA advocates saw OA as a lever for undermining the dominance of the large commercial publishers, by the mid-twenty-teens it is clear that these publishers have found ways to incorporate it into their overall strategy. In fact, it is the smaller society publishers that are less likely to have been able to incorporate OA into their business models.

Despite initial reservations on the part of many publishers, virtually every major STM publisher now provides OA options, either via "hybrid" journals—traditional subscription-based journals that provide the option for authors to make an individual article OA by paying a fee—or through fully OA journals where all of the content is available immediately upon publication. Hybrid journals are a particular source of contention, as well as a particular challenge to manage. Publishers have been accused of "double-dipping"; that is, charging to make some articles OA without discounting the overall journal subscription price in which those articles appear (RLUK 2013). Because of the aforementioned opacity in publishers' explanations of their finances, they have generally been unable to persuade all skeptics that such double-dipping does not routinely occur. In response to this, several publishers, including Thieme (Thieme 2017), Elsevier (Elsevier 2017), Nature (Nature 2017), Oxford University Press (Richardson 2008), among others, have published explanations demonstrating their commitment to adjusting prices in order to account for paid OA content.

While there is much debate about the varieties of OA and the proper terminology to use for those variants, in general, "gold OA" refers to articles in which the version of record is freely available from the date of publication. "Green OA" refers typically to an author's final accepted and peer-reviewed manuscript version deposited in a repository and made freely available after an embargo period, typically twelve months.

While "gold" OA is often equated with journals that charge a publication fee (typically referred to as APC, for "article processing charge"), this is not always the case. The Directory of Open Access Journals tracks fully open journals (i.e., "gold") that adhere to certain best practices (DOAJ 2017). In October 2016, they listed 9,231 journals from 129 countries. The majority of these are small journals that fund publication through other means—institutional subventions, a portion of society membership fees or other revenues, and the like. However, the most prominent and prestigious gold OA journals, especially in the STM fields, virtually all charge an APC. The major "legacy" STM publishers all have substantial portfolios of fully open gold OA journals.

Government policies in the United States, Canada, and Europe have furthered the cause of green OA. The 2008 United States National Institutes of Health (NIH) Public Access Policy requires that, for publications arising from work funded by NIH grants, at least the author's final peer-reviewed manuscript (if not the version of record) be deposited into PubMed Central at the time of acceptance of the article and made publicly available no later than twelve months after publication of the final version. Because this is required of the grant's principal investigator, NIH provides guidance for the investigators about publisher agreements they may sign in order to ensure that they are able to meet the requirement. Publishers that are reliant on papers based on

NIH-funded research have responded in a variety of ways. At a minimum, they have adjusted their publishing agreements to explicitly recognize the rights of the authors to make such a deposit, while leaving the actual work of depositing entirely with the author. On the other end of the continuum, some publishers manage the deposit entirely on behalf of their authors, handling all of the steps up to the final one, which requires the investigator to validate the deposit. The Canadian Institutes of Health Research also implemented a similar public access policy for researchers awarded funding after January 1, 2008, and maintains PubMed Central Canada (CIHR 2016).

Public access policies in both Canada and the United States have been extended to research beyond the health sciences. In 2013, the White House Office of Science and Technology Policy (OSTP) issued a memorandum requiring all federal funding agencies with annual research and development expenditures over $100 million to develop policies for making the data and peer-reviewed articles resulting from this funding publicly available after twelve months. With these requirements, the pressures on publishers to assist with compliance have increased. Some federal agencies are using PubMed Central, but others are using other repositories, adding to the complexity. In response to these challenges, a group of publishers, working with CrossRef, have developed CHORUS (which initially stood for Clearing House for the Open Research of the United States), a system that automates much of the process and links to the version of record.

In the United Kingdom, where government oversight of university re-search is much more centralized, deposit of a green version or publication in a gold OA journal has been required since 2013 for articles and proceedings that "acknowledge funding from the UK's Research Councils" (RCUK 2016). In the rest of Europe, a report from the European Research Council mandates that some version of articles based on publicly funded scientific research will be made open by 2020 (European Commission 2017).

It remains unclear what impact, if any, green OA may have on journal licensing. Very little solid research has been done on this question, so green OA advocates frequently argue that embargoes should be shorter, as there is no evidence that green OA has a negative impact on subscriptions. Others argue that this is only because we have not reached the point where virtually all of the content of particular journals is available as green OA, and, if that were to happen with relatively short embargoes, librarians would take that availability into account when making cancelation decisions. Nonetheless, and regardless of the extent to which some version of open access becomes the dominant mode of journal article publishing, publishers are modifying their business practices and programs in order to deal with it.

Predatory Publishing

One early criticism of an open-access model in which authors funded publication through fees for individual articles was that it would lead to abuse. Publishers would be incentivized to increase revenue by publishing as many articles as possible, regardless of quality. While proponents of OA tended to discount this, the problem of "predatory publishing" has become a matter of considerable concern.

The term "predatory publishing" was coined by University of Colorado, Denver, librarian Jeffrey Beall. Beall used to maintain a website, "Scholarly Open Access," and he created "Beall's list," a compendium of publishers he believed were "[p]otential, possible, or probable predatory scholarly open-access publishers." Publishers were considered "predatory" if they seemed to exist only to collect money rather than to provide appropriate peer review, editorial control, or the other qualities of scholarly journals. While low-quality and vanity presses have existed in the past, the rise of legitimate OA journals seems to have encouraged these predatory publishers to proliferate and cause confusion in the scientific community. While Beall's list was criticized for being too subjective and irrationally inimical to all open-access publishing, it served to shine a light on these possibly unethical practices (Berger and Cirasella 2015). Beall's list was taken offline in January 2017 due to "threats and politics" according to *Inside Higher Ed* (Straumsheim 2017). In response to confusion and questions from researchers, many academic library websites now include information on identifying predatory journals and, now that Beall's list is no longer available, provide reference to other tools that should be consulted when making judgments about the suitability or quality of a particular journal. One of these is the online document, published by the World Association of Medical Publishers after Beall's list was taken down, to provide in-depth guidance, criteria, and a set of questions to help stakeholders distinguish between legitimate and predatory journals (Laine and Winker 2017).

In August 2016, the U.S. Federal Trade Commission filed suit against OMICS, one of the publishers on Beall's list, asserting that it engaged in deceptive practices by not performing thorough peer review, not disclosing its fees, and holding articles for "ransom" when those fees were not met (FTC 2016). At the time of this writing the suit has only begun to make its way through the system. Only time will tell what impact predatory journals will have, and how the scholarly community will deal with them.

PUBLISHER ASSOCIATIONS, CONFERENCES, AND OTHER RESOURCES

This chapter has barely touched on the complexity of issues that surround the publishing landscape. The terrain remains very fluid. There can be no doubt that by the time this book is published, some of the statements, facts, and data presented here will already be out of date. Fortunately, while individual publishers may not be as transparent about their business practices and finances as librarians might find useful, there are a plethora of resources available. The following is a selected list of organizations, conferences, and resources that librarians can use to expand their knowledge of the world of publishing. Regardless of how publishing and libraries evolve over the next decade, they are inextricably bound together as partners in the scholarly communication enterprise. There is a great deal that librarians can learn that will make them more effective partners and more successful advocates for their communities, if they will only take the time.

Society for Scholarly Publishing
https://www.sspnet.org/

The Society for Scholarly Publishing (SSP) was founded in 1978 with the mission "to promote and advance communication among all sectors of the scholarly publication community through networking, information dissemination, and facilitation of new developments in the field." Although the membership is largely made up of people from publishing, they actively welcome librarians as members, offering a discounted rate and including librarians on their board of directors and various committees.

The Association of American Publishers/Professional and Scholarly Publishing Division
http://publishers.org/our-markets/professional-scholarly-publishing/

AAP is the primary trade group representing American publishers of all types. Their PSP Division focuses on publishers that work primarily in the scholarly and scientific publishing domain.

International Association of Scientific, Technical and Medical Publishers
http://www.stm-assoc.org/

Known simply as STM, this is the leading global trade association for academic and professional publishers, with over 120 members in twenty-one countries. They host a number of conferences and programs each year and publish a variety of position papers and analyses on their website.

The Charleston Conference: Issues in Book and Serial Acquisition
http://www.charlestonlibraryconference.com/

The Charleston Conference, held in November every year, was founded in 1980 as an informal gathering of librarians, publishers, and other interested individuals. It has since grown to annual attendance of well over 1,500 and the topics cover a very broad range of issues related to libraries and publishing.

Against the Grain
http://www.against-the-grain.com/

Published six times a year, *Against the Grain* contains articles of current interest for vendors, publishers, and librarians. It is made available for free to Charleston Conference attendees for a year or by subscription to anyone. ATG: The Podcast, is available free to anyone (http://atgthepod cast.libsyn.com/podcast), and episodes contain interviews with various thinkers in the library and publishing worlds as well as recorded sessions from the Charleston Conference.

UKSG
http://www.uksg.org/

Formerly the UK Serials Group, the annual UKSG conference is similar to the Charleston or SSP conferences in bringing together a wide variety of people interested in scholarly communication. In addition, UKSG hosts a number of smaller conferences and webinars throughout the year.

The Scholarly Kitchen
https://scholarlykitchen.sspnet.org/

The Scholarly Kitchen blog, hosted by SSP, has become a major source of discussion on all aspects of scholarly publishing. Although supported by SSP, it is editorially independent and the views expressed are strictly attributed only to the authors, or the "chefs" as the stable of posters are known. The Scholarly Kitchen includes a well-moderated comment section that is frequently as interesting, if not more so, than the posts themselves.

Retraction Watch
http://retractionwatch.com/

Started by a couple of science journalists, Retraction Watch has grown into an important source of voice tracking retractions in journal literature as well as associated issues. Their weekly roundup of stories related to publishing is an excellent source for keeping up with the latest news in the world of scholarly publishing.

Doody's Core Titles
https://www.doody.com/dct/

Launched in 2004 by Doody Enterprises, Doody's Core Titles was developed to replace the discontinued Brandon-Hill Lists, which had been a primary book selection tool for health sciences librarians since 1965. In addition to publishing lists of recommended titles, it also publishes reviews and articles relevant to the concerns of librarians charged with selecting materials for their libraries.

REFERENCES

Anderson, Kent. 2016. "Guest Post: Kent Anderson UPDATED — 96 Things Publishers Do (2016 edition)." *The Scholarly Kitchen* (blog), February 1. https://scholarlykitch en.sspnet.org/2016/02/01/guest-post-kent-anderson-updated-96-things-publishers-do-2016-edition/.

Berger, Monica, and Jill Cirasella. 2015. "Beyond Beall's List: Better Understanding Predatory Publishers." *College & Research Libraries News* 76, no. 3: 132–35. http://crln.acrl.org/content/76/3/132.short.

Carr, Patrick L. 2011. "The Commitment to Securing Perpetual Journal Access: A Survey of Academic Research Libraries." *Library Resources & Technical Services* 55: 4–16. doi: dx.doi.org/10.5860/lrts.55n1

CIHR (Canadian Institutes of Health Research). 2016. "Tri-Agency Open Access Policy on Publications." Last modified December 6. http://www.cihr-irsc.gc.ca/e/32005.html.

Clarke, Michael. 2010. "Why Hasn't Scientific Publishing Been Disrupted Already?" *The Scholarly Kitchen* (blog), January 4. https://scholarlykitchen.sspnet.org/2010/01/04/why-hasnt-scientific-publishing-been-disrupted-already/.

———. 2015. "The Changing Nature of Scale in STM and Scholarly Publishing." *The Scholarly Kitchen* (blog), June 25. https://scholarlykitchen.sspnet.org/2015/06/25/the-changing-nature-of-scale-in-stm-and-scholarly-publishing/.

DOAJ (Directory of Open Access Journals). 2017. Accessed April 3, 2017. https://doaj.org/.

Dobbins, John. 1996. "The Electronification of Academic Press: LACASIS Meeting Report." *Oasis* 33 (4): 1,7. http://www.asis.org/Chapters/lacasis/oasis/oasis_sum96.pdf.

Doody's Core Titles. 2017. Accessed April 3, 2017. http://www.doody.com/dct/default.asp.

Dorsey, E. Ray, Benjamin P. George, Elias J. Dayoub, and Bernard M. Ravina. 2011. "Finances of the Publishers of the Most Highly Cited US Medical Journals." *Journal of the Medical Library Association* 99 (3): 255–58. doi:10.3163/1536-5050.99.3.013.

Elsevier. 2017. "Pricing." Accessed April 3. https://www.elsevier.com/about/our-business/policies/pricing.

European Commission. 2017. *H2020 programme: Guidelines to the Rules on Open Access to Scientific Publications and Open Access to Research Data in Horizon 2020.* Version 3.2.

Accessed April 3. https://ec.europa.eu/research/participants/data/ref/h2020/grants_manual/hi/oa_pilot/h2020-hi-oa-pilot-guide_en.pdf.

Frazier, Kenneth. 2001. "The Librarians' Dilemma: Contemplating the Costs of the 'Big Deal.'" *D-Lib Magazine* 7 (3). http://www.dlib.org/dlib/march01/frazier/03frazier.html.

———. 2005. "What's the Big Deal?" *The Serials Librarian* 48 (1–2): 49–59. doi:10.1300/J123v48n01_06.

FTC (Federal Trade Commission). 2016. "FTC Charges Academic Journal Publisher OMICS Group Deceived Researchers." Posted August 26. https://www.ftc.gov/news-events/press-releases/2016/08/ftc-charges-academic-journal-publisher-omics-group-deceived.

Ismail, Matthew. 2017. "State of the 'Big Deal.'" *Against the Grain* 29 (1): 1,10.

Jerram, Peter. 2011. "2010 PLoS Progress Update." *The Official PLoS Blog,* July 20. http://blogs.plos.org/plos/2011/07/2010-plos-progress-update/.

Laine, Christine, and Margaret A. Winker. 2017. "Identifying Predatory or Pseudo-Journals." *WAME: World Association of Medical Editors.* Posted February 18. http://www.wame.org/identifying-predatory-or-pseudo-journals.

LPC (Library Publishing Coalition). 2017. Accessed April 3. https://www.librarypublishing.org/.

Millar, Michelle, and Thomas Schrier. 2015. "Digital or Printed Textbooks: Which Do Students Prefer and Why?" *Journal of Teaching in Travel & Tourism* 15: 166–85. doi: 10.1080/15313220.2015.1026474.

Nature. 2017. "Site License Price Adjustments for Hybrid Journals." *Open access at Natureresearch.* Accessed April 3. http://www.nature.com/openresearch/about-open-access/policies-journals/#Site_license_price_adjustments_for_hybrid_journals.

NISO (National Information Standards Organization). 2008. *Journal Article Versions (JAV): Recommendations of the NISO/ALPSP JAV Technical Working Group.* Baltimore: NISO.

O'Sullivan, Francine. 2013. "60 Things Academic Book Publishers Do." *Elgar blog,* October 23. https://elgar.blog/2013/10/23/60-things-academic-book-publishers-do-by-francine-osullivan/.

OED Online. 2017a. "publisher, n." Oxford University Press. Accessed February 23. http://www.oed.com/view/Entry/154076.

———. 2017b. "publishing, n." Oxford University Press. Accessed February 23. http://www.oed.com/view/Entry/154077.

Patterson, Mark, and Jennifer McLennan. 2016a. "Inside *eLife*: What It Costs to Publish." *eLife.* Posted August 11. https://elifesciences.org/elife-news/inside-elife-what-it-costs-publish.

———. 2016b. "Inside *eLife*: Setting a Fee for Publication." *eLife.* Posted September 29. https://elifesciences.org/elife-news/inside-elife-setting-fee-publication.

Perrin, Andrew. 2016. "Book Reading 2016." Pew Research Center. Posted September 1. http://www.pewinternet.org/2016/09/01/book-reading-2016/.

Pickett, Keith M. 2016. "Resource Format Preferences across the Medical Curriculum." *Journal of the Medical Library Association* 104: 193–96. doi:10.3163/1536-5050.104.3.003.

Richardson, Martin. 2008. "Oxford Open Prices Adjusted for Open Access Uptake." *Oxford Journals Update* 2, (Winter 2007/2008). http://www.oxfordjournals.org/for_librarians/oxford_open.pdf.

RCUK (Research Councils UK). 2016. "RCUK Policy on Open Access." Last modified December 5. http://www.rcuk.ac.uk/research/openaccess/policy/.

RLUK (Research Libraries UK). 2013. "Fair Prices for Article Processing Charges (APCs) in Hybrid Journals." http://www.rluk.ac.uk/wp-content/uploads/2014/02/RLUK-stance-on-double-dipping-Final-November-2013.pdf.

Squires, Steven J., ed. 2016. *Annual Statistics of Medical School Libraries in the United States and Canada.* 38th ed. Seattle, WA: Association of Academic Health Sciences Libraries.

Straumsheim, Carl. 2017. "No More 'Beall's List.'" *Inside Higher Ed.* January 18. https://www.insidehighered.com/news/2017/01/18/librarians-list-predatory-journals-reportedly-removed-due-threats-and-politics.

Strieb, Karla L., and Julia C Blixrud. 2013. "The State of Large-Publisher Bundles in 2012." *Research Library Issues* 282: 13–20. http://publications.arl.org/rli282/.

———. 2014. "Unwrapping the Bundle: An Examination of Research Libraries and the 'Big Deal.'" *portal: Libraries and the Academy* 14: 587–615. doi:10.1353/pla.2014.0027.

Tan, Teri. 2014. "College Students Still Prefer Print Textbooks." *PW: Publishers Weekly.* Posted July 8. http://www.publishersweekly.com/pw/by-topic/digital/content-and-e-books/article/63225-college-students-prefer-a-mix-of-print-and-digital-textbooks.html.

Thieme. 2017. "Thieme's Policy on Double-Dipping." *Thieme Open.* Accessed April 3. http://open.thieme.com/double-dipping.

ULS (University Library System, University of Pittsburgh). 2017. Accessed April 3. https://library.pitt.edu/e-journals.

Van Noorden, Richard. 2013. "Open Access: The True Cost of Science Publishing." *Nature* 495: 426–29. doi:10.1038/495426a.

Ware, Mark, and Michael Mabe. 2009. *The STM Report: An Overview of Scientific and Scholarly Journal Publishing.* Oxford: International Association of Scientific, Technical and Medical Publishers.

———. 2015. *The STM Report: An Overview of Scientific and Scholarly Journal Publishing.* The Hague: International Association of Scientific, Technical and Medical Publishers.

One Library's Story

*Putting Together a Collection to Support a
New Medical School*

Elizabeth R. Lorbeer and Joseph A. Costello

In 2006, the American Medical Association called for a 30 percent increase in medical school enrollment by 2015 to meet the growing demand for physicians in the United States (www.aamc.org/newsroom/newsreleases/2006/82904/060619.html). After decades of growth stagnation, planning commenced for several new medical schools. Western Michigan University Homer Stryker M.D. School of Medicine (WMed), a private medical school in Kalamazoo, Michigan, is one such school. Established in 2012, WMed confers the Doctor of Medicine (MD) degree as of 2018. WMed is a collaborative partnership between Western Michigan University (WMU) and Kalamazoo's two teaching hospitals: Ascension Borgess and Bronson Healthcare. WMed is affiliated with Western Michigan University but has autonomous governance and financial infrastructure.

During WMed's start-up, a dedicated academic medical library did not exist. Residency programs affiliated with the two teaching hospitals in Kalamazoo had existed for years, and both hospitals have libraries; however, the library collections and services are geared toward community health care providers and patients. Clinicians, residents, and newly hired faculty for WMed were initially expected to use the local hospital libraries and the university libraries of Western Michigan University. The medical school administration realized, however, that the university libraries and the hospital libraries were lacking the specialized collection, study space, and professional staff to support medical education and that access to appropriate resources would be essential for accreditation. Also, from an information technology perspective, it was not practical to offer students logins to disparate systems. It was decided in the early stages of the WMed start-up that a digital library was needed, with shared collections and services among the collaborative partnership. Toward this end, a founding library director was hired in 2013.

Building an entirely new, collaborative library from scratch is no easy task, even if it is fully digital. The timeline we were given required the presence of a functional digital library in nine months with delivery of library services within twelve months. The schedule, mapping to accreditation milestones, was aiming to support the educational needs of the first class by August 2014. A robust library also helps a school recruit, and support, new faculty. The start-up budget allowed the purchase of all core resources needed to support the first two years of WMed's medical education curriculum and the hiring of two professional librarians within the first year.

The greatest challenge in building the new WMed Library was the aggressive timeline. It was not possible, or practical, to install an integrated library and discovery system or an instance of an interlibrary loan system such as ILLiad. Our goals were to meet users' needs right away while predicting the information needs of new faculty, students, and programs in the future; so one of our most important initial, strategic decisions was that the components of the library we install, market, and maintain be nimble. To begin, we focused on these five core components to provide the basis of essential library services for opening day:

- An online website—hosted by Springshare's LibGuides
- Document delivery and resource-sharing—an instance of DOCLINE
- Unmediated account to purchase journal articles individually—Copyright Clearance Center Get It Now
- An institutional PubMed LinkOut account
- An electronic resource management tool—ProQuest Serial Solutions 360 Core to connect to third-party full text aggregated databases (e.g., EBSCO MEDLINE Complete, and ProQuest Health & Medical Collection) and open-access journals

A collection policy was written to establish boundaries for the collection, to provide a conceptual framework for the selection of materials, and to put in place some acquisitions practices. It specifically omits an archiving policy, as the digital library design is to supply content on demand rather than being a repository of materials.

To begin building collection content, we chose electronic book and database packages (e.g., AccessMedicine, ClinicalKey, Lippincott Williams & Wilkins [LWW] Health Library, and R2 Digital Library). These resources were added when faculty began arriving, allowing educators to assemble course content for the first two years of medical school, while offering a core collection to support undergraduate medical education on opening day. Our primary strategy for other types of resources was first to collaborate with our affiliated partners to share online collections. During start-up, both commercial and society press publishers were willing to add the medical school's IP ranges to the current electronic journal contracts held by the academic library at no cost because the numbers of medical school faculty (70) and the numbers of students in the first class (54) were so small. The number of employed faculty three years later has risen slightly to 111 full-time equivalent (FTE), with three enrolled classes (186 medical students). Since the medical school is small compared to other U.S. medical schools, and is the smallest school in the Midwest region, it's difficult to justify the purchase of large bundles of content. For titles not held by the academic campus library, the Abridged Index Medicus (AIM) core clinical journal titles list was consulted and a small journal collection of thirty-five medical titles was added in January 2014. Additionally, the hospital libraries and the medical library jointly license and share the LWW Total Access journal collection. Many of the journal titles replace departmental print subscriptions in the residency programs.

Whether or not we could add IP ranges to the e-book database vendor contracts of our academic and hospital partners varied. In most cases, there was a cost involved to include the medical school library, as these existing contracts were designed to exclude additional graduate degree programs. We were unable to identify a single publisher or vendor who was willing to merge the individual subscriptions among the hospital and academic libraries. So, instead, the medical library licenses with either the hospitals or the academic campus based on an interest in the resource among the partners. The library supplements its collection by using third-party document delivery services, primarily Get It Now, ReadCube, and Reprints Desk. These services allow library users to obtain articles directly from the publisher. DOCLINE is used to obtain articles through interlibrary loan, and the WMed library still relies on its partners (i.e., the university libraries and the hospital libraries) for the occasional interlibrary loan using ILLiad. Overall, the medical library favors adding new content to the collection through demand-driven services such as ProQuest Ebook Central and R2 Digital Library.

After opening day, a plan to provide students with iPads in their third year of study for clerkship programs emerged with an expectation that library resources be accessible via responsive web platforms and mobile applications. Therefore, we began work to ensure that the online presence of the library was designed for smartphone and tablet use. Not all of the electronic resources the library subscribes to work well in the mobile environment, but user-friendly solutions such as Third Iron's BrowZine, integrating a variety of journal subscriptions, help us promote mobile library access.

The initial collection was able to meet deadlines set forth by the dean. Collection growth since then has been carefully planned to be sustainable. Over time we have added more materials to support third-year clerkship rotations (e.g., Case Files Collection, LWW Health Library Clerkship Collection, and Med-U), exam preparation materials, and other databases. An unexpected development was a request by the medical students to have a few copies of their required textbooks available via print so that they could alternate between using print and electronic versions while studying. An initial investment of $3,000 was made to build a small print collection; and while a few books have gone missing, we think it has been worth the investment as students subsequently provided positive feedback in the latest school-wide satisfaction survey.

We knew that eventually we would want to implement a web-scale discovery service to effectively manage and search the 150,000+ electronic book titles and 66,000+ journals to which we wanted to provide access. Managing this many e-book titles from shared and demand-driven solutions, especially, was difficult using only Proquest Serial Solutions 360 Core and its A to Z list. At the same time as we were implementing 360 Core, WMU's academic library was amid discovery system evaluations. WMU eventually chose a product from a competing vendor (the Ex Libris Group). While it would have been nice for the medical library to share the discovery system with the main library, it was not feasible to restructure the online presence of the medical library when the Higher Learning Commission (HLC) and the Liaison Committee on Medical Education (LCME) site visits were coming up. We eventually investigated and implemented a web-scale discovery service from ProQuest. The purchase of Ex Libris by ProQuest has added another wrinkle to this story, and library representatives from both the academic and medical schools are watching how the two companies will merge their technologies and services.

The class size of WMed is purposefully small (no larger than eighty-four students) to allow learners to receive individual attention and work in close collaboration with medical educators in a team. Initial staffing of the library was one director to begin building the library collection and policies on her own. Originally, the library staff was to be composed of three professional librarians and two paraprofessionals; however, with the robust offerings of large-scale discovery systems and flexible platforms to host and manage content, it made more sense to substitute the two paraprofessional positions for a professional library digital strategist position to assist with improving our online presence. It may be true that without a large physical collection or the need for cataloging, circulation, and other such services, there is less need for paraprofessional staff. Our professional staff takes turns filling interlibrary loan and DOCLINE requests, answering the library's general email, and supporting outreach activities such as "Library Teas" and other themed wellness events.

The primary lessons we learned in designing and creating a new online library are that content solutions need to be simple enough for a small professional library staff to manage, while employing flexible technology that is cost-effective for the long term. What makes our online library especially successful is our ability to deliver custom services to each person. Our team can create access to new content in real time, deliver services, and provide instructional material to meet any emergent user need. As a developing medical school, we couldn't predict all faculty, administrator, or student needs, but, as our medical education program is continuously assessed, evaluated, and refined, we respond. We've created relationships with our users, who trust our capacity to help support a dynamic, positive learning environment, which ultimately enables us to deliver useful, prompt, and reliable content and services nearly any time, anywhere.

Chapter Two

Managing a Health Sciences Collection

Susan E. Swogger

COLLECTION DEVELOPMENT AND
COLLECTION MANAGEMENT

The joint practices of collection development and collection management are undergoing rapid change in concert with the evolving practices of library and information sciences and changes in the publishing industry. As discussed in chapter 1 of this book, health sciences libraries are at the forefront of much of this general industry change. Collection management in the health sciences library requires knowledge of and investment in enduring practices such as book or journal selection and deselection but also capacity for adaptation to proliferating new forms of content, evolving means for acquisition, and increasing pressure to demonstrate value. This chapter will discuss some aspects of current practical health sciences collection management practices in an environment shaped by shifting trends.

Collection development, with its emphasis on the selection and acquisition of new materials to build largely permanent library collections, was long the core of library practice. Hospital and other special biomedical libraries have always placed more emphasis on currency and may not have been able to house materials perpetually as academic libraries did, but they, too, in the past, emphasized acquisitions of individual materials for ownership. Print materials could be acquired, processed, and then relegated to the shelves and the custody of the public services staff, barring damage or loss. Minimal continuing investment by the collections staff was required. Collection development librarians at any of these types of libraries who made task charts illustrating their staff time investment would show a very large percentage of time devoted to reviewing individual book or journal descriptions and selecting for purchase such things in support of the institutional mission, typically described in a collection development policy. The idea of building a core library collection in support of the institutional mission remains a primary aspect of maintaining a library. However, the focus of collection development is shifting toward selecting groups of resources, or even providing users with the opportunity to select from groups of resources, based upon data analysis and direct user choice more frequently than the formerly predominant subjective librarian experience-based judgment. With this change has come an ever-increasing investment of energy in the requirements of collection management tasks.

The term collection management encompasses an array of tasks and processes aimed at the decision making necessary to effectively deal with existing collections. With the primarily print collections of the past, individual materials required specific investment of energy from a collection manager rarely, in well-established patterns, and often only in response to changing circumstances such as space needs or program developments (Quinn 2001). With a largely online collection comes a continuing and typically increasing investment of budget and time in maintaining access to resources. Whether an online resource a library holds comes with perpetual or temporary access, it requires a much heavier investment in evaluation and management from the collections staff than the equivalent tasks did for earlier majority-print collections, and this aspect of practice increasingly dominates staff and infrastructure investment (Quinn 2001).

The general library trend toward collection management as a more dominant concern than collection development is evident when reviewing the components of and activities required by the different parts of the collection.

THE CURRENT COLLECTION

Collections of resources in health sciences libraries typically consist of a mix of journals, point-of-care or clinical support tools, books, multimedia, and other supplementary materials such as anatomical models or charts. This has been the case for decades, but format and means of acquisition and access have changed considerably. While many academic and research health sciences libraries have legacy print collections either in house or in storage, these are typically added to sparingly—if at all—and the majority of newly purchased books and continuously subscribed journals in health sciences libraries are held in electronic format.

Libraries are also getting an ever-larger percentage of their collections via subscription or purchase of large groups of electronic journals or books rather than by individual selection of each title. Often, a library collection consists of as much, or more, electronic content that is leased or only temporarily available as that which is owned. Increasingly, publishers are creating omnibus resources that function like subscription access-only databases that offer all their monograph, reference, video, and journal content for a subject area like medicine in one setting with one subscription, most typically without providing the subscriber with permanent access to the included content. As is often the case, health sciences library collections have been at the forefront of this area of change, with early versions of such subscription models described in discussions of trends published in the late 1990s (Blansit and Connor 1999). Collection management in this setting focuses on maintaining access to these shifting and often overlapping mini-collections in conjunction with management of print and online resources with permanent ownership arrangements.

Effective development of this type of collection requires careful and continuous collection management, both to ensure that the ever-changing collections of journals within subscription packages still meet the needs of a library's user community *and* to deal with the shrinking value of library funding relative to the costs of library resources. Health sciences librarians, whether at universities or hospital chains, will always be able to find many more desirable resources than their budgets can accommodate. Current publishing and technology trends require that they are also always aware of and adaptive to new means of acquisition and new definitions of collections. The collection development or management librarian functions as the expert in these areas for his or her library.

COLLECTION DEVELOPMENT LIBRARIANS IN THE LIBRARY STRUCTURE

Collection development and management responsibilities have a wide variability in dispersal in different health sciences library structures. In health sciences libraries large enough to have multiple staff, it is not uncommon to have a single position responsible for most aspects of collection management, which may include some or all tasks relating to collection development. In this situation, the collection manager may act as coordinator for collection development responsibilities that are dispersed among multiple public services liaison staff specializing in different subject areas. Alternatively, the collection manager may have majority responsibility for collection development and collection management or supervise a specialist librarian who focuses on collection development alone. For many academic health sciences librarians, there is no separate health sciences library. These librarians are subject specialist librarians within a larger university library serving many subject areas. In those cases, it is typical for health sciences collection development responsibilities either to rest with a specialized health sciences selector or to be dispersed between several health sciences liaison librarians who report to a more general university library collection manager.

Hospital libraries without direct university affiliation are typically smaller by far than academic health sciences libraries and are less likely to have staff dedicated solely to collection management or development. It is not uncommon for hospital librarians to be solo librarians; in this case all professional responsibilities are combined into one position. Hospital librarians, also, have been at the forefront of the general move toward online collections for health sciences libraries and are increasingly likely to have shed all or most print collections or to be involved in rapidly evolving information and knowledge management services beyond resource provision, as Margaret Moylan Bandy (2015) alluded to in her 2014 Janet Doe Lecture at the Annual Conference of the Medical Library Association. Special librarians serving research institutes or pharmaceutical companies, in the increasingly rare cases where such institutions maintain a library, are also generally solo. As such, it is increasingly common for the majority of micro-level collection development aspects of the library to be outsourced to online resource vendors who produce subscribed databases of electronic journals and books, or even to the users themselves via a patron-driven acquisition model. In such a situation, the librarian's focus on collection management and development centers on ensuring that the most useful point-of-care clinical and other online groups of resources are available to their user communities.

Librarians with collection development and/or management responsibilities who do not work alone benefit from strong communication with every other person in the library who interacts even superficially with its user community and activities. Some librarians with collections responsibilities are also subject liaisons and part of the public service department and will naturally have much interaction with other public service librarians, but for collection managers who are not liaisons, input from liaisons is crucial. The public/user services staff and liaisons, with their knowledge of the user community and subject areas, are critical for identifying potential new acquisitions and for publicizing trials or newly purchased resources to the user community. Collections librarians also benefit by close coordination and strong working relationships with technical services librarians and staff.

If there is a separate acquisitions department in the library, acquisitions librarians and the staff of that department handle the actual details of purchasing library materials selected by the collections librarians. It is common to have dedicated staff with acquisitions responsibilities when a separate line of responsibility is necessary for auditing purposes, such as is typical for state or public libraries. In other libraries, collections and acquisitions responsibilities may rest in one position (Johnson 2004). Even in libraries where the positions must remain separate, there is a very high degree of cooperation, and it is common for both collections and acquisitions staff to be involved in communications with vendors and publishers as well as with the management of the budget.

Collection managers also regularly work closely with the accounting and budgeting divisions. It is critical for decision making to provide and show good stewardship of the library and institution's resources and to be cognizant of the institution's current and future financial position. A library is typically considered a major cost center for an institution, and it is not uncommon (and indeed can be very common) for a sudden freeze in spending to be demanded by the institutional administration. In many cases, library administration will choose to take one-time spending cuts out of library acquisitions budgets rather than resorting to lay-offs or other measures. Knowledge of current costs and likely increases in upcoming expenses in combination with regular evaluation of return on investment for library collections can help a librarian determine the healthiest sacrifices to make and justify the need to keep specific resources.

Some institutions have a separate electronic resources librarian who may be responsible for the details of tracking and linking of new and existing electronic subscriptions and purchases, while in many these responsibilities rest with the collection manager. In either case, such librarians will also need to communicate effectively with any web services, systems librarians, and information technology (IT) staff to ensure that electronic resources will be functional. There is no benefit to trialing or purchasing a resource that cannot run on a library or hospital's network; doing so will cause frustration and disappointment for both the library user community and any vendor partners. Equally, if there are any oddities about the resource and its functionality, IT staff must be part of the decision-making process. As this group will be expected to make the new resource work when it (inevitably) has difficulties, it is very important that they be involved in and aware of its setup and technical support information from the beginning.

Hospital librarians or academic librarians that are expected to make resources available on hospital networks might also have additional setup issues beyond the typical. Such networks often have very stringent security, commonly ban the streaming content that is increasingly included in online resources, and may include a high proportion of archaic and/or homegrown utilities. Any one of these issues may require some extra finesse on the part of the IT, e-resource, or systems staff; a close working relationship between collection development and such staff will help forestall frustration and speed the availability of resources to the library's community.

Finally, in large institutions like universities or even university systems, the collection manager or coordinator for the health sciences library should be in close contact with the head or heads of collections for other units of the entire university library system. Most typically, the health sciences library will share utilities such as the library catalog, discovery systems, interlibrary loan services, access to numerous electronic resources, and at least some percentage of budget with the university library system. Close communication will ensure that the needs of the health sciences library receive consideration in relevant decisions and prevent wasted duplication of resources or efforts.

COLLECTION DEVELOPMENT POLICIES, FORMAL AND DE FACTO

As is likely becoming clear to any reader, there are many moving parts involved in collection development. Well-thought-out plans and policies can help to smooth out decisions and make them understandable to all who are involved. The most formal of these is the collection development policy, or CDP. A collection development policy is a structured document that details the depth and scope of a library's collection. It acts as a blueprint for the building of the collection it describes and should be an important source of information about what a library considers to be its collecting responsibilities.

Some health sciences libraries have individual collection development policies for different subject areas (such as medicine, nursing, or pharmacy) or for distinct collections of high importance (such as audio-visual materials or special collections). Other health sciences libraries will have one broad collection development policy. Collection development policies are designed to be broadly inclusive and, ideally, to need minimal updating. It is not uncommon for decades to pass before a full update is made. However, many libraries in the early part of the twenty-first century are in the process of updating their policies to reflect the radical changes happening to both the formats included in their collections and the definition of collection itself, as discussed elsewhere in this book. In general, collection policies provide a broad, rather than specific, picture of what a library's collections might contain and are closely tied to the institutional mission.

Ideally, a library's collection development policy will give a knowledgeable reader an overview of a library's long-term subject interests as well as that library's identified user community and the format and type of resources collected. As valuable as this information is, many consider the most valuable aspect of such a policy to be the restraint that it provides. The International Federation of Library Associations and Institutions' 2001 *Guidelines for a Collection Development Policy using the Conspectus Model* explicitly states,

> The main reason to write a collection development policy is to prevent the
> library from being driven by events or by individual enthusiasms and from

purchasing a random set of resources, which may not support the mission of the library. (Biblarz et al. 2001)

As libraries must consider the needs of their entire user community when making large investments in resources, the collection development policy can be very helpful in explaining to requestors why their needs must be balanced with the needs of others. Conversely, policies can help librarians identify further interests and needs that might support the acquisition of a resource that was not initially obvious.

The vast majority of libraries will host their collection development policies online in a publicly accessible area, making them available both to the public and to any collection development librarians looking for insight. Collection development policies can provide valuable information about how a library supports its programs, and a new collection development librarian can use these for ideas. For example, a librarian tasked with supporting a new public health program might review collection development policies from several other libraries supporting already-established public health programs to see what subjects are included and what forms of support they receive. Collection development policies can also prove useful when a department or school is seeking information about library support, as may occur during an accreditation review or when justifying fiscal investment in the library.

Collection development policies are unique to the libraries they support, but most use some combination of classed model and narrative description of the library and its community. A classed model describes the collection using a hierarchical library classification scheme (such as the National Library of Medicine or Library of Congress Classification Schemes) along with collection depth indicator divisions to note the intensity of collecting for each subject area (Johnson 2004). The following are common collection depth indicator divisions (Biblarz et al. 2001, 7):

- 0 = out of scope
- 1 = minimal information level
- 2 = basic information level
- 3 = study or instructional support level
- 4 = research level
- 5 = comprehensive level

These depth indicators can help selectors decide whether their collection goals justify the expense of an obscure monograph or exclude it in preference for an undergraduate-level overview. They can also be used for in-depth collections analysis, using a method called the conspectus (Biblarz et al. 2001). Such reviews are much less common in the current era as the definition of the collection shifts away from materials individually selected by librarians, but the concept and procedures of this method can still be helpful for planning how to examine narrowly defined subject areas to support a new program, for a withdrawal project, or for an accreditation review. An example of a collection development policy is shown in table 2.1.

DE FACTO COLLECTION DEVELOPMENT POLICIES: APPROVAL PLANS, SUBSCRIPTION DATABASES, AND CONSORTIAL NETWORKS

Collection development policies are not the only documents or entities that reflect and inform the direction of collection building; indeed, there is some controversy as to their continuing value, and some libraries do not have them at all. Those that do not have traditional collection policies as shown above likely do have informal policies or guidelines addressing the kinds of resources that will be acquired. There are many other things that can function as de facto collection development policies; for example, approval plans on file with book jobbers, very large online subscription or aggregator resources with minimal customization such as Elsevier's ClinicalKey or EBSCO's e-book collections, or consortial resource collectives and collaborative collections relationships with other libraries. Each of these very different entities is similar to a collection development policy in some ways but differs from a collection policy in other ways, most prominently in that they are not completely controlled or even controlled at all by the library nor able to stand as statements of the library's mission as to traditional policies.

Approval plans are probably the most similar to traditional collection development policies in appearance but focus entirely on monographs and are much more frequently changed. Discussed in further detail below, they serve as a detailed contract between a library and a book vendor as to what will be purchased. These plans function as continuously active search algorithms acting within a book vendor's sales catalog database. An approval plan has a much greater level of detail than a collection development policy's subject outline and is typically much more frequently updated, though it is based upon the limits depicted in the policy itself. It will include exactly which categories of books, publishers, formats, subjects, languages, reading levels, and pricing are acceptable to the library, and any other designated limits. The approval plan's superior currency and apparent duplication of information in a collection policy leads some libraries to rely on it as the primary description of their collecting interests rather than a static, formal policy.

Very large subscription online resource collections, bulk e-book aggregator collections, participation in state or consortial resource collective buys, and relationships with other libraries also shape a library's collection. As

Table 2.1. Sample Collection Development Policy

Collection Development Policy

Mission Statement	The Nursing Library seeks to support the research, clinical, and educational interests of the Violet University.
Library User Community	1. Violet School of Nursing and clinic, composed of students, staff, and faculty
	2. Patients of the Violet Nursing clinic
	3. Violet University of the state of Violet-Green
Description of User Needs	The core community requires teaching, clinical, and research materials focused on nursing; consumer health and basic nursing materials are necessary for the broader secondary community.
Description of Programs	The School of Nursing focuses on undergraduate nursing programs, with graduate programs in advanced practice and public health nursing. There is a core concentration in nursing informatics.
Library Scope	The collection will focus on supporting the specific needs of the Violet Nursing School and on consumer health. Other health sciences areas will be collected at a basic level.
Cooperative/ Collaborative Factors	Main Library of Violet University provides a large collection of basic science and other materials also available to the Nursing Library. The library belongs to the Pink Consortium, which provides access to a large number of additional online resources and vendor relationships.
Format Considerations	All resources will be collected in electronic format if possible.
Chronological Coverage	All new acquisitions will be of recent publication; exceptions will only be made for the history of nursing subject area or in special circumstance.
Geographical Coverage	The collection will focus on materials produced in the United States with special emphasis on subjects focused on the state of Violet-Green.
Language Coverage	The collection will focus on English language materials. Consumer health materials will also be collected in French and Spanish when possible.
Gifts Policy	Gifts will be accepted in limited circumstance when fitting the scope of the library.
Retention Policy	The library will retain only materials that have circulated in the previous ten years; previous editions will be discarded when the new edition is acquired.

| **Special Collections** | There is a special collection of historical nursing materials for the state of Violet-Green. |

| **Subject Profiles** | These subjects are collected, at the described levels. |

0 = out of scope

1 = minimal information level

2 = basic information level

3 = study or instructional support level

4 = research level

5 = comprehensive level

QS Anatomy	2
WC Communicable Diseases	3
WY Nursing	3
WY 11 AW9—History of Nursing, State of Violet-Green	5
WY 28 Nursing Museums	0
WY 18 Nursing Education	2
WY 85 Nursing Ethics	4
WY 108 Public Health Nursing	3

these are curated and selected by an entity outside of the library, they will affect the collection available to users in potentially quite different directions than librarian selection based upon a formal CDP. For example, it is not uncommon for a health sciences library to subscribe to a collection of social sciences e-journals in order to acquire access to journals about public health. Though this package includes the desired journals that are core to the library's formal collection, it will also include titles that library staff would never select. Some of these resources will prove to be valuable to a user population increasingly interested in interdisciplinary work, but many will be of little benefit and, rarely, may be directly contrary to the qualities that the library would seek to include by choice. Bulk collections can add significant content to library offerings, but they tend to be relatively uninfluenced by the long-term collection-building mission or collection development policies of the subscribing libraries.

Most health sciences libraries have some degree of formalized relationships with other libraries, either in the same institution or in a library consortium, and many of these extend to shared purchases, subscription, or collections. For example, the majority of academic health sciences libraries are part of university library systems that include the full range of other academic subjects, and many at public institutions share online resources with quite different universities within a broader state system. Similarly, hospital libraries may serve a large hospital network containing both large and small hospitals with very different information needs. Most libraries also access some amount of content or negotiate shared contracts or pricing discounts by joining with other libraries in a group called a consortium. These can range from buying clubs to much more complex organizations that share library catalogs and resources. Being part of larger groups means that the library resources available to users include significant, and indeed even majority, percentages of content that was not selected to support a library's core goals and audience. This part of the accessible collection typically includes useful materials and is quite visible to the user community, but it is not bounded by the limits of the collection development policy.

Each of these entities shapes and impacts the library's collection but is minimally impacted by individual collection development choices. As such, while most fit a collection development policy's strictures on the macro level, many of their components might not on the micro level. Some librarians might choose to allow their combination of such resources to serve as an effective collection development policy and avoid the amount of time and effort that goes into creating this document. While this reduction in bureaucracy might be worthwhile, librarians that do this are forgoing the protection of a backstop against having the library and its mission redefined in response to short-term pressures and trends. At the very least, policies are important for defining whether a library participates in consortial deals or purchases large packages at all, whether the collection is online only, and whether ownership or rental is the preferred model for acquisition. The investment of time in reflection that writing a collection development policy requires provides the opportunity for librarians to formally describe their libraries and make thoughtful and purposeful redefinitions if necessary. Changes may occur, but they will be deliberate and not haphazard.

THE USER COMMUNITY

The assorted policies listed above are keys for librarians getting to know an existing library collection and thus how to expand it, but the most valuable resource for either collection development *or* collection management is close knowledge of the group of users that is expected to benefit from the library collection. Building a healthy bridge of communication with users is one of the most critical aspects of collection development, whether it is direct or routed through a liaison librarian, and this is explored in detail in chapter 4. Librarians are experts on resources and on the means of their acquisition, but users are the experts on what they need to gain from those resources. Their needs and interests will vary depending on who they are.

While user needs are unique to every setting, some broad generalizations can be made about which types and content levels of resources are most helpful to which users. For example, clinicians need current point-of-care resources, clinical references, procedures, and guidelines. Researchers, graduate students, and clinical faculty who also do research need access to the most current research published in journals and other primary research sources. Undergraduate students typically need a more introductory level of information of the sort found in textbooks, and graduate students also benefit by learning from advanced textbooks and scholarly monographs. Professional school students (as most health sciences students are) typically have a very structured curriculum with specific textbooks or readings that can be acquired by the library to support them. The subject areas and program aims supported by the library will also speak to varying user needs. Public health students may need access to government publications, medical humanities faculty may be more reliant on scholarly monographs than science faculty, teaching faculty will need resources discussing health science educational methods, and so on. The varying information needs of these different user groups drive which resources, types of resources, and formats of those resources best suit an individual library. As stated above, open communication with both librarian liaisons and faculty is critical to determine how these generalizations match a user community.

MONOGRAPH SELECTION

The most frequent selection decision most collection development librarians must make is individual monograph or textbook selection. Individual monographs, whether print or e-books, are typically less expensive than other resources and, when purchased for long-term retention in either format, require only a single outlay of money. These kinds of acquisitions are the least financially risky, with no long-term encumberment of budget, and it may be reasonable, rather than waiting for a request, to acquire them on a wide variety of subjects on speculation that they will find use. Subscription access to online monographs is a special case that has qualities similar to a journal or database subscription and will be discussed separately.

Although most current acquisitions activity focuses on e-books rather than print, many health sciences libraries are still acquiring some print books. There are a number of issues affecting this choice of format. In some cases, books are only available to libraries in print. This is common especially with undergraduate and some graduate textbooks, anecdotally because many publishers make much of their profit from selling them individually to students. For some libraries, it is desirable to acquire certain books in print (either instead of, or as well as, online) for permanent retention, possibly because the author is a member of the faculty, for interlibrary resource sharing purposes, or because members of the user community indicate a preference for certain types of books in print. Many e-book licenses do not permit resource sharing through interlibrary loan, which has long been a core ideal for most libraries (Schmidt 2013). Those that do typically allow sharing of individual chapters but not of whole books. Additionally, while the situation is rapidly improving, it is not uncommon for e-books to have inferior image quality or even be missing images that are available in the print editions. If an e-book is known to be required as a textbook, a library might even refuse to buy it, if there is no more than a single simultaneous user license available, in order to forestall frustration among the student users (and thus the electronic resources support staff). Certain types of books such as histories, biographies, memoirs, consumer health, or popular works meant for "long form" reading may also only be available in print or be more desirable to users in the print rather than electronic versions.

Any given e-books may be available on multiple platforms, or online hosts, whether on the publishers' own platforms or aggregator platforms that offer books from many publishers. Libraries can purchase e-books either directly from a publisher or through a mediator such as a book jobber or an aggregator platform, and the collection development librarian must make the decision of which best suits the needs of the library. In most cases, purchasing the e-book on the publisher's platform offers the best value: unlimited simultaneous users, lowest price, and the best access to supplemental materials. However, some e-books are only available from an aggregator or may be available at lower cost from the aggregator than the original publisher. Additionally, the library might prefer to offer a uniform online experience to its user community or dislike the terms of a license with a publisher.

Many other considerations for a librarian choosing e-book platforms are discussed in other chapters of this book: discoverability of the content, linking options, usability, format of the content, printing options, and accessibility. Collection managers will need close knowledge of the available e-book options and their qualities to make the best fiscal and user experience decisions, and they may find it helpful to create a locally ranked chart of which vendors are preferred based on their libraries' priorities to promote consistent, transparent purchasing. Fortunately, it is rarely necessary to check both publisher and aggregator options directly to find availability. Most book jobbers will inform the selector of available options. Additionally, some selection aids offer this information; for instance, Doody's Review Service provides information about the assorted online platforms on which any e-book is available.

The selection of new books of every type in anticipation of library needs, whether a sole focus or a minor part of a librarian's professional responsibility, requires making careful choices and exploring new subject areas. New collection development librarians will need to investigate even well-known subject areas from a new perspective and will need to repeat this investigation every time their areas of responsibility change or expand. A small or large targeted development project beyond the regular review of newly published book titles may be triggered by a new academic program, new research laboratory, new grant, clinical department, faculty member with specific research interest, curriculum overhaul, or course being planned. In many of these situations, the librarian must get to know the area beyond what is in the existing collection and acquisition plan. The following sources, accessible through a variety of means, can prove fruitful for consultation or inspiration in monograph or book collection development, though which are most useful will vary by institution and circumstance.

Faculty, Clinicians, and Researchers

- One-on-one discussions with faculty
- Faculty presentations and open lectures
- Classes
- Participation on committees and other university projects
- Course syllabi for directions and readings
- Recent publications lists for the institution

Institutional News

- News about grants, research, initiatives
- News about new hires and changes

Book Jobber/Approval Plan

- Approval plans reveal which subjects are of interest to the library or are left out of notifications
- Book jobbers send notification of new books according to a library's approval plan recorded interests
- Many book vendors offer bundled reviews as a service
- Some book vendors list number of other libraries purchasing books as a benchmark; this may reveal that a book is desirable or that it can be acquired easily via interlibrary loan
- Many book vendors offer subject-based selection lists

Book Reviews

- Book reviews in core journals—*NEJM, JAMA, Blood*, etc.—that the faculty will also be reading to anticipate requests

Basic Textbooks

• Basic overviews of the topic

Association Pages

• News, publications, major scholars listed on professional association sites
• Lists of conferences to attend nearby
• Suggested syllabi or curricula

Twitter and the Blogosphere

• Major scholars, foundations, professional associations, etc., in the subject area on Twitter
• Major blogs in the subject area

Librarian Peers

• Relevant MLA sections and SIGs (special interest groups)

    a. MLA Collection Development Section
    b. MLA subject-specific sections and SIGs

• Continuing education opportunities

    a. Regional Science Boot Camps for Librarians
    b. Courses offered by MLA and other organizations
    c. Conference attendance

• One-on-one help

Selection Aids and Core Lists or References

• Librarian-focused resource review services

    a. Doody's Core Titles in the Health Sciences (www.doody.com/dct): Curated database of core health sciences books for medical and nursing topics
    b. Resources for College Libraries (RCL) (http://rclweb.net/): Curated database of core and recommended books for undergraduate studies in many areas

    c. Thompson, Laurie L., Mori L. Higa, Esther Carrigan, and Rajia
       Tobia, eds. 2011. *The Medical Library Association's Master
       Guide to Authoritative Information Resources in the Health Sci-
       ences.* Medical Library Association Guides. New York: Neal-
       Schuman Publishers, Inc.
    d. *Charleston Advisor*: Journal for review of online e-book pack-
       ages and databases

Usage Statistics

- Usage statistics can show areas of high or low interest
- Usage statistics help one discern whether to buy a new edition of an
  owned book
- Usage and turnaway statistics help justify a purchase/refusal/cancela-
  tion

Approval Plans and Book Jobbers

Librarians may purchase print or e-books directly from their publishers, but
they are just as or more likely to use a mediator. Library "book jobber" is the
common name for a library book vendor that specializes in acting as middle-
man between a library and the many, many publishers that produce desirable
books (Nardini 2003). These companies save a considerable amount of time
for library staff by acting as a single point of contact for purchasing, by
negotiating discounts for libraries, and by presenting the collection development librarian with regular notifications of newly published books and their
e-book options that fit the library's approval plan. As mentioned above, such
plans communicate to the book jobber in exacting detail what formats, subjects, publishers, content levels, and types of books are acceptable to an
individual library. A very important collection management task is to keep
this plan updated with the library's most current interests and needs. In the
approval plan, librarians can set up standing orders for print books from a
particular series or request automatic acquisition of new books or editions.

Individual E-book Subscriptions

Some e-books are only available on a subscription basis, and some are available as either a purchase or a subscription but may be more desirable as a
subscription. Many such subscriptions work with an annual fee and automatic updates with newer editions as they are released. Sometimes a subscription
allows options with different costs for different levels of use or numbers of
simultaneous users. Sometimes there is a continual update with newer material. Continually updating resources based upon earlier print books have

typically functioned more as encyclopedic references, often with new content added directly following new discoveries or guidelines rather than waiting for new editions. The American Academy of Pediatrics' *Red Book Online* (published in print as the *Red Book 2015 Report of the Committee on Infectious Diseases*) is one such title, as is *Harrison's Online* (an updating version of the widely used textbook *Harrison's Principles of Internal Medicine*). Many of these individual titles have become the cores of expansive databases with additional videos, images, tools, news, and other supplementary content, taking full advantage of the opportunities provided by moving to this format. It is debatable whether they can even be considered "books" anymore, even if there is still a print version available (inevitably, with a much smaller amount of total content than the online version).

When an e-book is available either as an annual subscription or, at a much higher cost, as a perpetual access purchase, the collection manager must decide which option best serves the library. If a book has frequent new editions, it is often easier to get it on a subscription basis to ensure immediate access to the new edition and avoid having a collection of outdated e-books. Subscriptions also free up time and streamline purchasing for collection managers as did standing orders for print editions. If new editions are rarer, and the need and interest in the book is expected to be long-term, it may be best to purchase the book with perpetual access rights even if this is the more immediately expensive option. Sometimes budgetary concerns play a part in the decision. If a librarian has one-time money to spend immediately, a purchase might be possible whereas a subscription might not.

The subscription model with limited user concurrency was a common early acquisition model available for e-books, and health sciences libraries were regular adopters. It is not unusual for a library to have a few of these subscriptions in the annual expense column that have been there for a decade or more. Collection managers may want to review these old subscriptions, as they may be replaceable with much lower-cost perpetual-access purchases from aggregator vendors. The books may be duplicated in the library's collections, may no longer be needed at all, or, on the other hand, may show heavy usage, suggesting a need for additional user capacity.

E-book Packages and Patron-Driven Acquisitions

A collection development librarian must be aware of the rapidly changing array of options for resource acquisition, many of which were not possible scant years ago and which may vanish or change substantially in an equally short span of time. While individual book (or more likely e-book) selection still occurs, the bulk of recent monograph collection in health sciences libraries typically includes acquisition of a variety of package formats. In fact, in many cases, a health sciences library will have acquired a significant percentage of the most highly used and desired current monographs and textbooks in the omnibus subscription resources referred to elsewhere in this chapter, which are neither owned nor individually selected. While this chapter will discuss monograph, journal, and other collections independently, many products include multiple types of content, which can blur the lines for decision making. Selection of e-books in a package, whether an omnibus package or less complex e-book package, is quite different than that for individual titles.

Individual "just-in-case" selection of books by librarians, or selection at the micro level, is increasingly viewed as suboptimal as a sole collection-building strategy, as the heavier investment of time and money required is no longer viable for many libraries. Many of the selection aids described above, such as core title lists, presume a title-by-title purchase strategy that is in use only for a smaller and smaller subset of most collections. Relying on a combination of traditional expert selection at the micro level with collection development on a macro level allows librarians to provide access to vast collections of minimally mediated resources in addition to a small group of carefully curated specialist materials (Tyler et al. 2013).

When librarians invest in a large collection of e-books, they give up individual title selection even while still determining the possibilities available to the user by their choices of collection. In these cases, librarians use most of the same selection sources described for individual books but may rely more heavily on sources of reviews for whole e-book platforms and databases, such as those regularly published in *Medical Reference Services Quarterly* or the *Charleston Advisor*. There are four common models for acquiring access to large e-book collections, each with its own advantages and disadvantages. These are bulk purchase of a single publisher's e-book collection, subscription to an enhanced collection of resources including e-books from a single publisher, subscription to large aggregated collections of e-books from multiple publishers on a single platform, and pay-per-view patron- or demand-driven acquisition projects.

With the first model, a library pays for perpetual access to a collection of e-books directly from their publisher, on the publisher's platform or a platform licensed by the publisher (in the case of some societies). As noted for similarly acquired individual e-books, this model typically offers more generous terms of use for the books and more complete access to any supplementary materials than third-party aggregator options. In many cases, the library will purchase perpetual access to a year's release of new titles and then repeat this purchase in subsequent years. These collections are generally more expensive than any subscription equivalent but represent a single fee paid for long-term ownership. If ownership is important for a library, this model may be preferred. Such expenditures may be budgeted for on a recurring basis, just like a journal package or database subscription. Examples of e-books available for purchase with this model range from large packages of subject collections on Elsevier's ScienceDirect platform or on Springer Nature's SpringerLink to much smaller packages of e-books such as those from Thieme or the American Academy of Pediatrics. Most typically, the types of monographs available for purchase with this model tend to be clinical specialty or research-oriented books rather than textbooks or general clinical references, although there are exceptions.

The second model, subscription access to e-book collections on a publisher's own customized platform, is common and has been becoming more so for health sciences educational textbooks and clinical references. McGraw-Hill, Elsevier, Lippincott Williams & Wilkins, Thieme, and other prominent health sciences publishers offer access-only subscriptions that include all or most of their subject-relevant e-books, with additional videos, teaching, self-quizzing, and other useful content. Each of these omnibus resources includes a number of major reference books and textbooks with a long history of adoption by medical schools or hospitals. Most are positioned by publishers as one-stop clinical and teaching resources. Some also include access to e-journals and other resources as such significant percentages of the collection that they may not be directly comparable to other book collections. Some publishers, such as the American Academy of Pediatrics and Truven Health, make single encyclopedic references available on customized, enhanced e-book platforms that, though based on a single title, function far more like databases.

This model takes fuller advantage of the opportunities of the online environment to provide tools, media content, and other options that are impossible to include in a static print or e-book. However, such resources typically represent a recurring cost and are much more expensive than their print or static online equivalents. These resources do not provide perpetual access to included books and tend to require higher involvement than other resources do for electronic resources staff. Occasionally, publishers provide libraries with an option of models, with a higher fee for perpetual access to an e-book package and a lower, recurring fee for subscription access. This is ideal as it allows that option for libraries interested in ownership or who have available one-time money, while libraries that do not have that policy or mission can choose a lower but recurring cost.

A third model has the library pay an annual subscription fee to access books from many publishers on a single aggregated platform. To be desirable, such e-book packages may offer a large discount per title in exchange for a library agreeing to purchase all of a collection rather than some smaller piece of it. As these collections include more of the available titles, users have the opportunity to find everything they want without requiring a librarian to guess what they want.

The disadvantage of this model for the library is the typically high total cost and relatively low percentage of useful content. Most usage tends to be focused in a small percentage of the available books in these packages (Sprague and Hunter 2008). Additionally, with subscription-based access-only packages, whether from a publisher or an aggregator, it is not uncommon for titles to appear and disappear from the collection without much notice to the library (Georgas 2015). Libraries must invest staff time to handle these problems, to get notice of changes to update their catalogs, and to seek out alternative access to e-books or journals that will be missed. There is also a huge variation among platforms in both digital rights management (DRM) requirements, which limit how and who can use an e-book, and in functionality. Often the number of simultaneous users is limited in these aggregator collections, which can be a serious problem when a book is in high demand. As an aside, this last problem can be a useful tool for long-term collection development. Regular monitoring of turnaway reports and data can suggest which e-books should be purchased with a higher number of simultaneous users and/or perpetual access if possible. In recent years, many publishers that once allowed their content to be made available on these aggregator platforms have pulled their content out to make it available solely on their own platform. It is unclear how many important textbooks will be available on aggregator platforms in the future if this trend continues.

The fourth model, patron- or demand-driven acquisition, and its variations, also provides users with the chance to access a much larger number of possibilities than does traditional selection. It also offers users the chance to determine which books the library purchases for perpetual retention. A library makes an agreement with an aggregator or publisher to gain access to a very large collection of e-books and to pay some amount per use of the e-books by its users. After a book receives a set number of uses, a purchase is triggered and it is added to the library's permanent collection. These transactions can be seamless, or they can provide the librarian a chance to mediate or decline the purchase. While the library pays considerably more per book than it does with other means of acquisition, this model has the advantage of ensuring that all the books paid for are actually used (Schroeder, Wright, and Murdoch 2010). Librarians can limit the amount of money they are willing to pay annually, with the program set to automatically pause or cease when this amount is reached.

There are many variations on this practice. One "evidence-based collection development" model, for example, requires the library to prepay some amount of money for access to an entire e-book collection. At the end of a year, it gains perpetual access to a set number of e-books with demonstrated highest levels of use. Then there is an option to renew the contract for another year or lose access to everything else. This model is less risky for libraries than the longer-established model, as libraries pay only a specified amount up front. It seems likely to become increasingly popular, as the longer-established form of patron-driven acquisitions seems to be falling out of favor with publishers, with fewer and fewer books available in those pools. With each of these demand-driven models, librarians can use the collection development policies of the library to help set the parameters of the possibilities available to the user community (e.g., price, publication years, subjects, types of books, languages, publishers), but the users themselves choose which books they will use and therefore add to the library's permanent collection (Arougheti 2014).

STREAMING MEDIA SELECTION: FILMS, PODCASTS, AND MORE

There is an ever-increasing range of streaming and other media-based resources available and relevant to medical libraries. Many databases, publisher websites, e-journals, and e-books include considerable original streaming media or image resources as supplementary to their core content. While some of the most specialized of these are discussed below in the section on databases, much deliberate streaming media selection and acquisitions is like e-book selection. Streaming films or podcasts may be available for either purchase or subscription, either individually or as part of group packages, and there are patron-driven acquisitions models available from some vendors. Selectors often have multiple options for acquisition of films and multiple platforms available for groups of subject or topical films.

There are, however, some unique aspects to streaming media selection and management. Films, especially, are typically of most value in a teaching context for the health sciences and have little value in many cases once past a certain age or once no longer in use for a class. In part, probably, because both analog and digital audiovisual materials typically have had fragile physical forms, and the technology required to access them changes frequently, many non-specialized libraries do not place a high preservation or retention value on them (Campbell 2006). The nearly wholesale move to streaming versus physical media has not changed this priority, but it has made it easier for vendors to provide purchase opportunities that fit the way these materials are often used. Sometimes the only option is to subscribe to media content for brief periods—or even for single showings. For example, a currently prominent option for patron-driven acquisition of streaming content, Kanopy, triggers rentals of videos for a year or three years, rather than an outright purchase. A collection manager must be aware of these issues when making choices of films to acquire.

A special aspect of health sciences films and audio recordings is that, in many cases, health sciences procedures and methods so recorded are considered actively dangerous or unethical to use once past a certain date. Traditionally, such films might have been withdrawn and destroyed when housed on DVD, video, or filmstrip. For example, sound recordings from the Continuing Medical Education vendor Audio-Digest only qualify to earn CME credits for three years post release. Some libraries in turn have discarded their CDs past this date in order to keep currency of clinical information on par (Audio-Digest 2017). If streaming media resources are held on a subscription base, there is little effort required by the library; old videos are typically dropped from or replaced within the package by the vendor. The question of what to do with streaming media in the collection that is held in perpetuity as it becomes outdated is more controversial. Documentaries retain usefulness for a long time and may never need to be removed from the collection. Some procedure videos may look outdated, while the content is still fine. For videos that present procedures that are no longer current, some libraries may choose to suppress owned content as it becomes outdated, while others may try to label such videos as outdated and simply hope that users will be drawn to the record with the most recent date. The collection manager must be aware of and monitor current trends in this area.

JOURNAL SELECTION

As described in chapter 1 of this book, journal content has always been a focus of health sciences libraries, and it continues to be the largest portion of most collection budgets. The thirty-eighth edition of *Annual Statistics of Medical School Libraries in the United States and Canada* reports that collection expenditures for journals and serials take up almost 72 percent of academic health sciences library collection budgets (Squires 2016). As serials costs have increased while library budgets have shrunk or remained largely static, the percentage of budget dedicated to monographs appears to have shrunk in order to sustain investments in journals. A complicating factor for trying to understand these statistics are the large omnibus databases described above that contain multiple kinds of content and the e-book packages that may be treated like serials in library budgets. Nevertheless, rising journal costs are not a new trend. Any search of library literature over the past twenty years will reveal the tension between library budgets and increasing serials subscription costs, often in apocalyptic terms (Panitch and Michalak 2005). Health sciences libraries today increasingly rely on multiple sources for journal content in addition to traditional journal subscriptions.

Traditional journal selection practices are similar to traditional monograph selection practices. However, they have some special qualities that make the decision to acquire a new journal more consequential. Individual journals are typically far more expensive than individual e-books. It is not uncommon for an individual medical journal to cost several thousand dollars annually. Journals also represent a recurring cost commitment, meaning that every year, from their first subscription date, the library's overall available purchasing budget is limited by that same amount or more, as most go up in price annually—average price increase for journals in both 2015 and 2016 hovered around 6 percent, which is typical and projected to continue (Bosch and Henderson, 2016). Because of this, it is less usual to acquire a new journal at one person's request or in hopes that it might find favor. At some libraries, it is even necessary to follow a "cancel-to-add" policy—dropping an equal amount of current spending to add a new journal (Pedersen, Arcand, and Forbis 2014). It is typical at established libraries to acquire new titles only after much careful budget planning, in response to multiple requests or repeated interlibrary loan requests, or at the start of a new academic program. Health sciences libraries tend to rely much more heavily on "bulk-buy" or access-only acquisitions methods for new journals without proven histories of requests and activity. When a library is indeed ready to subscribe to an individual journal title, the following can provide sources of both inspiration and evaluation information. Not surprising, much of this is similar to the criteria used in consideration of new monographs, but there are some special aspects to journal selection.

Faculty, Clinicians, and Researchers

- Direct requests and recommendations
- Recent publications lists for the institution

Institutional News

- News about recent publications

Journal Rankings Lists

- Journal Citation Reports, now part of Clarivate Analytics' InCites platform, offers the impact factor, which is highly respected by faculty and sometimes important for tenure (requires a subscription)
- Scimago offers the SJR, or Scimago Journal & Country Rank, a rank of journal impact based upon citation data from Elsevier's Scopus database (free)

Interlibrary Loan Requests

- If a journal is requested several times, by different users, at different times, it could be a good candidate for subscription (Note: If the requests cluster around one user, it indicates a research project; if it is several users at the same time, it indicates an influential article. Neither of these indicate a need for subscription minus other evidence.)

New Programs

- High-impact journals for the new area
- Suggestions from the new faculty members

Core Journal Lists

- Some MLA subject-specific sections and SIGs offer these
- Some accrediting bodies offer these for specific areas
- Thompson, Laurie L., Mori L. Higa, Esther Carrigan, and Rajia Tobia, eds. 2011. *The Medical Library Association's Master Guide to Authoritative Information Resources in the Health Sciences.* Medical Library Association Guides. New York: Neal-Schuman Publishers, Inc.

Librarian Peers

- Relevant and subject-specific MLA sections and SIGs
- MLA Collection Development Section
- Continuing education opportunities

    a. Courses offered by MLA and other organizations
    b. Conference attendance

- One-on-one advice from peers

Usage Statistics

- Usage statistics can show areas of high or low interest
- Turnaway statistics help one discern whether to add a subscription to a particular journal
- Usage statistics can justify cancelations or shifts to alternate forms of access

The development of a new program or department at an institution can be one reason for needing to add multiple journal subscriptions. In this case, faculty or physician input and publishing activity, titles suggested by relevant accrediting bodies, other core title lists if available, and metric rankings such as impact factors are likely to be most useful in creating a short list of desirable new subscriptions. If the department or program is truly new, it can be helpful to review publications at other institutions with similar established departments or programs. For ranked journal title lists, most faculty and librarians are familiar with Journal Citation Reports and journal impact factors, now part of Clarivate Analytics' InCites platform. The impact factor was first developed as a measure of the influence of a journal for use as a library selection tool; this original purpose has evolved among faculty, librarians, and the publishing industry into a highly valued measure of the influence and impact of both journals and individual authors (Garfield 2006). While even its original creator considered its current enormous influence on faculty tenure and professional reputation problematic, and its benefit as an "objective measure" of quality is controversial, this is still a very common metric used in academia and by granting agencies (Garfield 2006; Bradshaw and Brook 2016). While alternate rankings and measures of impact such as those offered by Elsevier's Scimago Journal Rank or the h-index are becoming more widely known and accepted, impact factor is the metric most widely respected, and administrators will want to know that the new program or department will be supported by a library that provides access to the "best" journals by this metric (Bradshaw and Brook 2016).

Most large health sciences libraries use the services of subscription agents to order and pay for most if not all of their journals. A subscription agent such as EBSCO Subscription Services, W. T. Cox Information Services, Basch Subscriptions, or Harrassowitz GmbH & Co., to list a few commonly used by medical libraries, is the journal equivalent of the book jobber used for acquiring monographs. Like the book jobber, a subscription agent can simplify tasks for a collection manager. For a percentage fee, a subscription agent can help manage routine subscription and renewal processes relating to individual and package subscriptions; monitor such events as title or publisher changes, merges, and ceases; assist in reporting and information gathering; assist in negotiating and managing "Big Deals," and provide other useful services. The benefits and drawbacks to reliance on subscription agents are described in more detail in chapter 3.

Big Deals

Most health sciences libraries acquire large groups of journals all at once by entering into a "Big Deal." Big Deals provide access to all the titles in a publisher's package for a negotiated price that saves the library money over individual journal title subscriptions. There is inevitably a considerable amount of journal content included in the deal that the library has no interest in and would never acquire following its own collection development policy. This is not a problem when there is ample funding, but if the library needs to make budget cuts and wishes to cancel journal content to do so, the least useful journal titles are often locked into a Big Deal, resulting in more important titles needing to be cut. There is often a lack of flexibility to maintain subscriptions from smaller publishers when there are several Big Deals with the largest publishers (Pedersen, Arcand, and Forbis 2014). The publisher may add titles, remove titles, or change them without any input from the subscribing library; the contract will require that the library pays for these at least through the end of the contract cycle, and they are typically not able to remove them with any new negotiation.

If a library chooses to "break" a Big Deal, adding the desirable titles back is frequently prohibitively expensive, sometimes resulting in a situation where a library is paying the same amount for a fraction of the content. While Big Deals offer access to all titles in a publisher's package (which may be a subject package rather than an entire publishing catalog), they may or may not provide perpetual access to all of them. It is common for a Big Deal to provide perpetual access for a subset of core titles that is chosen by the library and rental-only access for the other titles. These titles will vanish from the library's collection if it cancels the Big Deal. Even so, some libraries find canceling preferable to being locked into a contract for years at a time. At present, the Big Deal remains a common and useful part of the library collections landscape—but it rests uneasily for many libraries. Collection managers must consider them carefully. They can offer great value if a library can afford them, but they are very difficult to withdraw from without hurting the user community. More on Big Deals can be found in chapters 1 and 3 of this book.

Aggregators

Another option for journal acquisition is via access-only aggregator platform subscription. Commonly referred to simply as "databases," collections of journals with full-text access are available for various subject areas. For example, EBSCO Information Services offers the database CINAHL Plus with Full Text, which is widely used to support nursing and other allied health areas; and the American Psychological Association offers PsycARTI-CLES along with the index PsycINFO, which provides access to their large collection of psychology and mental health journals. Sometimes it might be a more viable choice for a library to subscribe to one of these specialty databases to support a new program rather than adding a small number of permanent-access journal subscriptions at the same price. While this choice does not add anything to the long-term collection, it provides access to users at a much lower cost than a similar collection of individual journals with retention rights. Drawbacks to such databases of full-text journals include the fact that titles may come and go from such collections without input from the library, and there is no perpetual access to any of the included content after the contract ends. Another important consideration is that some titles within these databases are burdened with an embargo—a period typically ranging from a month to two years before new content is available.

Individual Article Acquisition by the Library

Chapter 1 discusses the rise of the individual article as an item for acquisition rather than an entire journal or journal volume or issue. As part of this trend, some health sciences libraries are forgoing subscription to some journals in favor of pay-per-view (PPV) access to articles through such services as Copyright Clearance Center's Get It Now. Unlike the pay-per-view aspects of patron-driven acquisition of e-books or films, there is no trigger to purchase the journal. Libraries instead pay for access to an article for one person, one time. No real collection in the traditional sense is built with this model, but the user community gains access to information needed to support their work. The great advantage of this model is that it provides access to a very large collection of journals and ensures that everything that is paid for is used. For many libraries, PPV can prove to be far less expensive than subscribing to all or even any of the journals that its users may need (Hendler and Gudenas 2016). Smaller libraries and many of the born-digital libraries that have arisen to serve new medical schools and hospitals particularly find this an attractive model, and pay-per-view may be coupled with interlibrary loan to provide robust access.

The fact that many articles in the health sciences are published open access or are required to be publicly available after an embargo date is increasingly a consideration for collection managers. More on the economics of open access is discussed in both chapters 1 and 3. While most users of health sciences libraries would not be satisfied if limited to only material that is over a year old, it may be a viable option for some libraries to rely on older open-access content, supplemented with interlibrary loan or pay-per-view access for newer articles, especially for topical areas with smaller groups of interested users. The collection manager must rely on knowledge of the budget and communication with the user community to determine the best choices and be willing to adjust this in the future if circumstances change or the chosen option proves inadequate.

DATABASE SELECTION

From a collection management perspective, databases typically represent recurring expenses for access-only content. Access-only collections of journals or journal abstracts from multiple publishers are commonly known as databases, as are a wide variety of other online resources and tools—users and staff will use this term for nearly anything that has a distinguishable identity that is accessed online. Their cost levels range widely, as would be expected with such a wide variety of types of resources. The least expensive tend to be focused on a single type of content or subject, while the most expensive tend to be clinical point-of-care resources or the omnibus type of resources discussed above that include journals, monographs, and other resources on one platform. Other interesting types of resources that can fall into this category include drug reference databases, indexing and abstracting services, exam review and preparation tools, and databases of medical images. Most medical library collections will include these general types of databases, which may overlap.

Clinical Point-of-Care Databases

- Collections of algorithms, calculators, practice-oriented references, images, etc., for use at the point of care by a clinical professional. Examples: UpToDate, DynaMed Plus, Pediatric Care Online

Research Content Databases

- Collections of abstracts, journal articles, books, and other content for use in research by students, clinicians, and faculty. Examples: PubMed, Scopus, Web of Science, PsycINFO, Cochrane Library

Research Support Databases and Resources

- Tools and collections of information for use in supporting and organizing research such as citation managers or metrics. Examples: PlumX, Zotero, EndNote, Mendeley, Journal Citation Reports

Reference Databases

- Encyclopedic references made up of publisher-curated information on particular subjects, which may include content-specific tools. Examples: Micromedex, Sage Research Methods

Education and Learning Support Databases

- Collections of textbooks, exam preparation resources, learning cases, and self-study resources. Examples: AccessMedicine, ExamMaster, Board Vitals

Library Functional Databases

- Description: References and tools to support library activities and functions. Examples: Doody's Review Service, QxMD, BrowZine

For the collection manager, many of these databases represent new types of resources that did not exist in the past and therefore are a challenge to fit into the budget. Many of them provide only temporary access to included content, while others provide different means of accessing or using content that is available elsewhere. While the user community will perceive and experience database content seamlessly as part of the library's collection, librarians may need to adapt and change both library technical services procedures and budgetary guidelines to best suit the special qualities of databases. Some of these new products may offer opportunity for collaboration with new partners both within and beyond the library—for example, with those managing clinical care in any affiliated hospital or clinic, with librarians outside of the health sciences, and with research support services units.

Trialing Databases

Because of the high recurring costs of many databases and, for some libraries, the lack of permanence of the content, collection management librarians often decide to perform extensive evaluation of these resources before deciding to subscribe. Librarians typically learn about new databases from vendor communications or while attending conferences, or receive a request for a database from a library user group. A first step might be to check review sources and trial the database in question privately, but, if possible, it is advisable to hold a public trial of the database and request feedback from the user community. This will provide data that can be shared to defend a decision to either acquire or reject a resource. Another benefit is that it publicizes the resource from the start of the library's interest, earning the user community's investment in the new resource. Particularly if a database has been requested by library users, holding a public trial so that they can test its usefulness reinforces a communicative and collaborative relationship between the library and the user community.

The collection management librarian (possibly in close coordination with the electronic resources librarian, if that is a separate position) initiates and coordinates database trials and carefully monitors their process and results. It is good practice for the collection management librarian to create a short summary of the benefits of the database, the qualities that make it unique, and its expected uses and audience to share with those expected to offer feedback. Not only can this serve as the library's record of trialed resources and as a start to any necessary cataloging activities, it can help users understand why they might be interested in it. While all vendors offer summaries and descriptions of their resources, and reviews from librarian or medical journals can also offer such summaries, descriptions personalized to the library and institution are often more useful to the user community. This process will also help determine if the database should be under consideration at all. In nearly all situations, it is best to trial a database only when there is a realistic chance of subscribing to it in order to maintain good relationships with both the vendors and the users involved. The collection development librarian should consider each of these questions before trialing a database:

- Is it affordable at the present time?
- Is it affordable on an ongoing basis?
- Who would use it and does this affect what available level of access is desirable?
- Does it support the core mission of the library?
- Does the vendor offer a license and terms of use acceptable to the library? If it is a vendor with an existing relationship, could this resource be added to an existing license or contract?
- Would adding it mean that other subscriptions could be dropped or materials withdrawn?
- Are there other interested parties that might be willing to cost-share (the main academic library, the hospital, etc.)?
- Is the resource available through a consortial arrangement that might lower the cost, or could it be suggested to a consortium for consideration?

The answers to any of these questions could change the timing of the database trial, the library's choices for available means of trial, or whether a trial need occur at all. Fortunately, once the library expresses interest, nearly all database vendors that typically work with libraries will offer free trial access to the entire institution for some span of time. It is important for the collection manager to request enough time for the user community to fully evaluate the database. If possible, a trial period of sixty to ninety days is desirable to give the targeted part of the user community time to examine it and use it in practice, but it is not uncommon for trials to be limited to a month or less. In some cases, it might be better to have it for an entire year for example, if the purpose of the database is so unique that it will require an intensive effort to publicize it or the users might need to have access for a longer period to truly test it (for example, it is needed for a course or for use in a lab). In that case, it is sometimes possible to negotiate a lower-cost subscription for an initial trial year, with a promise to jump up to the standard price the second year if it should prove its worth as a subscription. In many cases, the library will be able to secure the best terms for the new database by working through a consortium to subscribe. A consortium negotiates on behalf of its library members with a vendor for a lower-cost subscription; generally, with better terms available, the more libraries participate. Such an agreement can reduce the ability of the library to negotiate special terms such as extended trial periods, but the benefits often outweigh this drawback.

It can sometimes be possible to integrate a trialed e-journal or e-book database into the online collection with links and measure usage as the pri-

mary means of gaining feedback. This is only practicable for databases largely made up of the sorts of content that users will be able to find through links
in PubMed or other resources that they already use; in such a case, they will
find the content and use it—or decline to do so—through their usual online
research activities. Reviewing the usage statistics, judged in the context of
the expected size and character of the user community, can suggest whether
the database should be subscribed as is or the library might be better served
by adding only a component of it.

Many databases cannot be trialed in such a way effectively, especially if
they contain nontraditional content or are intended for clinical support. For
these types of databases, the trial must be more actively publicized. Librarians can publicize a trial as narrowly or widely as they choose. Sometimes it
makes sense only to involve a specific group of users, and other times it is
helpful to include the entire user community. In a publicity campaign, it is
important to provide easy options for offering feedback. Some common
means of both marketing and gathering feedback include posting on the
library and department websites or guides via learning management systems
such as Blackboard or Canvas; mass emails and posters, both physical and
virtual, in places that users gather; recruiting interested faculty to promote it
in classes or meetings; visiting department meetings; hosting focus groups
(with food provided); integrating the resource with any hospital or education-
al-access electronic health record installations; using library social media
accounts such as Twitter or Facebook; and coordinating with university or
hospital training or communications staff (Ritterbush 2012). More about involving users in assessment of resources through focus groups and other
methods is discussed in chapter 4.

Most vendors will happily provide marketing templates, posters, and
giveaways, or even send staff to help promote the resource. This can be very
helpful, but the collection management librarian will need to be aware of and
keep careful control over vendor activities surrounding the trial. In many
cases, hospital policy will not permit the use of giveaways, and any visiting
vendor representatives must be careful to follow such policies. Additionally,
librarians must review vendor communications before distribution to ensure
they are not in contradiction to a library's goals or policies. Feedback mechanisms should be clearly visible and both simple and swift to use; survey
utilities such as Qualtrics and SurveyMonkey are common, familiar to users,
simple to use, and provide straightforward analytical tools (Ritterbush 2012).
For best response, feedback surveys should be very brief, request specific
information relevant to the trial, and provide an option for users to request
updates on the results of the trial (Ritterbush 2012).

Just as important as gathering feedback is returning it to the user community. It is vital to be forthright about the decision-making processes and about
what should be expected by users who might become invested in the idea of

acquiring the resource in question. It is especially important to communicate the final decision and the reasoning behind it to any users who took the time to contribute feedback or offer requests. Even if the result is not what was hoped, library users will be far more likely to accept the outcome and feel that the relationship with the library is positive if they are given responses to their input and feel that it was valued.

LICENSING ISSUES

Electronic information resources consist of intellectual property subject to copyright law, and the owners of that property will nearly always require a license or other agreement to set terms for subscription and use. This license agreement will typically set more limits than copyright law does and is subject to contract law, meaning that its terms will always take precedence over any ideas of fair use (Dygert and Langendorfer 2014). This concept can be troublesome and confusing for the user community. Librarians must be aware of the exact terms of licenses and effectively communicate them to library users since they do not have copies of the licenses.

Before beginning a public trial or issuing the pay order for a new resource, collection management librarians or their teams must review licenses for acceptability of terms, secure approval for the terms and associated financial contract, or establish that the resource can be added to an existing master license from that vendor. Each library should establish a set of priorities and "deal-breakers" for licenses. Informed by these, librarians will often need to negotiate changes to the general terms of the license. In most libraries, the collection manager or an associated team negotiates or agrees to at least the initial terms of the license, sometimes with final approval required from an institutional legal representative. The collection manager sometimes has final signatory authority for placing the actual order to pay and sometimes must pass it along to someone else with that role. Negotiation strategies are discussed in depth in chapter 3.

There are several common types and models of licenses and licensing situations. Many library vendors or publishers offer multiple platforms, packages, or types of content. Sometimes these require multiple licenses, but often it is simpler for both vendor and customer to have one master license with amendments or components covering different resources. This sort of license, once established, is generally easy to amend to add new terms covering newly subscribed titles or collections. While licenses for such resources, especially if they include perpetual access rights to any covered content, can be quite complex, licenses for single databases or access-only content are relatively simple with minimal negotiation possible or required (Dygert and Langendorfer 2014).

The most typical library license will spell out who the licensor and licensee are, which addresses shall be used, a glossary of terms used in the document, authorized users and sites, authorized uses, responsibilities of both licensor and licensee, legal issues in case of a dispute, mutual obligations, content included, schedules of access and payment, interlibrary loan limitations or permissions, and terms of payment. While these are similar to a traditional academic license and a medical academic license, it is not uncommon for a medical academic license to have additional terms addressing clinical use. For example, many clinical resources are available at a much lower cost for educational use only, if no hospital or clinical professionals are included. Others will have terms describing how the resource might permissibly be integrated with hospital electronic heath record systems. Some of the potential "deal-breakers" that librarians at different institutions negotiate based on their priorities are walk-in community patron usage, interlibrary loan rights, use of materials in course management systems, and accessibility language. These considerations are discussed in more detail elsewhere in this book. Another common issue is indemnification. Many vendors include terms that require the licensee to indemnify them against legal issues, but most, if not all, public institutions are banned from agreeing to such requirements. It is also common for licenses to ask that terms be kept secret, which is also verboten for a public institution subject to public record requests. These terms and issues must be reviewed and amended as necessary. It is important to review every license renewal or amendment with care, no matter how familiar the vendor, since it is very common for terms to be changed.

Fortunately, there are many useful model library licenses and other resources available to both librarians and publishers, prominent among them LIBLICENSE Model License Agreement (Center for Research Libraries 2014) and the CRKN Model License (Canadian Research Knowledge Network 2016). Each of these offers detailed model licenses for use and consultation by librarians and publishers. Librarians will find that it is common for new, inexperienced, and smaller society publishers to lack understanding of the library environment and request too-restrictive terms in their licenses. It can be very helpful for libraries to be able to offer examples of useful terms and structure from these models (Taylor and Beh 2014).

The high requirements for staff time and expertise required by full-scale license review and negotiation can be quite burdensome for libraries *and* for publishers. It is not unknown (though certainly not good practice) for a license to sit on the desk of a busy collection manager for months before review and acceptance. As such, the National Information Standards Organization (NISO) Shared E-Resource Understanding (SERU) license alternative was developed to alleviate some of this burden and speed access to the resources for users. SERU agreements are far less time intensive and less prescriptive than license agreements; they seek to act as a "mutual understanding" between publishers and libraries rather than as formal legal documents, relying instead on copyright law and the principles laid out in the SERU statement (Rolnik, Lamoureux, and Smith 2008). Rather than using elaborate and specific legal terminology, SERU "describes a set of commonly agreed-upon expectations for using and providing electronic resources," which all parties involved in a SERU agreement decide to respect (NISO 2012). At this point, there are hundreds of publishers and libraries that have joined the registry of those who will accept SERU in at least some transactions (NISO 2017). While this kind of agreement does not suit every situation and cannot replace all license agreements even for participating libraries and publishers, many libraries choose to rely on it when possible.

DESELECTION AND WITHDRAWAL OF MATERIALS

Health sciences libraries have always had an interest in removing outdated materials promptly, whether simply from reference or circulation or from the library entirely. As most of the current collection moved entirely online, it also became very common for libraries of all types to reduce physical collections in favor of collaborative study or instructional spaces, or even to cede space to other departments of the university or hospital (Lynn et al. 2011). Online journals and journal backfile archives of older content have been established long enough to both greatly improve in technology and to build trust in the library community. Changes in pedagogical practices and rising student expenses also continue to drive use away from traditionally published textbooks toward the use of modules and readings from multiple textbooks, faculty-produced instructional materials, open educational resources, or other similar resources (Desai and Chilton 2016). These trends drive an increasing need for collection managers to engage in regular targeted or broad deselection projects, and this makes regular and targeted collection analysis (as detailed in chapter 4) to support these projects imperative.

Physical Item Weeding and Withdrawal

The collection manager is typically the person who spearheads any print material weeding or withdrawal project. This sort of library content reduction can be less impactful than an electronic journal or database cancelation as it removes content that is often outdated, unlike a journal cancelation that removes access to current and future content. However, any sort of large-scale reduction of the library's physical collection is likely to draw a negative emotional reaction from both library staff and the user community (Wajda 2006). Some libraries have handled this in the past by sneaking withdrawn books into the dumpster. This action is inevitably discovered, drawing bad publicity and inducing distress and mistrust among library users, and should be avoided. If a library is withdrawing an item not to discard but to sell, the response from the user community is also often deeply negative; so, if this is the path decided upon, this likely response should be anticipated (Wajda 2006). Performing a careful and transparent analysis of the collection areas to be reduced and communicating openly about the analysis and any positive goals driving the project is the best way to reduce this ill effect.

The easiest type of withdrawal project for the user community is one in which print journals, for which there is online access perpetually owned by the library, are being transferred to storage or withdrawn. Typically, health sciences library users have not used the print journals in years and are unlikely to care about withdrawal of the print, so long as they are informed of the impending removal and reminded of online accessibility (Lingle and Robinson 2009). At academic libraries, some faculty who have experience using the print editions may have tender feelings about the print volumes that should be considered but not overindulged. In such a case, early and nonconfrontational communication with these users can be critical in earning their eventual support of and even investment in the library's goals. Often the expression of willingness on the part of the library to bring back materials from storage if usage shows a demand can allay much concern; very rarely will this actually result in the need to return journals—and if it does, it's a useful demonstration of need. If a journal is being withdrawn altogether without any online access, it can be helpful to the user community to offer free interlibrary loan for titles that were once owned but no longer are. The type of collections analysis review mentioned above should also provide data that can be used in communications with users to support librarian decisions.

Librarians often have more concerns than library users about print journal withdrawal because they know that the quality of online backfiles can vary greatly. Some journal backfiles, particularly early ones, consist of poor-quality scans of the printed volumes and may be missing random content, including whole issues, articles, images, and supplementary content. Images may have been scanned in black and white with low-quality resolution. Backfile quality is improving over time, and some publishers have gone back to redo early scans, but low-quality backfiles are still sold to libraries at high prices. Concern about actual ownership of online content remains something that has not yet been fully tested; alarming stories about certain publishers removing access to "owned" content by removing access to the interface necessary to access it have been rife in recent years. This kind of concern can be addressed for some titles by library and publisher participation in shared archives intended to provide access even if the publisher vanishes, such as LOCKSS (Lots of Copies Keep Stuff Safe), CLOCKSS (Controlled Lots of Copies Keep Stuff Safe), or Portico, but this is not possible for every title or every library (Rais, Arthur, and Hanson 2010). This is the reason for the development of shared print repositories such as those described in chapter 5.

The existence and availability of such repositories is important for inspiring librarian confidence in print journal withdrawal or transfer projects. Nevertheless, despite these concerns, most librarians can easily withdraw entire shelf ranges of bound journal volumes to storage or withdraw them entirely and free up enormous amounts of space without real harm.

When it becomes clear that the library must free up significant floor space for new needs, bound journal volumes can be the best target, as the Health Sciences and Human Services Library (HS/HSL) at the University of Maryland, Baltimore, found when it chose to give up considerable space in a successful attempt to both meet university needs and control the inevitable impact on the library (Tooey 2010). Upon seeing the increasing need for space for new hospital and university programs, the library administration moved proactively to reduce its collection, free space, and avoid removal of unique and higher-use content by focusing on journals and a careful selection of monographs. The resulting collection was more streamlined to meet user practices, and the project placed the library as an active partner in university planning and decision making. As with many projects, a well-managed cancelation project can provide opportunity for fellowship and deeper enmeshment with the broader community.

Monograph weeding or withdrawal typically draws more emotion from library users and librarians, and it is much more time consuming. As with other major changes to the library collection, transparency and clear communication with users and staff are deeply important to reduce distress. If library materials disappear in any noticeable way, it is important to make it known where they are going or what the terms of their removal might be. For example, if a large number of books are being transferred to storage, librarians can post clear notices in the physical building and online to this effect and inform users how books can be retrieved. If books are being withdrawn because they are outdated or duplicated, librarians can make this known and make it clear how to request those or other books through interlibrary loan or for repurchase. If books are being removed to add something desirable like new study rooms or collaborative spaces, librarians should highlight this fact prominently.

There are as many ways to determine how to withdraw or transfer print books as there are libraries, but the basic process generally begins with circulation statistics and/or a review of currency. The first consideration for either should be the primary end goal; typically, either to maintain collection currency or to reduce collection size. Each of these goals will require a systematic analysis of the collection for the qualities that would make a book a good candidate for withdrawal, but the second is typically less frequent and may require adjustment to reach a targeted quantity or shelf footage number. If it is necessary to reduce the collection by a specific volume count, it is best to begin reducing the collection by select qualities first and then broaden the criteria as necessary to reach the right numbers, as the University Libraries of Loma Linda University did (Lingle and Robinson 2009). In that case, the libraries began by identifying print books and bound volumes with these criteria: print holdings duplicated by stable electronic access, print holdings duplicated elsewhere in the library system, and print materials with low usage (Lingle and Robinson 2009). To reach their goal of reducing space, they then reviewed resources for the amount of space required per title, the number of external interlibrary loan requests, and availability of the materials at regional or national levels (Lingle and Robinson 2009). In their case, this information encouraged them to keep some materials identified for removal by their first criteria.

In the earlier described space-motivated reduction, the University of Maryland at Baltimore's Health Sciences Library used the common practice of moving monographs published before a certain date without recent circulation to storage, while removing duplicates and out-of-scope materials (Tooey 2010). This author was also involved in a similar project at the University of North Carolina at Chapel Hill's Health Sciences Library, using similar criteria. Each of these libraries also brought back materials from storage upon user request. If possible, small exceptions should be made on request from the start of the project as an act of goodwill—it is common for faculty to approach the library staff when they observe the scale of the reduction. Two more stories of major print collection downsizing projects in health sciences libraries are included elsewhere in this book.

Some types of books contain information that becomes rapidly or even dangerously outdated, and most reference or textbooks produce regular new editions. Managing this should be a continual part of a collection manager's job. Most hospital libraries and smaller academic libraries have always done this regularly as a matter of course, often reviewing and weeding their entire print collection ruthlessly. Many large academic libraries have attempted to keep comprehensive collections, including editions stretching into the far past, but this is changing. Larger-scale weeds in academic libraries are far more common in current practice than they have been in the past, as the most valuable use of library space moves away from warehousing collections.

In the twenty-first century, it becomes far harder for libraries to justify keeping "just-in-case" books or even books that are considered core to a particular subject but see low use. Most health sciences libraries will not benefit by keeping more than the most recent two editions of such books on site, if that. As more and more libraries move to primarily online monograph collections, it is becoming increasingly common to have a current online edition and a print copy on the shelves that is two or more editions older. Unless the collection development policy requires otherwise, it is often a good idea to routinely weed these older editions or move them to a historical collection, particularly if they contain outdated medical procedural or pharmaceutical prescribing information. If the collection development policy does require otherwise, it may be time to revise it. However, if the library aims to keep a small print collection of critical reference materials in case of a disaster involving loss of power, the current edition must be purchased in print, even if it duplicates an online edition.

Even as acceptance of electronic journal backfiles as permanent replacements for print volumes has grown, it seems likely that e-books with perpetual access will become accepted as replacements for print books on the library shelves. This is already the case in many health sciences libraries that do not maintain historical collections. Medical textbooks are an excellent target for weeding since many of them have bulky editions that may have recently become available online with or without perpetual access. Each library will have to decide whether to buy or keep print at all based on its priorities, but the existence of larger-scale print repositories makes many libraries more comfortable with the decision to discard print.

Deselection of E-books and Owned Streaming Media

With the increasing preponderance of e-books in the health sciences collection, many libraries find themselves with multiple older electronic editions of clinical reference textbooks and other older e-books that would have been withdrawn following standard practices if they had been print books. Some libraries do not regularly weed outdated print books, and this may have little ill effect on their user community beyond reduction of available shelf space, but this is not necessarily the case for e-books. Choosing between editions of e-books is more problematic than with print books for many users both because there can be more variation between different electronic versions of the same edition, and because e-books lack the easy visual context clues that print books show for outdated content. While catalog records do show dates, they cannot show dust. Additionally, in many cases, libraries will acquire access to an e-book on multiple platforms, either as part of several different aggregated collections or deliberately for specific features—which is unlikely to be expected by users accustomed to the rarity of print volume duplication. Vendor-provided cataloging records are also notoriously poor in quality, though necessary to manage library workload, and using them often results in different editions or versions of the same e-book appearing in duplicate or misleadingly out of order in results lists (Walters 2013). Additionally, some discovery systems present the results of a book title search in order of "popularity" or by source platform rather than "most recent edition at the top," so that old editions end up at the top of the results list and the new edition is well below other titles that are only remotely similar. Multiple e-book records for the same book in the library catalog can appear in random order with no obvious difference for the end user (Walters 2013). Libraries must decide how to handle these situations, which will frequently occur without notice to the librarian.

Some librarians choose to let users try their luck and hope that they pick the most optimal record, some do a manual search for each newly added e-book and combine records to include all versions of an e-book in one, and some suppress all but the preferred version. Some may simply add a note to the e-book's catalog record stating that it is an outdated edition. Suppression of a catalog record, or hiding it from the publicly visible catalog, is the closest thing to withdrawal that is possible in most cases for owned e-books. Print books can be removed and discarded, but e-books are housed on another entity's server. If users have saved a link directly to the e-book rather than to the catalog record, in most circumstances, they will still be able to go directly into the older e-book. While this is an issue with all academic books, it is arguably a much more serious one for medical books, especially if a library supports clinical practice. Outdated content can be deadly. As this is such a serious concern, many libraries choose to maintain a short list of references that must receive manual attention to avoid having older content promoted—whether this means manually adjusting the catalog record to ensure that new editions display first or even suppressing the older titles. This can be most beneficial with pharmaceutical prescriber's guides, vaccination schedules, therapeutic guidelines and procedures manuals, and clinical references highly valued by the institution. Publishers are aware of this issue, and one major benefit of subscription to a typical e-book collection without perpetual access is that they will handle it nearly automatically for the library. Many publishers remove older e-books from their platforms as they upload new editions and then typically offer updated MARC records files via their websites and the various commercial e-resources workflow management services. If a library purchases perpetual access to some titles that it also has short-term access to as part of a subscription package, the technical services department must take care to ensure that records for owned content do not disappear with the removal of the subscription content, unless desired. There is otherwise little direct technical intervention required for this type of withdrawal circumstance. However, the automated removal and addition of content is likely to impact an academic community at the beginning of each term—faculty are not generally pleased when a required textbook that they are accustomed to assigning suddenly has a failing link. The electronic resources, collection management, or liaison librarian must anticipate their concerns and update them with current links and explanations of this issue as needed.

The situation is similar for purchased access to streaming media files. While outdated VHS cassettes or DVDs would be swiftly identified and discarded as they break or circulate (or fail to circulate), streaming files tend to sit unnoticed in the library collection. In many cases, this is a more critical issue than even the problem of the library catalog sending users to the older version of e-books, because of the high proportion of health sciences films that focus on medical procedures and continuing education. It can cause real harm to patients if clinical users rely on outdated examples and explanations of treatments and techniques. In the case of streaming content that is included in the catalog, this can be handled as described above for e-books. At the 2017 Charleston Conference, a long-standing and valuable conference focusing on every aspect of library collections held annually in Charleston, South Carolina, the special concerns affecting medical videos were a topic of discussion, and this seems likely to continue to evolve and change as an area of practice.

Journal and Database Subscription Cancelation Reviews

While reducing monograph purchases for a year or two in response to budget cuts or other priorities is relatively simple, academic health sciences libraries have around 93 percent of their budgets tied up in recurring expenses, many of them contract bound (Squires 2016). This situation is likely similar or even more so for hospital and smaller libraries. To handle significant reductions in the budget, it is necessary to cut subscriptions. Even in years without formal budget reductions, many libraries take a "one in, one out" stance on new subscriptions, as referred to above, or must find a way to reduce subscription expenditures (Bosch and Henderson 2016). This is because it is increasingly common for libraries to use some version of a zero-based budget model for continuing resource expenses. More on budgeting models is included in chapter 3. In short, for this model, the budget must be built around projected actual costs rather than a flat increase based on the past (Linn 2007). In practice, this often means that each expense must be justified. When done well, this can be a very effective means of ensuring that the collection continues to be relevant. In difficult budgetary times, this can be the only means to acquire new resources for repositioning the collection toward new priorities.

Evaluation of subscriptions for potential cancelation typically includes looking at both usage and the context of that usage. The majority of electronic resources provide usage statistics using the COUNTER Code of Practice, a publicly available standard (COUNTER 2017). This ensures that similar resources can be compared using the same data created using the same policies. Unfortunately, the standard does not always work well for unique types of resources. For these, usage statistics are often available using a different, publisher-created standard. This must be considered when comparing these resources to others. Usage data direct from the publishers is generally more reliable than data gathered by other means. Most libraries provide multiple access points for every online resource: library catalogs, discovery layers, links on subject guides, link resolvers from databases, ProQuest360, Google Scholar, links coded within learning management systems, and journal discovery apps such as BrowZine or Read by QxMD; these generate additional data, but each can give only a picture of access via that avenue. The only source showing all usage is the vendor or publisher platform that hosts it. The collection management librarian is in an ideal position to be aware of and manage usage data for all the access points of interest for owned or subscribed content and to interpret what each subset of overall usage for a resource may mean.

Despite the existence of an established standard, it is impossible to create one complete report showing all usage for all materials in a library using the same measures. There are some distinct differences in the qualities of different types of materials useful for evaluation. For example, e-journals should be expected to show a much higher level of usage than e-books, as they include far more content and are continuously updated. It is also generally acknowledged that e-books typically show higher usage than print book circulation; however, as e-book usage reports generally measure use by chapter or view, which is impossible to measure for print books, this is not truly an equivalent comparison. COUNTER offers several different reports suited to types of resources, but even these require the collection development librarian's close knowledge of the context of the library and its resources for interpretation. Librarians typically find that resources within large databases will vary dramatically in usage, but the decision of whether to keep or cancel must be made about the database as a whole. Is it worth subscribing to an entire database to get access to one enormously popular e-book? Or can that e-book be acquired singly for a lower cost? It is difficult to make decisions by comparing unique databases with different purposes and patterns of use, such as a drug database with an exam preparation resource. In these cases, all that can be examined is usage for each database, and it may be more useful to compare the usage of these databases with their own usage in past years.

Cost per use is an important metric for evaluation that considers both annual usage and subscription costs. Cost per use is calculated by dividing the payment for a resource by the number of times that resource was used. A low cost per use means that the resource is well used. If the cost per use is high enough for a journal, it may be more fiscally responsible to acquire desired articles via interlibrary loan than to pay for an annual subscription. On the other hand, if the cost per use is low for a particular database, further review may not be necessary—it has proved its value to the user community. This method cannot provide contextual information, such as which users may have been most interested in the resource, or whether it was most valuable for research, clinical, or training purposes, but it permits basic comparisons of identical data between like types of resources. Cost per use is most valuable for the initial triage of journal and serials review, as there is more similarity in structure, means of access, and pattern of use between different journals than between resources in any other category. A single spreadsheet can show cost per use and other useful comparative data for all subscribed journals and can easily be adjusted or sorted or show additional notes for review at a single glance.

The collection manager must apply context to this data for all resource types. As mentioned above, databases are so often so different from each other that they cannot be truly compared by usage alone; contextual information about their intended user populations and other qualities is critical to consider in concert with their cost per use. Though journals tend to be more similar, they can differ in the size of expected audience, average costs in a field, the numbers of articles available per issue and year, contract length and licensing terms, and so on, all of which are important to be aware of in order to achieve a fiscally responsible and even-handed cancelation list. It is critical to avoid penalizing disciplines because the number of faculty is small, the average journal cost is higher, or their journals are newer and thus have fewer articles to show use. Sometimes these factors may mean that it is wiser to cancel a journal with a low cost per use than one with a higher cost per use, particularly in cases where the higher cost per use title also has higher usage overall. If the journal subscription fee is low, it is likely to have a lower cost per use than some much more heavily used ones. The journal may also be of high importance but to a small audience, whereas another journal may have higher use because it is of secondary interest to a much bigger audience.

In light of the above, it is often useful for a library to create a standard list of context determination questions to consider for every resource that has either low usage or high cost per use to trigger a cancelation possibility evaluation. The following are some examples of context that may be important to consider when evaluating a journal or database for cancelation:

Audience

- Is it high impact for an important audience?
- Is the expected audience small or large?
- Is its content suitable for the library's user community?
- Is the content unique for a user group (for example, it is the only exam preparation database the library provides)?

Vendor and Platform Issues

- Can it be canceled at this time under the terms of its contract? (If a journal or database is part of a Big Deal, it may only be cancelable at a specific point or may not be cancelable at all so long as the deal is active.)

- Would canceling it negatively impact other contracts with the vendor?
- Is it bundled with something else that should not be canceled?
- Is it available freely elsewhere (e.g., PubMed Central, open access, a subscribed aggregator)?

    a. If so, does the library need perpetual access or is access-only sufficient?
    b. If so, is there an embargo that is unacceptable?
    c. If so, is the alternate access complete or is there missing content?

- Are there frequent access problems, or does it have missing content?
- Does it work with the library's other electronic systems?

Journal Issues

- Is it a new journal that hasn't had enough time to generate robust usage?
- Has the journal changed publishers so that usage statistics may be on multiple publisher platforms depending on the dates?
- Is the journal available on multiple platforms or from aggregators as well as publisher platforms, dividing the usage statistics?
- Does the subscription include access to older content?

Canceling a large database or collection of e-books or journals can be traumatic for an institution that has come to rely on the content. Often the content is not findable elsewhere, books or journals may not be available for individual subscription or purchase outside of the database or deal, and users must rely on pay-per-view or interlibrary loan options (which are higher effort and lower immediacy for users). It can be done successfully, however, as evidenced by the University of California's story in this book of canceling ClinicalKey.

Transparency of decision making about something so impactful as the removal of library content is very important for good communication with the user community. In many cases, users will be both understanding of the need to cut the budget and willing to help. An important factor in gaining cooperation can be an open process for and willingness to bring back titles that prove to be missed some period after cancelation—whether this is indicated by an excess of interlibrary loan requests or formal requests from faculty (Degener and Swogger 2012). Some libraries will offer lists of potential cancelations to relevant departments and request their feedback. Others will seek feedback from the entire community, which they may or may not weigh differently depending on the source of feedback and resource in question. Many give opportunities for comment to anyone who might be willing to give it (Degener and Swogger 2012).

On the other hand, some librarians find that asking for user input in a cancelation project can be frustrating because their users do not understand the actual costs and requirements of the collection or the strictures caused by acquiring resources using a package deal, or value the use of materials by people different from themselves. Librarians at the University of New Mexico also found that it was important not to weigh quantitative results from their survey of users about journal cancelation too highly in their review because of the unbalanced response rate from different colleges and departments—again, context was critical for effective evaluation (Nash and McElfresh 2016). Librarians cannot let the most vocal users have more influence on decisions than is warranted and will need to use institutional knowledge and librarian expertise as well as data in decision making.

CONCLUSION

As is clear from the variety of topics included in this chapter and in this book, collection development and collection management are broad areas that include a wide divergence of tasks and concerns. Keeping a solid focus on the information and communications needs of the user community and the available resources to meet them is far more important than the actual tools and routes used to connect them—these will change and evolve rapidly in even the next few years, but the need for well-informed management by librarians will remain.

REFERENCES

Arougheti, Stephen. 2014. "Keeping Up With . . . Patron Driven Acquisitions." Association of College & Research Libraries (ACRL). http://www.ala.org/acrl/publications/keeping_up_with/pda.

Audio-Digest Foundation. 2017. "Audio-Digest Foundation: About ADF: Accreditation FAQs." Audio-Digest Foundation. Accessed March 13. http://www.audio-digest.org/CME-Accreditation-FAQ.

Bandy, Margaret Moylan. 2015. "Pivoting: Leveraging Opportunities in a Turbulent Health Care Environment." *Journal of the Medical Library Association* 103 (1): 3–13. doi:10.3163/1536-5050.103.1.002.

Biblarz, Dora, Marie-Joelle Tarin, Jim Vicker, and Trix Bakker. 2001. "Guidelines for a Collection Development Policy Using the Conspectus Model." International Federation of Library Associations. http://www.ifla.org/files/assets/acquisition-collection-development/publications/gcdp-en.pdf.

Blansit, B. D., and E. Connor. 1999. "Making Sense of the Electronic Resource Marketplace: Trends in Health-Related Electronic Resources." *Bulletin of the Medical Library Association* 87 (3): 243–50. http://www.ncbi.nlm.nih.gov/pmc/articles/PMC226578/.

Bosch, Stephen, and Kittie Henderson. 2016. "Fracking the Ecosystem: Periodicals Price Survey 2016." *Library Journal* 141 (7): 32–38. Posted April 21. http://lj.libraryjournal.com/2016/04/publishing/fracking-the-ecosystem-periodicals-price-survey-2016/.

Bradshaw, Corey J. A., and Barry W. Brook. 2016. "How to Rank Journals." *PLOS ONE* 11 (3): e0149852. doi:10.1371/journal.pone.0149852.

Campbell, Brad. 2006. "Preservation Services for Audio Visual Media Material: An Inquiry into Current and Future Models." Thesis. New York: New York University. https://www.nyu.edu/tisch/preservation/program/student_work/2006spring/06s_thesis_campbell.pdf.

Canadian Research Knowledge Network. 2016. "CRKN Model License." Canadian Research Knowledge Network. http://www.crkn-rcdr.ca/sites/crkn/files/2016-09/crkn_model_license_2016_final.pdf.

Center for Research Libraries. 2014. "Liblicense Model License Agreement with Commentary." Center for Research Libraries. http://liblicense.crl.edu/wp-content/uploads/2015/05/modellicensenew2014revmay2015.pdf.

COUNTER. 2017 "Project COUNTER—Consistent, Credible, Comparable." COUNTER. Accessed March 22. https://www.projectcounter.org/.

Degener, Christie, and Susan Swogger. 2012. "The (All Too Familiar!) Journal Cancellation Review: Proven Techniques for Eliciting Quality Feedback." Paper presented at the 21st North Carolina Serials Conference, Chapel Hill, NC. http://nccuslis.org/conted/serials2012/SerialsDocs/Swogger_Degener.pptx.

Desai, Rishi, and Julie Chilton. 2016. "Open Educational Resources in Medical Education: Applying Learning Science to Medical Education." YouTube video, 53:07. Libraries in Medical Education. Online webinar posted June 15. https://cc.readytalk.com/cc/s/meetingArchive?eventId=a7fchgfeq7hw.

Dygert, Claire, and Jeanne M. Langendorfer. 2014. "Fundamentals of E-Resource Licensing." *The Serials Librarian* 66 (1–4): 289–97. doi:10.1080/0361526X.2014.881236.

Garfield, Eugene. 2006. "The History and Meaning of the Journal Impact Factor." *JAMA* 295 (1): 90–93. doi:10.1001/jama.295.1.90.

Georgas, Helen. 2015. "The Case of the Disappearing E-Book: Academic Libraries and Subscription Packages." *College & Research Libraries* 77 (11): 883–98. 702. http://crl.acrl.org/content/early/2015/02/05/crl14-702.

Hendler, Gail Y., and Jean Gudenas. 2016. "Developing Collections with Get It Now: A Pilot Project for a Hybrid Collection." *Medical Reference Services Quarterly* 35 (4): 363–71. doi:10.1080/02763869.2016.1220751.

Johnson, Peggy. 2004. *Fundamentals of Collection Development and Management*. Chicago, IL: American Library Association.

Lingle, Virginia A., and Cynthia K. Robinson. 2009. "Conversion of an Academic Health Sciences Library to a Near-Total Electronic Library: Part 2." *Journal of Electronic Resources in Medical Libraries* 6 (4): 279–93. doi:10.1080/15424060903364750.

Linn, Mott. 2007. "Budget Systems Used in Allocating Resources to Libraries." *The Bottom Line: Managing Library Finances* 20 (1): 20–29. doi:10.1108/08880450710747425.

Lynn, Valerie A., Marie FitzSimmons, and Cynthia K. Robinson. 2011. "Special Report: Symposium on Transformational Change in Health Sciences Libraries: Space, Collections, and Roles." *Journal of the Medical Library Association:* 99 (1): 82–87. doi:10.3163/1536-5050.99.1.014.

Nardini, Robert. 2003. "Approval Plans." In *Encyclopedia of Library and Information Science*, 133–38. New York: Marcel Dekker. https://pdfs.semanticscholar.org/c9e7/83ed0385c2716131f85d03937cb0f4c4ab01.pdf.

Nash, Jacob L., and Karen R. McElfresh. 2016. "A Journal Cancellation Survey and Resulting Impact on Interlibrary Loan." *Journal of the Medical Library Association* 104 (4): 296–301. doi:10.3163/1536-5050.104.4.008.

NISO (National Information Standards Organization). 2012. "SERU: A Shared Electronic Resource Understanding." *Recommended Practice of the National Information Standards Organization* RP-7-2012. Baltimore, MD: National Information Standards Organization. http://www.niso.org/publications/rp/RP-7-2012_SERU.pdf.

———. 2017. "SERU Registry." National Information Standards Organization. Accessed May 5. http://www.niso.org/workrooms/seru/registry/.

Panitch, Judith, and Sarah Michalak. 2005. "The Serials Crisis: A White Paper for the UNC-Chapel Hill Scholarly Communications Convocation." Chapel Hill, NC: University of North Carolina. http://www.unc.edu/scholcomdig/whitepapers/panitch-michalak.html.

Pedersen, Wayne A., Janet Arcand, and Mark Forbis. 2014. "The Big Deal, Interlibrary Loan, and Building the User-Centered Journal Collection: A Case Study." *Serials Review* 40 (4): 242–50. doi:10.1080/00987913.2014.975650.

Quinn, Brian. 2001. "The Impact of Aggregator Packages on Collection Management." *Collection Management* 25 (3): 53–74. doi:10.1300/J105v25n03_05.

Rais, Shirley, Michael A. Arthur, and Michael J. Hanson. 2010. "Creating Core Title Lists for Print Subscription Retention and Storage/Weeding." *The Serials Librarian* 58 (1–4): 244–49. doi:10.1080/03615261003625984.

Ritterbush, Jon. 2012. "Trials by Juries: Suggested Practices for Database Trials." *Journal of Electronic Resources Librarianship* 24 (3): 240–43. doi:10.1080/1941126X.2012.706149.

Rolnik, Zachary, Selden Lamoureux, and Kelly A. Smith. 2008. "Alternatives to Licensing of E-Resources." *The Serials Librarian* 54 (3–4): 281–87. doi:10.1080/03615260801974271.

Schmidt, LeEtta M. 2013. "From the Editor: E-Books Building the New Subscription Library." *Journal of Interlibrary Loan, Document Delivery & Electronic Reserve* 23 (1): 1–3. doi: 10.1080/1072303X.2012.759636.

Schroeder, Rebecca, Tom Wright, and Robert Murdoch. 2010. "Patron Driven Acquisitions: The Future of Collection Development?" *Proceedings of the Charleston Library Conference.* doi:10.5703/1288284314834.

Sprague, Nancy, and Ben Hunter. 2008. "Assessing E-Books: Taking a Closer Look at E-Book Statistics." *Library Collections, Acquisitions, and Technical Services* 32 (3–4): 150–57. doi:10.1016/j.lcats.2008.12.005.

Squires, Steven J., ed. 2016. *Annual Statistics of Medical School Libraries in the United States and Canada.* 38th ed. Seattle, WA: Association of Academic Health Science Libraries.

Taylor, Liane, and Eugenia Beh. 2014. "Model Licenses and License Templates: Present and Future." *The Serials Librarian* 66 (1–4): 92–95. doi:10.1080/0361526X.2014.879027.

Thompson, Laurie L., Mori L. Higa, Esther Carrigan, and Rajia Tobia, eds. 2011. *The Medical Library Association's Master Guide to Authoritative Information Resources in the Health Sciences.* Medical Library Association Guides. New York: Neal-Schuman Publishers, Inc.

Tooey, Mary Joan (M. J.). 2010. "Renovated, Repurposed, and Still 'One Sweet Library': A Case Study on Loss of Space from the Health Sciences and Human Services Library, University of Maryland, Baltimore." *Journal of the Medical Library Association* 98 (1): 40–43. doi:10.3163/1536-5050.98.1.014.

Tyler, David C., Christina Falci, Joyce C. Melvin, MaryLou Epp, and Anita M. Kreps. 2013. "Patron-Driven Acquisition and Circulation at an Academic Library: Interaction Effects and Circulation Performance of Print Books Acquired via Librarians' Orders, Approval Plans, and Patrons' Interlibrary Loan Requests." *Collection Management* 38 (1): 3–32 doi:10.1080/01462679.2012.730494.

Wajda, Carrie Netzer. 2006. "Selection, Deaccessioning, and the Public Image of Information Professionals: Learning from the Mistakes of the Past." *Library Student Journal* 1 (November): 1–9.

Walters, William H. 2013. "E-Books in Academic Libraries: Challenges for Discovery and Access." *Serials Review* 39 (2): 97–104. doi:10.1016/j.serrev.2013.04.014.

One Library's Story

Duke University Medical Center Librarians Learn to Embrace Weeding Projects

Emma Cryer Heet

Located in the geographic center of Duke University's Medical Campus in Durham, North Carolina, the Duke University Medical Center Library and Archives serves approximately twenty thousand core patrons in the Duke University Health System: three hospitals, over four hundred diagnostic clinics, a school of medicine, school of nursing, physician assistant program, physical therapy program, and graduate programs in the basic medical sciences. The collection goes back to the 1930s with the founding of the School of Medicine. During the early decades of the 2000s, we have found, as have several other health sciences libraries, that our physically centralized location comes at a steep price. Space is at a premium in medical centers and can disappear at very short notice. Our story begins first with a mandated relocation of around 50 percent of our print collection.

In 2007, the Duke School of Medicine asked the library to clear the entire top stacks floor of our four-story building to make way for the Department of Medicine Oncology. We were given a very compressed timeline of three months to complete the task of weeding almost twenty-two thousand linear feet of print volumes. At the outset, our on-site volume count was 284,367. Approximately 18 percent of these volumes were withdrawn from the library altogether, for which a local recycling company was contracted. Forty-nine percent of our on-site volumes were relocated to an off-site storage facility known as the Library Service Center (LSC), shared with the Duke University Libraries, the University of North Carolina at Chapel Hill, and several other local libraries. We leveraged the plentiful storage space and article scanning and delivery services of the LSC to avoid withdrawing more than 25 percent of our print collection. With so little time and even less experience in weeding, the project was tense and hurried, workflows were less than ideal, and mistakes were made.

Our first step in the planning process was to create assessment criteria for off-site storage, on-site storage, and withdrawal. A small staff of five, primarily drawn from collections, access services, and administration, were in charge of this stage of preliminary planning. For monographs, we considered circulation data, local and national holdings, Brandon Hill title lists, and publication dates. We pulled the inventory and circulation counts from our integrated library system, and we consulted WorldCat for the holdings information.

The primary criteria for keeping books on-site during the first weeding project were publication date, high use, and recent use. If a book was used more than five times in the last five years, the book remained in the library. Books published within the last five years, regardless of use, were also kept in the library. Criteria for off-site storage was more flexible; we kept all first editions of books and every first, fifth, tenth, and so on editions of core textbooks. We stored many books that had been used heavily in the past but had little to no recent usage. We stored all books that represented the only copy held within the Triangle Research Libraries Network (TRLN), a collaborative group of four university library systems located in North Carolina's Research Triangle, and we kept books that may not have circulated but appeared to be rare according to WorldCat. Books older than five years that had seen no use and were duplicate TRLN copies were heavily weeded.

For journals, we analyzed electronic holdings, determining whether online access was perpetual or leased, and compared print holdings with those of our local consortial partners. TRLN adheres to a single-copy journal storage policy in the LSC, and we ensured we did not store duplicate journal volumes by checking our union catalog. We were the first TRLN library to move large runs of print journals to the LSC, so we erred on the side of keeping every title for which we held the most complete print holdings within the consortium. When we had explicitly purchased and licensed perpetual archival rights for the online version of a journal for which another TRLN library maintained duplicate print holdings, we withdrew our print volumes. In some cases, we kept gap-filling volumes on-site to complete the full runs of other libraries' journal holdings.

After the quick planning process, we developed workflows for staff members to follow to expedite the evaluation process. For monograph evaluation we assigned seventeen staff members to review call number ranges within their disciplinary specialties. We gave the evaluators spreadsheets organized by call number with circulation data and asked them to add WorldCat holdings information themselves. We trained everyone in the application of the selection criteria to encourage consistency, but the project had to be completed so quickly that there was a lot of room for evaluator discretion and no time for oversight. Each librarian marked the spines of volumes with chalk markers to indicate whether they should be withdrawn, relocated to the LSC, or kept on-site. A commercial moving company was contracted to pack and move the volumes and to dismantle the shelving.

Because this was our first experience with weeding on a large scale, we found many aspects of the project to be quite challenging. The biggest difficulty during this first weeding project was estimating how much shelving would be needed to house the remaining on-site collection. Staff had to measure and count volumes to develop a plan that the commercial moving company could follow. We ended up requiring more shelving on-site than we had calculated, which resulted in crowded stacks for three years until our next weeding project. With experience, we have refined the shelving estimation process and now leave 1.5 feet free on every shelf to create space for growth.

A second challenge we faced was an enormous clean-up phase in technical services once the physical move was completed. We underestimated how much labor would go into verifying volume counts and editing holdings records in several databases to reflect our increasingly complex location codes. We had to rely on staff at the LSC to check books into their inventory system before we could change locations in our library system with confidence. Months into the clean-up project, we discovered that one truck that had been directed to take books to the LSC had, in fact, taken them to the recycling facility, and this accident made many staff members resentful of the hurried weeding timeline. Fortunately, our timeline for the clean-up phase of the weeding project was more flexible, and we were able to train several access services staff members to assist with the withdrawal workflow.

A third unforeseen challenge, identified during the clean-up phase of the project, was inconsistency in the application of the weeding criteria. Some librarians were very lenient about what should be withdrawn, and some were very severe. The result of these inconsistencies was an on-site collection that appeared weighted in favor of certain specialties. We have been able to rebalance the on-site collection in subsequent weeding projects, and are mindful to keep the most frequently used books on-site regardless of subject area. In more recent weeding projects, we have used far fewer than seventeen evaluators, which has helped with consistency. Our current weeding workflow has collections staff reviewing the decisions of each evaluator once spines have been marked; we now weed at a leisurely pace for a more coherent analysis with checks and balances.

Our patrons, for the most part, have heartily embraced the changes to our space. One result of moving all of our print journals off-site was the development of a new document delivery service; articles requested from our print journals are scanned within twenty-four hours and delivered to Duke patrons as PDFs. The scanning service is extremely popular since patrons now spend less effort to acquire these articles than they did when the collection was on-site. The occasional patron will still visit the library and lament the lack of a large print collection on-site, and, as librarians, we sympathize with their nostalgia; but the collaborative teaching and learning spaces we gained from our weeding projects are used far more often than our print book collection.

As our library has evolved since 2007, we have graduated from the stigmatized view we once held of weeding our print collection to embrace the flexibility of our newly reclaimed physical spaces and off-site storage facility. Many lessons from that first harried weeding project have informed later projects initiated by us instead of an outside entity. We want to move more volumes off-site to free up valuable library space for our patrons and services. During 2016, we started two more weeding projects. We weeded for withdrawal (using Better World Books) the monographs we originally moved off-site in 2007, using eight years of circulation data and updated evaluation criteria to aid our decision-making process. Of our 33,000 monographic volumes stored at the LSC, only 2,200 have circulated since 2008. We applied more stringent criteria refined from our last monographic weed in 2011 to cull these books once more. The space we freed up at the LSC will be filled with some of our non-circulating special collections, which we want to house in a more secure location than we currently have on-site. Removing security restrictions from the patron spaces where those special collections are currently held in our library will also allow us to open up access from one of our reading rooms to an outdoor terrace where we house a medical garden and patron seating.

We are also weeding our remaining print journals housed in the LSC as part of a larger consortial project within TRLN that is moving from a lengthy planning stage to execution. The TRLN Collaborative Print Retention Project includes a single-copy storage policy for print journals, so we are working with the other TRLN libraries to weed and merge our holdings in order to preserve as many unique print journal titles as we can in our shared off-site storage at the LSC. Simultaneously, as we identify and preserve our journal holdings within TRLN, we are committing many of these journal titles to the Association of Southeastern Research Libraries' Scholars Trust, our larger regional cooperative journal retention program. The weeding projects undertaken with our trusted consortial partners greatly increase the benefits of these projects, transforming the gains from a simple reduction of stacks space and an increase in patron space to a long-term preservation strategy at local and national levels.

Chapter Three

Managing a Collection Budget

Steven W. Sowards and Joseph J. Harzbecker, Jr.

The goal of the collection management process outlined in chapter 2 is to meet the needs of the institution; the materials or collection budget sets benchmarks to guide the planning to do so; and the acquisitions accounting process gives regular feedback about progress through the fiscal year. Reaching that goal involves balancing several factors through budgeting and related approaches to collection management, and the correct balance can vary depending on the kind of library and its mission. Those factors can include meeting current needs of local users, addressing long-term needs, and/or preserving the scholarly record independent of short-term and local variations in use. Local strategy may adopt different priorities to accomplish these purposes for effectiveness (the ability to meet demand) and efficiency (meeting demand at the lowest realistic cost and in an acceptable length of time). Strategically, a health sciences library may employ varied levels of collection access that affect the budget: locally owned and housed collections (physical or digital); licensed resources, for which ongoing or even "perpetual" access is guaranteed by contract; resources provided via partnerships, consortial sharing, and interlibrary loan (ILL) borrowing; and on-demand commercial document delivery of resources. If the health sciences library is part of a larger library system, the local strategy employed may be in cooperation with the larger institution.

WHAT DOES THE MATERIALS BUDGET PAY FOR?

A health sciences collection budget consists of funds devoted to providing library users with necessary resources in all formats. Many of the types of resources available are discussed in detail in chapter 2. By far, the largest proportion of the collection budget of most health sciences libraries of all types is devoted to subscriptions of journals/serials and databases. For U.S. and Canadian medical school libraries in the Association of Academic Health Sciences Libraries (AAHSL), it is typically around 93 percent (Squires 2017). That number could be even higher for special and hospital libraries. A much smaller percentage of health sciences library budgets goes toward monographs. Every library is different, and what is included in the budget partly depends on the terms of cooperation with other libraries, but the range of resources typically purchased by health sciences collection budgets includes these:

- Journals and other serial subscriptions in print and e-formats
- Omnibus resources containing a mix of e-books, e-journals, streaming video, and other content
- Databases of various types: point-of-care tools, literature and abstract databases, exam preparation tools, collections of full text e-books, and reference and drug databases
- Monographs in print and e-book formats
- Reference works in print and e-formats
- Streaming video or DVDs
- Collections of data
- Finding aids (the online catalog, indexing and abstracting tools, or discovery layers)

This list contains both subscription resources (that have continuing costs from year to year) and one-time-cost resources. Journals, omnibus resources, other databases, and finding aids tend to be subscriptions. Monographs and reference works in e-formats and streaming video can be either subscriptions or one-time purchases, whereas their physical counterparts are, of course, always one-time purchases. Complicating the statistics is the fact that e-journal backfiles and backfile packages are generally also one-time purchases. More on the significance of the two types of purchases for the collection budget will be discussed later in this chapter.

At some health sciences libraries, the collection budget may pay for any of these auxiliary services and tools as well:

- MARC records for the catalog
- Electronic resource management tools (such as ProQuest 360 or Serial Solutions)
- Research support tools like citation managers and organization tools
- Preservation (including binding)
- Repair and conservation

- Support of trusted third-party repositories for preservation of digital content
- Scanning and digitization
- Open-access initiatives or article processing charges
- Outsourced production of needed materials (such as microfilming)
- Interlibrary loan
- On-demand document delivery or pay-per-view services
- Fees for memberships that provide access to resources
- Consortial dues that confer collection benefits
- Fees from vendors or agents
- Shelf-ready processing costs
- Shipping and delivery costs
- Ongoing access fees for databases or purchased packages
- Apps for mobile access to online content
- Collection analysis tools

In general, a collection budget does not pay for the following:

- Salaries and wages
- Supplies and services
- Physical plant and overhead
- Equipment like personal computers or shelving
- Professional development, travel, and training for librarians and staff

Whether or not unusual costs are assigned to the materials budget or the operating budget matters less than clarity and consistency about what is expected and must be paid for. What is covered will be unique for every institution and depends on whether the health sciences library is a stand-alone library or part of a larger system of libraries, and whether the operating and collection budgets are administered as separate enterprises. As with the other collection materials, some of these items are subscriptions and others are one-time costs, and this difference will be reflected in the budgeting for them.

DECIDING THE SIZE OF THE MATERIALS BUDGET

The size of the overall collection budget is unlikely to be set by the collection manager, though that person may play a role in planning and proposals. In most cases, the health sciences library director will receive an allocation of money from the library's larger institution: the university library, the medical college, hospital administration, or some other central authority. This yearly allocation generally makes up the largest portion of income for the library. In some cases, the institution allocates funds separately for operations and for collection development. In other cases, the library director must determine the share of money to go into collections versus operations. The collection budget is a significant portion of the entire budget for health sciences libraries. AAHSL libraries reported that collection expenditures accounted for more than half of their annual recurring costs (mean value 55.5 percent). This tended to be true for both small and large medical school libraries, and the collection budgets of these libraries ranged from around $415,000 to $5.6 million per year (Squires 2017). Only a few outliers reported personnel budgets that were significantly higher than their collection budgets.

In most academic institutions, the fiscal year for budgeting will correspond to the academic year: July 1 to June 30. However, other starting dates are possible. Hospitals and companies will likely have a fiscal year corresponding to the calendar year. Many publishers also operate on a calendar-year fiscal year (January 1 to December 31), and this can have an impact on the timing of discounts, sales, and renewals. Traditionally, annual periodical subscriptions and journal volumes correspond to one calendar year and are paid in the preceding fall months. Many vendors do allow a grace period of as much as two months for libraries that need to push a renewal into the next fiscal year.

Planning for the fiscal year is likely to begin well in advance of the starting date. The collection manager in charge of the budget needs to know the new allocations by the first day of the new spending year or shortly thereafter to guide spending as the year begins. Because, as noted above, 93 percent or more of the collection budget may be devoted to subscriptions, and subscription prices tend to rise every year (perhaps around 5 to 7 percent, but that is variable), it is important for the collection manager to have as much advance notice as possible if the new allocation will not match this rise in order to plan for reassignment of funds and to halt subscription renewals that cannot be paid for. If outside funding agencies—such as a state legislature—fail to meet budgeting deadlines for a university, this can seriously disrupt the ability to plan the budget or to manage expenditures to meet core needs and take advantage of discount opportunities.

Methods of Developing Budgets

There are two common methods for deciding the size of the library's collection budget, and, with both of them, collection managers are usually asked for input about needed funding levels for the coming year. In academic libraries, the collection budget manager may meet with the library director. Hospital librarians in charge of collection budgets may meet with administrators about the upcoming year's budget. This process may include justification for ongoing costs such as subscriptions and for anticipated new funds.

The collection budget manager will want to have done some "homework" about possible price increases by consulting with some of the biggest vendors beforehand.

The easiest method for library budget planning is "baseline budgeting," which begins with the level of allocation or expenditure from the previous fiscal year as a starting point, with modifications, increases, or reductions based on known or forecast price changes, the expectation of institutional demand for new resources, and changes in the user population (including its size and changes in mission, units, or programs). At its simplest, each budget line would be increased or decreased proportionally to reflect the change in funding for the coming year (for example, an increase of 5 to 7 percent across all lines). In reality, setting new fund levels is not that simple, even with a rising budget. Costs will rise faster in some areas, new initiatives may require support, and some lines of the budget may prove to need less additional funding. In the case of budget cuts and static budgets, the defects in a purely mechanical, across-the-board reduction will be even more obvious: strategic thinking and data-driven decision making will yield better results and be more easily justified. Furthermore, strategic attention to minimum effective levels of funding is especially necessary in a budget-cut situation. (If you have four cars, and you must remove four tires, better to take all four from one car than one tire from each car.) It is better to identify and properly support certain key resources than to render ineffective a longer list of resources by providing insufficient funding. Those same factors should be at work—but are often less obvious—when budget increases are possible: at what funding level will support for a new mission be "enough"?

"Zero-based budgeting" is another approach to planning that reverses the process of traditional baseline budgeting. This method begins with a blank slate: no past expenditure is assumed to continue without scrutiny, and each intended expenditure must be justified in advance. Presenting a rationale for new spending, whether specific items or along strategic lines, to the library director or administrators outside the library is stressful; making the same determinations internally, however, can be an opportunity for clarity and planning. Given the central role of journal subscriptions and standing orders for a health sciences library, this approach can lead to repetitive and unproductive questioning of payment for core resources. It is also difficult to predict demand for significant new resources very far in advance of publisher announcements. While this method risks wasting time when applied to essential resources, it does have the virtue of forcing examination of choices.

Zero-based budgeting may demand identification of every hoped-for resource in advance. However, some desirable resources may not be recognized or even published until mid-year. If the librarian cannot identify and justify funds for purchase of a resource until after it is on the market, two inefficiencies will reduce the quality of library service. First, library users may have to wait until the beginning of the next fiscal year for new funds to appear, and their access to information will lag relative to peers. Second, the library will forfeit the opportunity to purchase new resources at prepublication rates or other early discounts, so that library materials budget funds do not stretch as far as they could. As a compromise, the zero-based budget might include some discretionary funds for opportunistic selection.

In practice, budgets may be created through a mixture of baseline and zero-based budgeting. Obvious recurring needs such as journal subscription renewals may be supported, but other needs and especially funding for entirely new resources may be subject to analysis, justification, and forecasts about use. In some cases, special funds may be assigned for one-time purchase of resources (such as an online journal backfile), but will not enter the baseline budget for the following fiscal year.

Forecasting Price Increases

Collection managers at large libraries will not be able to discuss price increases with each and every vendor prior to proposing a budget. These managers can turn to a variety of sources that aim to forecast increases in costs, which can be useful either for budget justification or for internal planning to anticipate need. Historically, for health sciences libraries, the greatest driver of increased materials budget costs has been the increase in serials costs. At one time, annual price increases of 10 percent or more were common for the "A-list" science and medical journals that were least likely to be canceled. The forecasting tool of greatest reliability for local conditions is the past record of each library's costs combined with any contractual commitments to specific multi-year pricing or caps on price increases negotiated with publishers. There are also several published annual forecasts of serials cost increases. *Library Journal* publishes a "Periodicals Price Survey" each April that reviews trends, contains tables showing average journal prices for various fields of study, analyzes average price increases, and briefly projects cost changes for the coming year (Bosch and Henderson 2016). The Library and Book Trade Almanac publishes the " Library Materials Price Index (LMPI)" or "Prices of U.S. and Foreign Published Materials" report prepared by the Association for Library Collections and Technical Services (ALCTS) of the American Library Association (Barr 2016). After a one-year embargo, figures are freely available on the ALCTS website (www.ala.org/alcts/resources/collect/serials/spi). This is a lengthy document and covers both serials and monographs.

While there has been some moderation in the increase in annual costs for individual journals, several trends continue to make budgets for subscriptions difficult to balance. One is the launch of numerous entirely new journals, either as new titles from competing publishers in established fields or as journals covering new fields of study. The other trend is demand for information in new formats that were not formerly available for sale. These include some of the database and omnibus resource subscriptions that now dominate the budgets of some kinds of health sciences libraries like hospital libraries. These types of resources can have yearly increases that eclipse the journal subscriptions. There are also now e-book packages, streaming video packages, interactive image sources, new diagnostic and point-of-care tools, exam preparation resources, data compilations, and mobile app versions of databases available as a separate purchase.

A wide variety of other factors can drive up costs, some outside of the library's control. Some increases in cost reflect the models under which various products are priced. An institution may experience increased usage of a product because of new programs or new areas of research, which might alert the publisher to the need for a new pricing assessment. For products that are priced based on full-time equivalent (FTE) user counts or other gauges of the size of the reading audience, costs may increase as an institution grows. Many electronic products also are priced per site, with one "site" defined as a single location such as a campus or hospital. If an institution expands to include more sites, some publishers may require additional payment. Currency fluctuations can also be a problem for libraries. When a country's currency drops in relation to other currencies, subscription costs could unexpectedly rise. To avoid this situation, it is best to insist on contracts and payments exclusively in one's own currency when possible. Besides these outside elements, there may be pressures internally to spend more. If access to a resource is limited to a set number of simultaneous users, there may be pressure to purchase additional capacity (sometimes called "seats") if turnaway numbers are high and there are user complaints.

Other Sources of Income

While the largest source of income for health sciences libraries is usually the yearly allocation from the institution, other sources may provide funds to supplement the baseline budget, such as one-time allocations, "soft money" sources such as grants, or less predictable funding sources such as the yield on endowments or one-time gifts. These funds might be tracked outside of or parallel to the regular materials budget. Most institutions have overall development guidelines that dictate what portion of endowment yield can be spent each year: typically this reflects the wish to build up the endowment against inflation, and to even out the yield across several years. Thus, in a year with high endowment yield of perhaps 7 percent, the amount assigned to spend could be only 4 percent; but in a later year with low yield of perhaps 2 percent, the system may support spending that is a bit higher than the most recent annual return. Paying for important subscriptions or standing orders out of these funds is risky. If the funding ends or is reduced, subscriptions will have to be cut or funds reassigned from other areas of the budget. However, these other sources can be useful for one-time spending. In the case of donations and gifts, health sciences collection managers should work with their institution's or library system's development office. There is often a high threshold ($50,000 or more in the United States) for establishing a true endowment that will yield 5 percent in income each year. Smaller donations, however, can be combined and added to existing umbrella library endowments, or spent on one-time choices. With any donation, knowing the intent of the donor is crucial, and this should be recorded in writing. Librarians will want to avoid donor requirements that involve very narrow spending limits, time-intensive procedures, or restrictions on how the library handles materials purchased (such as separate shelving areas or bans on withdrawing materials when they are no longer useful).

Another occasional source of funds may be unspent money from the preceding fiscal year. Whether a library is permitted to hold funds as "carry forward" to the next year will vary by institutional rules and/or state laws (if the institution relies on state funding). When it is allowed, some amount of funds may be carried forward to pay for materials on order that were not invoiced by the end of the fiscal year, or funds may even be saved for future purchases. Allowing this kind of savings prevents the wasteful need to use-or-lose funds late in the year. In some cases, an institution may allow funds to build up over several years toward an agreed-upon major purchase. Flexibility of this kind also means that library staff do not have to spend the budget down to an exact zero balance each June, which can mean wasting time juggling small orders that add up to a set sum or racing to get invoices in-house and paid. Acquisitions units in larger libraries will know that a certain proportion of orders placed late in the year will not be invoiced in time to permit payment with funds from the fiscal year that is ending and will plan accordingly, holding some orders for a few days, for example, to shift payment into the new fiscal year. To plan well, the collection manager will need to know the institutional rules on this score and keep in mind that carry-forward money is a one-and-done resource.

ALLOCATIONS: DIVIDING UP THE BUDGET TO MEET NEEDS

Some kinds of allocation—that is, distribution of funds within the materials budget for set purposes—may happen when the budget is being proposed. For one, the funding body may specify that certain funds be assigned to specific purposes, particularly if the library had to propose specific goals or justify the budget. Secondly, funds needed for renewals are, to some extent, pre-committed: subscriptions must be paid, or access is lost. Third, and on their own initiatives, managers of collection budgets may have goals or purchases in mind. Further allocations will take place when the new budget is in place.

For accuracy in forecasting, planning, spending, and reporting on materials budget funds, collection funds will be assigned to one of several lines, each devoted to a specific purpose. The allocation of money to those lines can be highly uneven in amount, reflecting the scope of needed resources and the way in which materials are marketed and sold. The division into separate lines will be unique for every library and may reflect the units being served (such as a department or college), subject areas or specialties (such as medicine or nursing), formats (serials versus monographs), funding sources (lines tied to specific endowments or grants), functions (journal binding or memberships), approval plans, or other local needs. It is wise to have a capstone reserve line as well, to address contingencies, opportunities, and problem solving.

For effective control, it is best for only one individual to be assigned oversight and spending authority for each line within the budget. Doing so prevents uncoordinated spending decisions that inadvertently may be in conflict. In a smaller library, one individual may manage and authorize use of all lines in the budget; in a larger library, several librarians may operate in their own realms. These librarians may have authority to spend up to certain capped limits per item, as well as being limited to a maximum spending level for the line; individual orders exceeding those limits will require higher-level review and approval. While budget lines are guidelines and can be modified to reflect evolving needs during the fiscal year, the collection budget manager should be involved in any decision to shift funds from one allocation to another.

The number of subordinate lines within the budget can vary widely, reflecting institutional culture and size. There may be further subdivisions as well, reflecting different formats or patterns of acquisitions spending. For example, within broad subject funds, such as for medicine or nursing, it is useful to track separately the funds assigned to serial renewals and other standing orders, as opposed to firm orders for individual items subject to a single payment, or approval plan or blanket order payments that go to agents selecting monographs from a profile (Clendenning, Martin, and McKenzie 2005).

Deciding the actual level of funding in each line for a new fiscal year is one of the key functions of the collection manager. There are a number of approaches. Once again, both zero-based and baseline models come into play. Allocation formulas might be used in larger libraries, especially academic libraries that serve many different subject areas. These formulas employ numerical counts and weighting to portray the intensity of demand for library resources across institutional units. Canepi reviews some of the diverse factors that have been employed in allocation formulas by academic libraries (Canepi 2007). Here are some factors typically considered when assessing a specific area of study:

- Cost of materials (such as average journal subscription price)
- Number of enrolled students, majors, and faculty
- Number of credit hours generated by enrollment
- Circulation or other usage reports for relevant materials
- Level of interlibrary loan activity
- Number of faculty publications or grants

In favor of allocation formulas are several factors: decisions are based on data and facts, rather than intuition; when calculated annually, the results can reflect new and current trends at the institution. Arguing against their use are other factors: the selection of numerical elements and their weighting is arbitrary; patterns of publication, enrollment, and library use may differ from field of study to field of study; many vendor products (such as the omnibus resources, databases, or packages of e-books or e-journals) are interdisciplinary in subject and in type of resource and don't fit neatly into budget lines; conclusions based on past years' figures are always backward-looking, rather than forward-looking; and logically calculated results from the formula may be unrealistic or politically unacceptable.

While formulas may not always be practical, most health sciences libraries will wish for budget allocations that reflect the trends and priorities of the institution they serve. When greater investment by the parent institution takes place in one area, reflecting either current deep levels of activity or aspirational goals, it behooves the library to reflect this in its own investments. If available, institution-wide budget figures can be revealing, especially when compared year-over-year and over an extended period of time, such as five to ten years. If overall investment in a department or program has doubled in that time, for instance, perhaps the library materials budget should reflect that increase.

Collection development policy statements can play a role in budgeting. These written commitments to levels of intensity in collection building as described in chapter 2 can help guide budget-making decisions over time. These documents can be descriptive (if the collection is sufficient for instruction but not research, it is best to say so), but also can be helpful when aspirational: if the institution's goal is research in a particular area of study, matching that "Level 4" goal with actual spending can guide decisions on funding. These texts help staff to keep priorities in sight, and can be useful when explaining decisions and priorities to library users or funding bodies.

Stakeholders outside the library and library users are likely to want some input on collection budget allocation and spending choices. The collection manager will need to balance desirable external input and engagement with internal decision making based on data and a larger-picture viewpoint. Input on needs will often come from librarians that have direct contact with the library users, such as liaison librarians in an academic environment. In some cases, there will be a formal library committee to offer input.

ACQUISITIONS OR PURCHASING DEPARTMENTS

As noted in chapter 2, the collection manager in a health sciences library that is part of a large library or library system will need to communicate and work with library staff in units outside of the collection unit. There may be a separate acquisitions unit within the health sciences library or within the larger library system. Acquisitions staff handle the actual purchases once collection managers have made their selections. They communicate with the vendors, book jobbers, and serials agents to place orders, handle and pay the invoices, receive notifications of access, receive physical materials, and keep track of encumbrances, expenditures, and free balances often through an integrated library system. Acquisitions units should send regular reports to collection managers.

Large organizations may have a purchasing department outside of the library for identification, purchase, and delivery of most items. However, libraries typically operate in an autonomous manner from these central purchasing departments. Central purchasing departments exist to compare prices and negotiate efficient low-cost sources for purchases, but most library resources are sold on a sole-source basis: that is, only one publisher or vendor can supply a specific book or journal. Competitive bidding and other comparative processes do not match well with the library-publishing marketplace. The large number of purchases at relatively low prices (such as individual books often costing less than $100) also distinguishes library acquisitions and budget management from many other institutional purchases. The increasingly digital nature of scholarly publishing separates the acquisition of information from that of, say, paper or latex gloves: this may lead to special kinds of reporting to the university auditor since funds are being expended on intangible assets that may, by design only, be available for a set length of time.

Libraries may only need to involve their institutional central purchasing department for very large-scale purchases such as an entire integrated library system (ILS) or a discovery tool, markets in which several vendors compete with similar products. For health sciences libraries that are part of larger library systems, this process would likely take place at the larger library administrative level. Health sciences librarians may be asked for their input on the products, however, so it is good for them to be aware of the process.

Central purchasing departments generally operate using an RFI (Request for Information) or RFP (Request for Proposals) process to secure the best deals. Vendors are invited to submit responses to a detailed statement of needs, and those responses are scored against the list of requirements, with price in mind. An RFP generally will call for a closed-quote bid from the vendors, while the RFI only seeks descriptions of how well the product matches desired criteria, and may precede an RFP.

USING AN INTEGRATED LIBRARY SYSTEM AS A BUDGET TOOL

Budget allocations mark the beginning of the selection-acquisitions-spending year. Most health sciences collection managers will work with and maintain spreadsheets to keep track of their allocations for different types of resources or subject areas. Once decided, specific budget amounts will be entered into an institutional accounting program. For hospital and other special libraries, this may be outside of the library, and the accounting in that system for library subscriptions and purchases may be very simple—perhaps just "library materials budget"—and the collection manager would keep track of spending in the library for various purposes only on a spreadsheet.

Larger libraries, such as academic libraries, typically have an integrated library system (ILS) for tracking purchasing. As orders are processed, acquisitions accounting staff will maintain records in the ILS of funds spent and funds available. To guide selection of health science resources, collection managers should work with acquisitions unit staff to identify and explain the features of any reports. Those reports may include online "real-time" tracking of expenditure within each line in the budget, but such reports may lag in their coverage of items in process (not yet encumbered). While the ILS of a larger library system will have many functions that aren't crucial to health sciences librarians' work with collections, it is good for those collection managers to know the options. There may be ways to produce reports on usage or spending that can guide future selection, based on accurate current spending information. Those larger health sciences libraries that do not use their ILS for tracking purchasing will likely use some kind of system that incorporates similar accounting practices.

A typical ILS can accommodate some local design choices for tracking and reporting on lines or other parts of the overall funding pool. A library may wish to have detailed reporting according to format type (such as periodicals, e-materials, or media), fields of study or practice (such as nursing or pharmacy), branch location (if a system has multiple sites), format (print versus electronic), or some combination of these factors. The ILS should be able to handle hundreds of separate lines if necessary.

Other elements of the ILS may be hardwired to reflect general practices in acquisitions and accounting. There may be some scope to change identification labels or display terms. An ILS may break down fund allocation and expenditure by types of payment, and how those payments affect accounting for action during the year. Categories could include the following:

- *Serials renewals* for all kinds of standing orders, subscriptions, and continuing costs.
- *Firm orders* for any one-time purchase.
- *Blanket orders* for approval plan payments. These orders typically pay for the same kinds of materials acquired by firm order but represent payments to a vendor or agent.
- *New serials*, that is, newly added subscriptions, almost always paid for with funds reassigned from other parts of the budget (reserves, firm orders, or cancelations). Some ILS products therefore track funds assigned to new subscriptions, at least during the initial payment (after which, funds will roll over into *serials renewal*).

Within a designated line of a budget (such as funds meant for monographs for public health), the ILS should be able to track spending. In a typical accounting module, funds move along a continuum.

- *Allocation* represents funds assigned in the original budget, possibly modified by transfers during the year.
- *Expenditure* shows funds already paid by the library to the vendor.
- *Encumbrance* keeps track of funds committed for purchases but that have not yet been "expended" either because the invoice has not been received or because the order has not been fully processed in technical services.
- *Cash balance* shows how much of the funds from the "allocation" remain on hand after "expenditure."
- *Free balance* is a better figure for guiding selection decisions because it shows how many funds are uncommitted. These are funds from the "allocation" that have not yet been assigned to either "expenditure" or "encumbrance."

Budget figures in the ILS will give real-time information, reflecting all changes and spending to date. For planning purposes, it is crucial to record the initial beginning-of-year allocation to all lines, and the final expenditure and encumbrance. Recording regular snapshots during the year—perhaps monthly—can be useful for year-over-year comparisons; for example, to see whether spending through March of the current year is running ahead of or behind spending in the previous March. The acquisitions accounting unit may provide some of these reports.

SERIALS RENEWAL AND SUBSCRIPTIONS

It has already been noted that subscriptions to journals, databases, omnibus resources, and some other types of materials make up by far the largest part of the collection expenditures for health sciences libraries of all types and sizes. For health sciences libraries that support medical schools in the United States and Canada, many of which are very large and have long histories, that mean percentage is 93 percent of the budget, with around 71 percent going toward journal subscriptions and 22 percent toward database subscriptions (Squires 2017). Libraries supporting teaching but not research, some hospital libraries, and some smaller health sciences libraries may find that their largest serial expenditure is on databases, management tools, and aggregated content.

Most journals follow a volume-year format that begins in January, so subscription payments (direct to the publisher or through an agent) are due in the preceding fall months. However, rolling renewal dates are possible for many items. Rarely, a multi-year deal may call for payment in advance that covers several years. Because a multi-year payment disturbs the regular renewal cycle and assignment of funds to roll over each year, this kind of exception is best limited to cases of attractive pricing. These types of exceptions require watchful accounting practices to make sure that renewals do not fall through the cracks.

Advance payments for journal subscriptions are a matter of some tension since the 2014 bankruptcy of Swets, a major serials agent. Periodical publishers operate on a basis of customer payment in advance. At one time it was common for libraries to pay a portion of their periodical renewal cost in advance to their agent, sometimes in return for a sliding-scale discount. In the Swets bankruptcy, payments from libraries already in the hands of the agent were never delivered to publishers, leaving both libraries and publishers holding the bag. Many libraries therefore have limited or eliminated their exposure to advance payments to agents, and, in the aftermath of that event, there has been much discussion of lessons learned and the continuing utility of using agents (Davis et al. 2016; Erb and Hunter 2015; Ferguson 2015).

Dealing with serials subscriptions is a complex business and the health sciences collection manager in a large organization may be working with others such as an electronic resources librarian or a more centralized chief collection officer. A wealth of other factors determine what a library will pay. Any of these models or a combination may be used by the vendor and may or may not be negotiable:

- Flat rate prices.
- Prices based on full-time equivalents, or "FTE," as a measure of the size of an institution, which may relate to student enrollment or to workforce

size or the size of a specific unit or department. Some publishers put maximum caps on FTE, such as "FTE of 40,000 or higher."

- Prices based on other measures of institution size or type as a predictor of usage or budget. Carnegie Classifications are widely used for doctoral institutions; these reflect intensity of research activity and not just head count, with R1 as the highest level. Indiana University now presents a "Basic Classification Description" on behalf of the Carnegie Commission on Higher Education (Indiana University Center for Postsecondary Research 2017).
- Prices based on whether an institution has a medical school or a hospital.
- Prices based on number of beds in a hospital.
- Prices based on a chosen number of simultaneous online users, beginning with single "seat" access. More seats can be added, sometimes by preset counts such as two to five or six to nine.
- Prices to "own" a digital resource are higher than to rent access, perhaps five to ten times the annual rate for leasing. Ownership generally means negotiated rights for "perpetual access" rather than local ownership and management of text.
- Prices based on actual use. In some cases, there is a dollar charge for each download, or the annual rental cost may reflect past and projected levels of usage as tracked by the publisher. Sometimes prepaid coupons or tokens are expended to track use.
- Consortial prices in which all members of a group of libraries enjoy a discount price are generally negotiated on a case-by-case basis. The vendor may tie levels of discounting to the extent of consortium participation. Some consortial deals will be offered to each library separately, while others may be centrally negotiated and managed.
- Discount prices may also be negotiated and will be unique to each situation. Discounts may reflect the extent of past purchases for "good customers" or may be available on a one-off basis as a promotion, including "early adopter" prices.
- Multi-year commitment prices may be available. In rare instances, the publisher may ask for payment up front for more than one year; this can be challenging to the library budget.

It is safe to say that a forward-looking materials budget in the health sciences will always anticipate the addition of new serials. The challenge is to find funds for those new subscriptions, which almost always could consume more new money than is allocated for the new year. There are several potential sources for those funds: cancelation of existing subscriptions, transfer of money from monograph or other one-time funds, fiscal reserves, outside funds, or carry-forward funds. It is also possible to use money from endowments and donations or from one-time money or "soft" money, although funding subscriptions through these fluctuating sources of funds can be risky. Of course, successful price negotiation on products and their sales model can build savings into the ongoing cost of materials.

If the library's goal, for instance, is to provide the "best" (or most-used) one hundred journals or the best journals to be had for a certain amount of money, then cancelations are necessary to keep within a budget. When a new journal is more promising than a title already on subscription (and has a comparable cost), canceling one title to pay for the other makes sense. Unfortunately, the situation is rarely this simple. Researchers and practitioners in the health sciences are interested in an ever-widening circle of journals and new databases. The need for new resources rarely means a reduction in interest in established resources unless an institution has made radical changes in focus, such as eliminating a particular department or residency program. In some cases, it may be possible to cancel a journal and rely on interlibrary loan or document delivery to meet occasional need, and that may be a good plan for libraries with a limited focus. For larger libraries, the CONTU "rule of five" can rapidly lead to expensive copyright clearance costs to deliver articles to desktops. At the end of the day, those ILL expenses may offset much of the savings, and the library will have forfeited the opportunity to build its own collection and the efficiencies of meeting repeated demand for the same journal articles from its own holdings. In addition, "Big Deals" with journal publishers (discussed more below) may prevent cancelation of individual journal titles.

It is tempting to pay for new subscriptions with money that previously had been earmarked for monographs or one-time purchases. This works in the short run but only postpones the day of reckoning, while also weakening any part of the collection that relies on monographs. Money spent on each additional standing order reduces next year's budget for one-time purchases until that budget eventually ceases to exist. While some libraries may have little need for monographs, the lack of any money not already tied up in subscriptions means that the only recourse is cancelation if price increases are higher than budget increases. More on this is described below in the section on budget cuts.

Endowments and other donations are also tempting sources with which to pay standing order costs, but they are not reliable in the long run. Economic downturns can reduce the yield on endowments unexpectedly, and force payment onto other parts of the budget. Acquisition of one-time resources is a better option for use of those funds.

Outside funds are sometimes offered to the library from other institutional units or administrators to secure new subscriptions. Like endowments and gifts, these remain "soft funds" and should not be relied on. A change in department chair or a budget cut can abruptly end the funding. In addition, the unit contributing funds may, with some justification, feel entitled to special treatment by the library or believe that only members of that unit should enjoy access to the new resource. Like donations, outside funds can be very useful for one-time purchases such as large online journal backfiles.

Many administrators outside the library may not understand the importance of supporting a serious, consistent, and ongoing commitment to pay for subscriptions in order to obtain the best pricing and to build a collection that users can rely on year after year. They also tend to underestimate the staff time required to start new subscriptions, cancel them, and start them up again, or the cost of losing discounts that have been "grandfathered" into agreements. A presentation by the library concerned to funding authorities may be a better way to produce ongoing benefits in the baseline budget. If a unit is truly committed to assisting the library, it is best to see if institutional accounting can register a permanent transfer of funds from one baseline to the other.

The "Big Deal" and Its Role in the Collection Budget

Any actions that can be taken to control serials subscription costs are welcome. One controversial method is the so-called "Big Deal" that brings access to all publications of a given publisher. Big Deals became popular in the late 1990s and were supported by the move to online journal publication. Under a typical Big Deal, a library with subscriptions to some journals from a given publisher pays an additional cost (sometimes called a "top-up fee") for access to that publisher's remaining unsubscribed journals, at an annual cost well below the normal subscription cost. Journals added under the Big Deal are rented and not owned; that is, if the deal eventually lapses, the library would lose access to current and past issues of those added journals (but would continue to have access to content that was purchased). Consortia may manage Big Deal contracts for groups of libraries.

Big Deals have been widely adopted by libraries because of their advantages. There is simplicity in knowing that all the content from a given publisher is available, and this may reduce the need to have an agent manage title lists. If the library agrees to a multi-year agreement, the publisher should guarantee a cap on annual price increases, which will help the library both to predict and to reduce future expenses. For example, in a three-year deal, the annual cap on inflation across the total bundle might be 5 percent; for a five-year deal, the cap might be 4.5 percent or even 4 percent.

The most visible attraction of a Big Deal is the ability to provide substantially more titles for an institution at a fraction of the normal cost. In some cases, twice as many journals may be available, although this will vary. A study evaluating Big Deals that compared prices paid with citation data as a statistic of usage found that the cost-effectiveness of such bundles varied greatly by publisher and type of institution, with some publishers offering much better deals and discounts to certain types of libraries (Bergstrom et al. 2014). The same study concluded that negotiation can make a considerable difference as well, with some libraries obtaining better prices, possibly due to harder bargaining, but also probably due to historical spends, price caps, and other negotiated aspects of the pricing.

Big Deals can be most cost-effective when the base of institutional library users is large and varied, because the number of journals without readership may be very small. They can make sense for a large university library with extensive degree and research programs. They can be even more cost-effective for a university library system, such as the California Digital Library, or for consortia that include a number of different types of libraries. Some Big Deals have been negotiated for entire countries. Health sciences libraries benefit from the Big Deals negotiated by these larger groups of which they are a part.

Publishers would not offer Big Deals unless they saw advantages to themselves. The immediate attraction of the Big Deal is the increase in payment from the library through the "top-up" fee. Simplicity in managing the subscription list for a library is also a plus, and so is better "circulation" for a publisher's less popular titles. In addition, under the all-in terms of the Big Deal, the library gives up the right to cancel specific journals as a tool to save money. If cuts must be made in serial expenditure, either the entire Big Deal will have to be torn up (most Big Deal agreements provide an escape hatch, in case of financial exigency) or the savings will have to be found by canceling journals from other publishers. If multiple Big Deals are in place, the list of journals eligible for cancelation can be limited.

It is this final feature of the Big Deal—the inability to address cost increases through title-level cancelations—that has led to the greatest criticism of these plans. As early as 2001, Kenneth Frazier at the University of Wisconsin–Madison pointed out negative results of these plans (Frazier 2001). Libraries forfeit their ability to make title-level selection decisions about journals and add unwanted or less-wanted titles to their collections. Contracts with major publishers push the industry closer to monopoly, as smaller publishers may be more at risk when cancelations have to be made, and libraries lose bargaining power.

Depending on one's definition of "Big Deal," research libraries in the United States have either pulled away from them, or they remain fairly widespread. This was confirmed in a 2017 *Against the Grain* issue dedicated to the "State of the 'Big Deal'" wherein some collection managers talked about giving up Big Deals, but others said that Big Deals were still financially the best option for their libraries (Ismail 2017). In one example, the head of collections at the library at University of Wisconsin–Madison, Doug Way, wrote that his institution's principled opposition to Big Deals had not led to an improved or sustainable budgetary situation, and that one of his first projects upon arriving at that institution was to institute some Big Deals (Way 2017). The study evaluating Big Deals showed that, in 2012, most libraries in the Association of Research Libraries (ARL) did not have deals for full title lists from the major commercial publishers (Bergstrom et al. 2014). Only 20 percent reported having the full title list from Elsevier and 16 percent the full list from Wiley. Furthermore, these percentages had dropped from 25 percent and 29 percent in 2006, respectively (in many cases, due to budget stress during the Great Recession). Another report of this same study, however, pointed out that that 92 percent of ARL libraries licensed a "large publisher bundle" from Elsevier and 96 percent had one from Wiley (Strieb and Blixrud 2014). Some of this difference could be because the original Big Deals from such companies were for full title lists, but, as companies have acquired or launched new journals over time, those journals have not always been automatically added into the Big Deals. So, over time, the Big Deals have become less comprehensive. Smaller publisher Big Deals tend to remain full title lists. The Association of Academic Health Sciences Libraries (AAHSL) Services and Resources Survey from 2014 (available online only for analysis with membership login) indicates that fewer of those medical school libraries than the ARL libraries have package deals (AAHSL 2014). Definitions remain confusing, but it appears that perhaps over 60 percent of such libraries had large packages from Elsevier and/or Wiley. This may indicate that medical school libraries that are not part of larger universities or consortia may be choosing smaller, more subject-targeted packages supplemented by document delivery instead.

Within a Big Deal, the library may have the right to switch journals back and forth between the "owned" side of the title list and the "rented" or courtesy-access side so long as total spent remains the same. Usage figures will allow collection managers to identify the most-used titles; the 80/20 rule will tend to apply. Annual content in the "owned" journals will remain part of the library collection if the Big Deal has to be dropped later, while the courtesy titles and their backfiles will no longer be available. Fine-tuning the "owned" list over time can reduce the negative impact of future budget cuts, if those cuts force the library to drop a Big Deal.

Tactics to Reduce the Impact of Serials Cost Inflation

When library directors and institutional overseers review the work of their collection managers, reductions in standing order costs are a high priority. This can place the collection manager in a tough position: on the one side, administration would like to see reduced journal costs, which suggests cancelations; on the other side, health sciences library users regularly ask for the addition of new journals and databases, not fewer. Several methods can provide some relief.

First, journal cost increases reflect not only the absolute number of titles on order but also the rate of annual cost growth ("inflation"). For numerous reasons, canceling journals is a negative option: it may be difficult in a Big Deal climate, and is likely to deny researchers materials that they need. As previously noted, multi-year agreements with publishers should include favorable caps on annual price increases. This may or may not be tied to a Big Deal and can involve a single title or resource.

A second tactic is to link limits on annual subscription cost increases to other purchases from the same publisher. For example, there may be one-time funding available to buy digitized journal backfiles. If the publisher realizes this additional income as part of their overall bottom line, the library may be able to secure reduced subscription cost increases.

A third tactic seeks to introduce new costs or price increases over time. When entirely new subscription products come into play or a vendor creates a new pricing model, the added cost can be prohibitive. It is to the vendor's advantage to add the library to its long-term list of subscribers, and so it may be possible to secure deep discounting over several years, with access while the library gets additional funding in place. For example, the library may not have funds right away for a new product that will cost an added $30,000 per year. The collection manager can suggest that costs are ramped up over time: perhaps $10,000 in the first fiscal year, $20,000 in the second fiscal year, and the full $30,000 only in the third fiscal year. The publisher may seek a multi-year commitment (without cancelation), but locking in these prices is helpful to the library as well. The same tactic can be used to handle a price increase.

A fourth tactic involves consortial leverage. When a group of libraries negotiates together with a publisher, concessions on price or terms of use may be possible. There is efficiency for the publisher through negotiation with a single entity, rather than duplicate negotiation with a dozen or more libraries, in both staff time and the size of the bottom line payment.

DOCUMENT DELIVERY AND INTERLIBRARY LOAN AS ELEMENTS IN THE COLLECTION BUDGET PLAN

Document delivery and interlibrary loan (ILL) costs are likely to be a portion of many health sciences library budgets, whether there are budget cuts or not. These costs can be budgeted as operations or collection expenditures, or both. Because judicious use of article delivery options can help curtail journal subscription costs, the collection budget manager has an interest in these activities. Budgeting for these services can be challenging, especially when a service offered is new and the library budget manager does not yet know how popular it will be. Budgeting will also be influenced by the library's decisions on whether or not to charge patrons for these services and whether patrons will be limited as to the number of requests they can make in a certain time period. Many smaller and specialized libraries, including new "born-digital" health sciences libraries, are relying on considerable just-in-time purchasing of articles rather than building large collections of journals for the future. However, more and more established health sciences libraries are also experimenting with using such services for a selected group of journals either as a reaction to budget cuts or simply to maximize resources.

On-demand purchasing of articles, especially for a limited number of library users or subject area needs, can often be much less costly than journal subscriptions. Article pay-per-view can involve purchasing directly from the publisher or through a document delivery service. The Copyright Clearance Center is a leading supplier of document delivery with services such as RightFind for companies and Get It Now for academic libraries. Often libraries can receive lower rates from such services than they can receive directly from the publisher. Such services can be set up for requestors to order directly or for requests to be mediated by the library as if they were interlibrary loan requests. The University of Nebraska Medical Center's McGoogan Library of Medicine compared their interlibrary loan copyright payments within a certain time period with the costs of pay-per-view for the same articles and found they would save money using pay-per-view (Brown 2012). Other libraries are offering a Get It Now service that is unmediated, either by linking from article databases (Suhr 2013) or by listing the journals available through the service on the health sciences library website. Budgeting for such on-demand services will involve educated guesses about the extent of use and annual costs, at least during the first years that the service is offered.

ILL of those same articles can be less costly but requires more investment in staff time. Libraries that borrow are expected also to lend, and libraries may incur some costs joining consortia and reciprocal borrowing groups. If a health sciences library is part of a larger university library, interlibrary services may be budgeted for and run centrally, but stand-alone health sciences libraries will likely need to budget staff and resources for such services. National Network of Libraries of Medicine Resource Libraries are available in each region of the United States to provide documents to other libraries in their regions, but they may charge for these services. There are also the CONTU guidelines for ILL that limit the number of articles that can be obtained without paying copyright fees. Tracking those "free" articles will have a cost in staff time and, when a library starts to incur high copyright fees because of repeated ILL of articles from the same journal, pay-per-view services can be a more cost-effective choice.

For libraries that are building collections but have limited funds, ILL costs may be weighed against subscription costs to determine the utility of a potential new subscription from a fiscal point of view. For example, if library users submit thirty ILL requests in a year for articles from a given journal, and if one accepts the often-used figure of $30 per transaction (representing sunk costs as well as copyright permission and fees), then one can project $900 as the annual cost for access. If a subscription to that same journal would cost less than $900 per year, it is worth considering; if the subscription cost is well above $900, then ILL remains the better choice from a financial perspective. The per-article cost for Get It Now and other commercial document delivery services falls in a similar range, around $30 per transaction.

Finally, some libraries are experimenting with a patron-driven model for journal article acquisition that can be more cost-effective than any of the above options and holds some promise for the future (more on patron-driven acquisition for monographs is below; England and Anderson 2013). Read-Cube Access is an instantaneous on-demand system that allows a tiered pricing system, rather than only one price, as on-demand purchase systems charge. The tiered price is based on permanence of access that the user requires, with short-term rental and cloud access being less expensive than PDF download. As of this writing it is only available for journals from a limited number of publishers.

OPEN ACCESS AND THE COLLECTION BUDGET

Open access (OA) as a publishing model is discussed in chapter 1 of this book. At present, it is more frequently encountered in the journal market and, for those journals of interest to health sciences libraries, usually involves a payment model of author publishing charges (APCs, also known as "article processing charges") rather than library subscriptions. For many libraries, there is no immediate cost because their users do not tend to be the authors, but libraries at institutions that support research leading to publication will need to think about the role of the campus library when authors ask for help to meet these APC costs.

APCs have the potential to become another disruptive element in library materials budgets: what is free to the reader may not be free for the institution. Some libraries have devoted modest sums to open-access APC payments on a pilot or experimental basis. However, there is the prospect of an entirely new model for journal publishing in which university funds are no longer directed to publishers via subscriptions to defray the cost of journals, but instead through APCs (while open access offers content to all global readers). The 12th Berlin Open Access Congress, held in December 2015, explored exactly this proposition and called for "a swift and efficient transition of scholarly publishing to open access" by 2020 (Max Planck Digital Library 2016). However, when the so-called "Pay It Forward" project and report from the University of California–Davis and the California Digital Libraries investigated the consequences of redirecting library materials budgets at North American research libraries to OA APC payments, the authors concluded that those budgets were insufficient to pay the necessary costs (University of California Libraries 2016). In other words, without an infusion of added funds from grants or other sources, an "all-OA" model would not solve library budget problems but instead would compete for funds and undercut libraries' abilities to pay for the full range of resources sought by users. An open letter to the academic community of October 2016 from the director of libraries at UCLA also addresses problems in the model (Steel 2016).

One reason why the projected costs for universities of paying APCs rather than subscription prices are so high is that a relative handful of research institutions house the majority of authors whose work makes its way into the article literature. Meanwhile, there are many institutions interested in the research literature that do not produce as much of that literature. A major example of this for the health sciences is pharmaceutical companies. While researchers at such companies may do some publishing, publishing is not as important for them, and much of the research is kept out of the literature so that patents can be filed. For-profit companies often pay higher journal subscription prices than academic institutions, but would pay very little in the OA environment, essentially becoming "free riders."

The health sciences library that serves researchers will have to conform to institutional plans and priorities around paying APCs. Some institutions have supported open-access publishing through memberships with such publishers as BioMed Central, but currently most memberships are at the "supporting" level, which pays only a fraction of the full APC. Now few, if any, institutions have drawn conclusions about whether APCs should be the responsibility of their libraries versus the responsibility of individual authors and their grants. Librarians should be prepared to assist their institutions in understanding the potential fiscal implications of a large-scale move to OA on this model for serials.

ONE-TIME PURCHASES

One-time purchases, also sometimes called firm orders, make up a smaller share of the overall budget but involve a wide range of resources. These include individual books, individual e-books, DVDs, bundles of e-books or streaming videos, some electronic reference works, backfiles of journal content, backfiles of book series content, and collections of data. To add to the complexity, some one-time purchases of digital content come with annual fees attached. Those may be smaller fees associated with ongoing maintenance costs at the vendor site, or larger sums if significant new content is added each year to a resource.

In contrast to subscriptions and standing orders, budgeting for one-time purchases is relatively simple: individual titles or packages will be chosen until the money is gone. Many academic libraries will use an approval plan (or "blanket order") for print monographic purchases. The burden of title-by-title selection is outsourced to an agent; in return for a fee, that agent consults a detailed approval profile prepared by the client library and delivers all books that meet the stated criteria. In these cases, budgeting will generally involve forecasting the amount that will be purchased based on the previous year. Since many health sciences libraries have significantly cut their spending on print books, there may be less scope for approval plans; great care will be needed in reviewing them since each monograph selection is significant. They can still save time for librarians, however. For instance, a very specific and narrow approval plan might be set up to allow a library to receive only the most important medical textbooks for a small print reserve collection (Czechowski 2008).

One-time purchases are also a good use for donations, one-time gifts of money, endowments, and other such sources that may be variable. When there is a lot of money, the collection manager can make investments in materials that will be permanently owned—for instance, purchasing a large journal package backfile or a collection of e-books, or paying the higher one-time ownership price for an electronic reference work rather than the lower subscription price (if both models are available). Such additions ensure that continuing access to materials will not be lost if a budget cut leads to a reduction in funds for annual payments. The collection manager will want to be on good terms with the institution's development officer. There may be situations in which gift money is available unexpectedly and only if it can be spent rapidly. For these occasions, collection managers should always maintain a wish list with resources at several price points, in case a development officer calls with an offer. One-time gift money may arrive late in the calendar year, as donors use charitable deductions to prepare for tax payments.

Financial Reserves in the Collection Budget

All collection managers should pace their spending during the year for flexibility, and it is prudent for them to build significant reserves into the materials budget each year. At least 5 percent of the total is both realistic and effective. Reserves play a key role in the library materials budget. It is impossible to predict all upcoming expenses for a fiscal year: new products may be released, attractive discounts may be available, or additional resources may be needed to solve problems or meet unexpected needs. Reserve funds are best spent on one-time purchases; if funds are redirected from reserves into standing orders, it will be harder and harder to build the next year's reserve. It is tempting to reduce the reserve allocation during "bad" budget years, but in fact, those reserves will be most in demand to solve problems at those times.

That 5 percent reserve can consist of several parts. Some portion should be available for immediate spending, with no strings attached: this is especially necessary for problem solving. There may be reasons to park money provisionally in a central reserve for purchase of materials outside normal channels and fund lines. For example, it may be known that a new resource with a high price—such as a major reference work—will be on the market later in the fiscal year. Holding those funds in a reserve line can prevent spending the necessary money inadvertently. This approach overlaps with another feature of central reserves: contingency funds. The exact cost of some products and services may not be known when the year begins and the budget is set, or may vary unpredictably from year to year, or may turn out not to be a cost at all during a given year. Placing enough money in reserve to cover plausible maximum costs will prevent mini crises later. At some point later in the year, when the real cost becomes clear, excess contingency funds can be spent as "free" reserves, perhaps for end-of-year one-time purchases when some publishers offer good discounts, or perhaps for problem solving.

Patron-Driven Acquisitions Models

"Patron-driven acquisitions" (PDA), sometimes called "demand-driven acquisitions" (DDA), is a marketing and resource selection method that relies on reader behavior to drive some one-time selection decisions for online resources, typically e-books or streaming videos (although a model for journal articles is described above with document delivery). The PDA approach leads to selection based on actual usage. Health sciences libraries have experimented with many different types of PDA programs and found pros and cons for different models (Bahnsen et al. 2014). In a typical PDA plan, a large set of selected item records will be loaded into the library catalog for discovery by library patrons. When patrons activate or download individual texts in sufficient numbers, this triggers either purchase of the resource by the library automatically or notification of interest to a librarian who makes an evaluation of whether to purchase. The latter mediated model is less risky financially since librarians have more control.

Additional costs often accrue in PDA plans. Many plans set actual purchase at three or four uses, but may charge a "short-term loan" fee for each use before the purchasing trigger. In recent years, these "STL" fees have been rising, and a library may find that it has paid far more than the list price for a book after a series of STL charges followed by eventual purchase. Some publishers are beginning to offer plans (sometimes called "evidence-based acquisition") that reduce the uncertainty and excess cost that accompanied the original PDA models, essentially allowing rental usage of a large set of materials for a set fee, with librarian-mediated selection for perpetual owner-ship at the end of the year of a subset of titles based on actual usage.

In a large institution, successful PDA management may require effort from multiple library staff members. Librarians involved in selection deci-sions will need to compare and choose among competing publisher or vendor plans and identify the exact set of records wanted; technical services librar-ians will need to load MARC records into the catalog; and acquisitions accounting staff will need to monitor expenditures.

Similar to document delivery services, because demand is unpredictable (especially in the first year of a PDA program), it is tricky to assign the right level of funding in the budget. If too many funds are assigned, they will go unspent at year's end. If too few are assigned, the deposit account that pays for PDA purchases will run out of money mid-year, either disappointing readers when e-books are not available or forcing the library to assign other funds to meet the need. The number of titles that will be selected by patrons will likely depend on how closely librarians can match the books included in the program to user needs. Many PDA programs from such aggregators as ebrary or EBSCO are very interdisciplinary and may be run by an entire university library or a consortium. There may be few books of interest for the health sciences. On the other hand, vendors like Rittenhouse that offer a PDA program that includes books from Doody's Core Titles are likely to generate a much higher rate of health sciences library patron selection.

During times of budget constraints, monographic funds and other such funds for one-time purchases are usually the first casualty for health sciences libraries. Many libraries may turn to demand-driven models of e-book pur-chasing to make the most of a very small book budget. Smaller health sci-ences libraries have found that a combination of user-driven e-book purchas-ing with pay-per-view options to fulfill journal article requests is an effective way to offer the collection their patrons want at the lowest price (Arnold 2015).

BUDGET CUTS

Increasing costs and decreasing financial resources will trigger the need for cuts to balance the budget, sometimes across the entire collection budget, sometimes in selected areas. The situations will vary depending on whether cuts will be temporary or ongoing; whether the cut is announced and imple-mented before the budget is crafted or imposed in the middle of a fiscal year when some funds have been spent (a callback); and whether a cut during a given fiscal year will affect all future baseline budget levels or represents only a temporary callback of funds, with restoration of normal funding in the following year. Input from stakeholders and library users will likely be sought, but there should be one ultimate authority in the library guiding the decisions about cuts to ensure a balanced, effective outcome.

For health sciences libraries, with so much of the collection budget tied up in serials, any budget in which funds fall short of the level needed to offset growth in serials costs is essentially a budget cut. It is crucial to address the problem through early well-planned decisions before runaway costs distort the budget (and thereby distort delivery of services). The most common danger in these situations is disproportionate growth of the serials portion of the budget ("serials inflation") at the expense of other resources while only postponing inevitable cuts.

A hypothetical and simplified $100,000 annual materials budget in table 3.1 illustrates the impact when serials inflation of 5 percent per year is not addressed, while the library receives a flat materials budget. The same kind of progression would take place if the library saw 2 percent increases but 7 percent serials inflation; with wider discrepancies, the impact will take place even faster.

In the first fiscal year, 5 percent of the budget is assigned as a reserve, 90 percent of the remaining funds are spent on journals and other serials, and 10 percent of the remaining funds on monographs and other one-time purchases. In the second fiscal year, without any serials cancelations, almost half of the monograph budget has been lost (to pay for increased serials costs), so that much of the reserve will have to meet ordinary monographic purchase needs. In the third fiscal year, the monograph budget has been all but wiped out; even using all of the reserve for one-time needs will produce a weaker monograph collection than desired. In the fourth fiscal year, too little remains in reserve to accomplish anything, either in terms of monographs or other important one-time purchases. In the fifth fiscal year, the budget can no longer be balanced because runaway serials costs now exceed available funds; serials cancelations that should have been initiated during Year Two can no longer be avoided, while in the meantime the monograph collection has been badly damaged and opportunities have been lost through loss of flexibility in use of the reserve. In Year Two and each subsequent year, 5 percent of the serials list should have been canceled (about one title in every

Table 3.1.   Impact of 5% Serials Inflation on a Flat Annual Collections Budget

Fiscal Year	Serials	Monographs	Reserves	Total
FY01	$85,500	$9,500	$5,000	$100,000
FY02	$89,775	$5,225	$5,000	$100,000
FY03	$94,264	$736	$5,000	$100,000
FY04	$98,977	0	$1,023	$100,000
FY05	$103,926	0	(-$3,926)	$100,000

twenty). These cancelations will be painful, but as illustrated, that pain can be postponed only by a few years in any case.

If the cut is temporary, however, and all funds will be restored in the following fiscal year, the collection manager, so far as possible, will try to protect subscriptions and make up shortfalls from monographic funds and reserves. There are several reasons for this. It is very costly in personnel time to cancel a list of serials only to turn around and reinstate them the following year. Loss of journal content will be particularly frustrating for many health sciences library users. Favorable license terms may also be lost. The timing of serials cancelations also matters. If a cancelation decision takes place too late in the year after many subscriptions have already been renewed, any savings may not be seen until the next fiscal year. Collection managers should not be afraid to ask vendors for special consideration. Rather than lose committed revenue, publishers may be willing to make arrangements to help the library during a one-time shortfall, perhaps in return for a promise to maintain subscriptions in the next year.

If a budget cut is going to be permanent and subscription cancelations are needed, collection assessment and rational decision making are especially critical. Strategies for targeted deselection are discussed in chapter 2 of this book. Cost-per-use data will be especially important in these cases because cancelations of low-use, low-in-cost resources will not yield the savings needed very quickly. The collection budget manager will need to note which parts of the budget are tied up in multi-year or consortial agreements. Generally, these will have contingency clauses allowing cancelation in case of financial exigency. Collection managers will want to contact the major vendors to see if special terms can be worked out, keeping in mind that vendors will want to minimize loss of revenue. One cut may be followed by another in the next year. It is important for collection managers not to use up all one-time funds and to keep some balance and extra money set aside. When funds are scarce, there will be more problems and emergencies that dictate assigning more funds, not less, to reserves.

During and after the Great Recession of 2008–2009, a number of libraries had no choice but to reduce costs and invoke exigency clauses to break Big Deals. To meet demand for articles found in journals no longer available, many turned to ILL and to pay-per-view document delivery services. At the University of Alabama's Lister Hill Library for the Health Sciences, a pay-per-view service replaced Big Deals (Lorbeer and Mitchell 2011). By applying principles of just-in-time delivery, mediated use of the service, prepaid deposits with vendors to secure discount prices, greater reliance on aggregators, and promotion of ILL to patrons, library patrons still had access to necessary information despite a reduced budget. Another smaller health sciences library faced with declining budgets replaced twenty-four journal subscriptions from one large publisher with pay-per-view tokens from the same publisher. While the costs to the budget were essentially the same, the pay-per-view model gave patrons access to 764 journals instead of just 24 and was deemed a better way for the library to meet patrons needs (Fought 2014). Publishers may be willing to negotiate terms of reduced access when faced with a Big Deal cancelation through financial exigency. The "top-up fee" method can be viewed as an in-house pay-per-view service for articles from that publisher, with a predetermined cost based on forecasts of use (knowing that cost in advance assists library budgeting). Rather than give up this revenue completely, the publisher may suggest other compromises.

NEGOTIATION WITH VENDORS AS A PART OF BUDGET WORK

Basics of Negotiation

Negotiation toward a "deal" can be seen in two ways: as a zero-sum game with winners and losers; or as a collaborative process in which both sides come to understand where their interests overlap, allowing a win-win solution. In reality, both models shed light on the process. It is also possible to stumble into lose-lose results.

The library may be part of an institutional culture that leans toward one model of negotiation or the other; those local cultures can influence how hard-nosed the negotiating style will be. There is no fundamental reason to insist on one style or the other, and librarians should determine their preference in a self-aware manner, and possibly on a case-by-case basis. When two individuals meet, the outcome may be a boxing match or it may be a waltz; what is important for the negotiator is to keep the library's goals in mind and adjust behavior to take the path most likely to meet those goals.

That said, a model built around a zero-sum, win-lose approach can expose the library to some hard knocks since it is difficult to win all the time. This is especially relevant for interaction with key publishers because the library will return to negotiate with the same firms (and often the same sales representatives) over and over again, sometimes on an annual basis. Securing a triumphant win in one fiscal year does not guarantee another win when the next fiscal year rolls around, and the "defeated" publisher may be motivated to win back their previous losses by taking a harder line. If a library and a publisher can identify overlapping areas of agreement, that foundation can smooth the path to an acceptable outcome. Fatigue can be a factor as well; hard-nosed negotiating consumes more time and energy. There can be specific situations in which the library needs to take the hard line in order to meet crucial goals, and it is better to apply time and energy to those cases than to expend resources unnecessarily for the sake of style or reputation. Librarians should also keep in mind that it may take as much work to save $1,000 related to Product A as it does to save $10,000 related to Product B. If time is limited, it makes sense to focus on Product B, for the better return.

If the budget represents targets or goals for spending to serve various subject or format areas, then negotiation is a key method to reach those goals when it comes to digital resources. Print books (and most single e-books) will have a set list price, and, while there may be discount opportunities, that price will not change due to the size of the purchasing library and its user count, or due to other factors such as multi-year commitments. For bundles of digital content, such as journal Big Deals, omnibus products, or packages of e-books, those factors do come into play; different libraries will pay different prices. These purchases are often the largest expenditure in the materials budget, and, therefore, negotiation on prices is crucial to deliver the most content possible with available funds. Negotiation of licenses for terms of use will also be important for all digital resources, regardless of pricing, and that topic is covered in chapter 2.

Negotiation can take place in a variety of settings: during personal visits to the library by a sales representative, at conferences, by phone, or by email. At some points in negotiation, the freedom of verbal give-and-take is helpful—neither side may wish to commit certain points to writing—and, at other times, having a written record of the exact offer is crucial. Obviously, at the end of the process, there needs to be a written agreement or contract, in some cases accompanied by an annex or addendum or other auxiliary documents. Printed copies of assurances and statements made by email should be retained as well. A verbal promise from a sales representative is easily forgotten as time passes, and the individual in that role may leave for another position. The successor will rely on written statements. Retaining complete files for agreements is an important activity. While it is handy to keep digital copies of email exchanges, these are subject to loss in a variety of ways. It is best to print and retain hard copy or at least backed-up PDF copies of messages that indicate terms of use or pricing, as well as signed agreements and addenda. Lapsed agreements may be kept separate from live agreements in the files, but keeping those outdated records will allow the collection manager to review changes in price and terms over time.

Numerous books, workshops, and conferences can assist a collection manager in learning about and understanding the negotiation process. As negotiators, librarians will find the style that allows them to accomplish their goals: understanding the library's needs, understanding what the vendor can offer, determining that compromises can be made and what requirements are deal-breakers, and figuring out what specific terms will secure the best access for the lowest cost. Library professional associations, such as the Association for Library Collections and Technical Services of the American Library Association, sometimes offer workshops or webinars about negotiating. Two generally available resources on the subject are *Getting to Yes:*

Negotiating Agreement without Giving In (Fisher, Ury, and Patton 2011) and *Negotiation: Closing Deals, Settling Disputes, and Making Team Decisions* (Hames 2012). For library-related advice, Janet L. Flowers offers "Specific Tips for Negotiations with Library Materials Vendors Depending upon Acquisitions Method" (Flowers 2004).

Health sciences collection managers will need to determine their roles in their own organizations. In some libraries, the health sciences collection manager will negotiate and sign all electronic resource licenses; in others, that authority is delegated to the library director, or the director is the final signer of contracts. In some organizations, such as large university libraries, there may be a central chief collection officer to negotiate major deals for the entire library system. Officers from the legal office may be involved, although this can be inefficient. Institutional legal units will have oversight of many contracts, but the large number of library-vendor agreements for licensed authenticated use of online tools, terms-of-use documents, exchanges of commitments by email, and other written records may lead to delegation of authority to the library. If legal oversight is needed for routine purchases, acquisition may take place too slowly to respond to offers with deadlines or urgent requests.

Negotiation will also reflect the needs and characteristics of vendors and publishers. The largest global scientific publishers are for-profit corporations, often with publicly traded stock. This means that short-term return-on-investment, not support for scholarship, is their number one priority. Senior managers may have no background in the health sciences, scholarship, higher education, or health care. This situation can lead to aggressive pricing models if investors are dissatisfied with profits; without investor funds, the publisher may not be able to excel or even survive. In 2015, reports about Reed Elsevier cited "an operating profit margin of 34 per cent—almost four times the average profit margin of groups in the FTSE 100" (Cookson 2015). Corporate mergers or actions by venture capitalists can impose added debt on a for-profit company, triggering price increases that do not reflect usage or library realities. Privately owned publishers and society publishers (for example, the American Society for Microbiology or the Massachusetts Medical Society, publisher of the *New England Journal of Medicine*) may operate with different priorities; this does not necessarily mean that their pricing is less aggressive. Academic subscribers may not be the most important clients for a society; if there is a commercial market for its publications, prices may be driven higher. Societies also may view subscription income as a way to subsidize annual membership fees or conference attendance fees as a service to their members.

It is helpful for librarians to understand the basic facts about a company with which they are working. For example, does their fiscal year end in July or December? This may determine the timing of sales offers. What is the range of products from the vendor? Scholarly journals may bring in a larger or smaller share of overall revenue. In some cases, librarians may find that products from different divisions of the same vendor are competing for the same library funds (journals versus monographs versus indexes, for example). Is the company active on a global basis? Practices, assumptions, copyright expectations, and compliance with laws and regulations may vary with geography. What is the role of the assigned sales representative? Some sales representatives have assigned geographical territories, while others cover types of institutions, such as the academic market or the corporate market. Some will have narrow sales responsibilities, while others will function as the point of contact for all inquiries with the company (including resolving technical access problems). Anderson and colleagues (Anderson, White, and Burke 2005) and Gruenberg (Gruenberg 2015) provide additional perspectives on working with vendors.

Features of Sound Negotiation

Regardless of personal or institutional style, seven features of sound negotiation are constants. First, clarity in designating the institution's spokesperson is crucial. While various persons may be authorized to ask for information or product trials, when serious negotiation takes place, the library should speak through a single voice. Library staff who are not authorized to negotiate agreements should be careful during any earlier contact not to suggest prices or terms, because their statements may be misinterpreted by the vendor as authoritative. It is destructive to the negotiation process if either side experiences new demands late in the process. If eventual formal terms of agreement disagree with earlier informal comments, there can be confusion and a loss of credibility.

Second, if possible, the actual give-and-take should be handled by intermediaries, not by the ultimate decision makers on either side. This allows the spokespersons to speak candidly and to explore ideas without overcommitting their organizations, since their statements are always conditional and subject to confirmation by a more senior figure. For instance, the health sciences collection manager may be the designated librarian to reach out to during negotiation, while the library director exercises final authority to approve and sign an agreement. Sales representatives almost always take pricing and terms of use back to a manager for formal approval (a practice most have seen when buying a car). Note that this separation of roles may not be possible in the case of solo librarians or hospital library directors who manage their collections.

Third, while negotiators can talk imaginatively in the early stages of negotiation, to explore possible compromises, exceptions, or additions to initial terms, terms they offer later in the discussion should not be presented unless they know the organization can and will accept them. Failing to honor statements undercuts the power of negotiation, and this is true for both sides. For the same reason, bluffs are bad practice. If librarians threaten to walk away from a deal, they should be sure that they mean it and that library administration and the institution will back them up. Once a threat is shown to be an empty bluff, negotiating leverage is badly weakened. Clarity about limits is important and is one reason that the negotiator needs to have scope for confidential discussion with the ultimate authority during the talks.

Fourth, negotiators need to be very clear in their own minds about which products are mandatory for the library and which are optional. For products that are mandatory, negotiators may not be able to walk away from the deal. Negotiation would need to focus on improved pricing or terms of use, perhaps in return for a larger agreement. For optional products, the negotiator has more freedom to walk away from an unacceptable agreement, keeping the door open for another round of discussion in the next fiscal year. If the seller sees diminished prospects for sales, other deals may be forthcoming. For instance, the sales representative may add new content to what is under consideration or offer a discount on added content to offset high prices for the main purchase.

Fifth, negotiators need to be very familiar with a company's products and the products of similar or competing companies. This will allow them to indicate perhaps a better offer from another company or to discuss why the features of a product might warrant a higher price.

Sixth, negotiators will need to remember that no matter how unhappy they are with quoted terms and prices, these terms are usually offered on a confidential basis. In some cases, a librarian may hear informal reports about offers to other libraries; while it can be helpful to have some idea about the vendor's willingness to be flexible, simple comparison of offers is less instructive than it may seem at first glance. The specific values that go into the pricing can vary based on all the factors discussed earlier in this chapter. Many publisher agreements include nondisclosure clauses that keep the terms and prices agreed upon confidential. For many publicly funded libraries, of course, all agreements may be subject to Freedom of Information Act (FOIA) requests.

Finally, librarians should understand that their sales representatives can be their best ally at the vendor company. It is in the sales representative's best interest to reach an agreement. Sales representatives may work on commission, need to reach sales targets, or be eligible for bonuses. If librarians have constructive ideas to redesign a challenging offer, the sales representatives are best equipped to interpret those ideas to management at their company. A good sales representative will not want to "leave money on the table" by failing to devise a sales strategy that matches the funds your library can afford to pay at a given time. The ability to communicate quickly, clearly, and safely with the sales representative is an asset. Relationships that continue for multiple years are valuable, and, by developing these, collection managers may waste less time explaining what the library sees as priorities, will see fewer unrealistic proposals, will get better answers to questions, and will have better awareness of new products that will match the library's needs. In some ways, the sale representative functions as a library-to-vendor intermediary in the same way that a liaison librarian functions as a library-to-faculty intermediary in a university library. Sales representatives will move from publisher to publisher during their careers but often will remain visible in a given market. A good relationship with a sales representative can continue even after a move to a different vendor.

Opportunities for Negotiating

End-of-year spending can be an opportunity for negotiating significant savings, especially for one-time purchases. The timing of special sales may reflect the end of the fiscal year for the library or for the publisher. The former wishes to spend out the budget and the latter wishes to reach higher sales targets. Collection managers can take advantage of end-of-year offers by knowing how much reserve money the library can spend, knowing when the publisher is likely to make offers, having a wish list on hand, having prior agreement on general license terms with key vendors, and coordinating with their own acquisitions department. It will be important to understand whether the publisher requires full payment by some date (such as December 31 or June 30) or whether a commitment by email is sufficient, and how long it will take for invoices to be generated by the publisher, delivered to the library, and paid by library and institutional entities.

A huge price increase for a subscription product or a bad budget year are two other opportunities for negotiating. The library's ultimate negotiating weapon is to withhold payment, including cancelation of subscriptions. In a truly bad budget year, this tactic becomes easier. If the money is simply not available to pay for more than three out of four products, publishers can find themselves in a "musical chairs" situation, which may prompt some relief (no seller wants to be the one left without a chair). Publishers may even end up competing against themselves if they have several product lines and the library can only pay for one. As noted above, bluffing is never a good idea and especially not in a cancelation situation. Once a library's bluff is called, it becomes harder to use any future budget situation as a bargaining chip. It is not necessary for librarians to show all their cards, of course, but an indication that funds are lean or not can help guide a publisher away from wasting everyone's time with an offer that is out of reach.

When considering the impact of new subscriptions, cancelations, or threats of cancelations, librarians should also keep in mind that patrons will care less about why the library dropped a product and more about losing access to their favorite resources. In terms of politics and goodwill, it is far easier never to have offered a resource than it is to take a resource away after the community has come to rely on it. For this reason, offers for temporary access or even widespread trial access can create problems for the library.

Relationships with Vendors

The topic of candor raises the issue of personal relationships with vendors, publishers, and their representatives. Librarians who work with collections will encounter a wide range of styles from sales representatives and customer service personnel of the companies with which they deal. Some vendors interact almost entirely by email; others are eager to visit campuses. Contact with some vendors is limited to a single renewal decision each year and an invoice. Other vendors may offer an array of products and be involved in multiple transactions. Not every visit is purely a sales call; there may be interest in understanding institutional strategy for collection building, budget trends, or emerging needs. There may be interest as well in trends at the national level. Library collection managers may know more about the range of publisher activities than do many staff at individual publishers, who tend to operate in their own silos. While discussion of these issues ultimately aims at selling product, smart publishers realize that it is easier to sell resources that meet the core goals of the customer. Librarians have opportunities with vendors to influence product design, features, or content. In some cases, this kind of relationship can advance to full participation in beta testing of new offerings.

There can be utilitarian value in having a close relationship with sales representatives of key publishers as well. In a variety of situations, time and trouble can be saved with a single point of contact at what may be a large company. The representative can put librarians in touch with the right people to help with loss of access or broken links, or with technical staff to help set up, modify, or customize a complicated resource.

Collection managers should be thoughtful about limits on their contacts with sales representatives, however. They may be offered a wide range of semi-social contacts and will need to draw their own conclusions about what is good for their organizations. As they make hard decisions about spending in a competitive marketplace, all parties should be confident that they are credible and objective decision makers. Giving up time in the work day for vendor visits or telephone sales calls is necessary for collection managers to stay informed, and visiting exhibit booths at conferences is important. Accepting a cup of coffee while talking with a vendor is not a breach of ethics. Many vendors invite collection managers to conference receptions, and that also is largely an acceptable social function. When vendors offer to buy a meal, librarians should exercise good judgment. Sometimes meals are combined with informational presentations, and some may help nurture good contacts with key sales staff, but librarians should be aware of the potential sense of obligation that comes with accepting that hospitality. The same caution applies to free tickets to sporting events or all-expense-paid junkets. The greater the expenditure and the smaller the informational content, the more risk for librarians of ending up in a position that may be hard to justify later. In some cases, institutional policy or even state law may limit the personal goods or services one can receive from a company. Physicians operate under even more stringent ethical, regulatory, and policy guidelines in their interactions with vendors, such as pharmaceutical companies, and some hospital librarians may be required to abide by very strict institutional restrictions. Many institutions, however, expect librarians to develop their own set of ethical guidelines regarding vendor gifts, parties, or meals.

It is worth noting that vendor representatives can display a range of ethical behavior as well. Some will "hustle" an organization more than others by contacting the library director, for instance, in search of a "yes" answer when the collection manager may have said "no." Some will contact library users directly and urge them to pressure the library. This can be frustrating when it involves professionals or faculty, but it is especially egregious if involving students. Some vendors will go over the head of the library director in the belief that higher administrators will command a purchase. This kind of interference should be ignored at all levels. In general, effective sales representatives instead will cultivate a good relationship with appropriate librarians and, by learning about the organization, determine which products are most likely to sell.

CONCLUSION

Managing the materials budget for a health sciences library collection is a complicated, sometimes frustrating, but often rewarding process. This work accomplishes a key step in translating institutional goals into the actual acquisition of resources. For librarians who enjoy problem solving, attention to details, and strategic thinking, there are significant satisfactions. The budget manager can (and should) get to know any librarians at the organization who have subject specialties or are involved in liaison and through them gain insights into trends and emerging interests across the entire institution and its library users. Over time, there is the opportunity to support the institution, shape the library's collection, steward funds, and nudge the world of scholarly publishing in new directions by interacting with publisher representatives and rewarding "good" initiatives with subscription and purchase payments.

REFERENCES

AAHSL (Association of Academic Health Sciences Libraries). 2014. *Annual Statistics of Medical School Libraries in the United States and Canada.* 37th edition: Services and Resources Survey. Association of Academic Health Sciences Libraries. http://aahsl.ccr.buffalo.edu/.

Anderson, Rick, Jane F. White, and David Burke. 2005. "How to Be a Good Customer." *The Serials Librarian* 48 (3–4): 321–26. doi:10.1300/J123v48n03_15.

Arnold, Susan J. 2015. "Patron-Driven Acquisitions: Cost-Effective Strategies in Uncertain Economic Times." *Doody's Collection Development Monthly.*

Bahnsen, Wendy, Yumin Jiang, Ramune Kubilius, Emma O'Hagan, and Andrea Twiss-Brooks. 2014. "Collecting and Acquiring in Earnest (The 14th Annual Health Sciences Lively Lunch)." *Proceedings of the Charleston Library Conference*: 152–55. doi:10.5703/1288284315582.

Barr, Catherine, ed. 2016. *Library and Book Trade Almanac.* Medford, NJ: Information Today, Inc.

Bergstrom, Theodore C., Paul N. Courant, R. Preston McAfee, and Michael A. Williams. 2014. "Evaluating Big Deal Journal Bundles." *Proceedings of the National Academy of Sciences* 111 (26): 9425–9430. doi:10.1073/pnas.1403006111.

Bosch, Stephen, and Kittie Henderson. 2016. "Fracking the Ecosystem: Periodicals Price Survey 2016." *Library Journal* 141 (7): 32–38.

Brown, Heather L. 2012. "Pay-Per-View in Interlibrary Loan: A Case Study." *Journal of the Medical Library Association* 100 (2): 98–103.

Canepi, Kitti. 2007. "Fund Allocation Formula Analysis: Determining Elements for Best Practices in Libraries." *Library Collections, Acquisitions, and Technical Services* 31 (1): 12–24. doi:10.1016/j.lcats.2007.03.002.

Clendenning, Lynda Fuller, J. Kay Martin, and Gail McKenzie. 2005. "Secrets for Managing Materials Budget Allocations: A Brief Guide for Collection Managers." *Library Collections, Acquisitions, and Technical Services* 29 (1): 99–108. doi:10.1016/j.lcats.2005.01.003.

Cookson, Robert. 2015. "Elsevier Leads the Business the Internet Could Not Kill." *Financial Times*, November 15.

Czechowski, Leslie. 2008. "Edging toward Perfection: Analysis of a New Approval Plan in a Health Sciences Library." *Library Collections, Acquisitions, and Technical Services* 32 (2): 107–11. doi:10.1016/j.lcats.2008.08.016.

Davis, Susan, Deberah England, Tina Feick, Kimberly Steinle, and Erika Ripley. 2016. "Why Using a Subscription Agent Makes Good Sense." *The Serials Librarian* 70 (1–4): 277–87. doi:10.1080/0361526X.2016.1157739.

England, Mark, and Rick Anderson. 2013. "Patron-Driven Acquisition of Journal Articles Using ReadCube at the University of Utah." *Insights* 26 (3): 267–71. doi:10.1629/20487754.77.

Erb, Rachel Augello, and Nancy Hunter. 2015. "Prelude, Tumult, Aftermath: An Academic Library Perspective on the Swets B. V. Bankruptcy." *The Serials Librarian* 69 (3–4): 277–84. doi:10.1080/0361526X.2015.1118423.

Ferguson, Christine L. 2015. "Learning From the Swets Fallout." *Serials Review* 41 (3): 190–93. doi:10.1080/00987913.2015.1068153.

Fisher, Roger, William Ury, and Bruce Patton. 2011. *Getting to Yes: Negotiating Agreement Without Giving In.* 3rd ed. New York: Penguin Books.

Flowers, Janet L. 2004. "Specific Tips for Negotiations with Library Materials Vendors depending upon Acquisitions Method." *Library Collections, Acquisitions, & Technical Services* 28 (4):433–48. doi:10.1016/j.lcats.2004.08.003.

Fought, R. L. 2014. "Breaking Inertia: Increasing Access to Journals during a Period of Declining Budgets: A Case Study." *Journal of the Medical Library Association* 102 (3): 192–96. doi:10.3163/1536-5050.102.3.009.

Frazier, Kenneth. 2001. "The Librarians' Dilemma: Contemplating the Costs of the 'Big Deal.'" *D-Lib Magazine* 7 (3). doi:10.1045/march2001-frazier.

Gruenberg, Michael. 2015. "Both Sides Now: Vendors and Librarians—Managing the Negotiating Process with Library Vendors." *Against the Grain* 26 (6): 84–85.

Hames, David D. 2012. *Negotiation: Closing Deals, Settling Disputes, and Making Team Decisions*. Los Angeles: SAGE Publications.

Indiana University Center for Postsecondary Research. 2017. "Carnegie Classification of Institutions of Higher Education: Basic Classification Description." Indiana University Center for Postsecondary Research, accessed March 15. http://carnegieclassifications.iu.edu/clas sification_descriptions/basic.php.

Ismail, Matthew. 2017. "State of the 'Big Deal.'" *Against the Grain* 29 (1): 1, 10.

Lorbeer, Elizabeth L., and Nicole Mitchell. 2011. "Sustainable Collections: The Pay-Per-View Model, in Reports and Papers from the 10th Annual Midsouth eResource Symposium." *The Serials Librarian* 63 (2): 173–77. doi:10.1080/0361526X.2012.700778.

Max Planck Digital Library. 2016. "Open Access 2020." Max Planck Digital Library. https://oa2020.org.

Squires, Steven J. 2017. *Annual Statistics of Medical School Libraries in the United States and Canada, 2015–2016*. 39th ed. Seattle, WA: Association of Academic Health Sciences Libraries.

Steel, Virginia 2016. "An Open Letter to the Academic Community." https://www.library.ucla.edu/sites/default/files/Ginny-Steel_open-letter_OA2020-PIF_October-2016.pdf.

Strieb, Karla L., and Julia C Blixrud. 2014. "Unwrapping the Bundle: An Examination of Research Libraries and the 'Big Deal.'" *portal: Libraries and the Academy* 14 (4): 587–615. doi:10.1353/pla.2014.0027.

Suhr, Karl F. 2013. "Get It Now: One Library's Experience with Implementing and Using the Unmediated Version of the Copyright Clearance Center's Document Delivery Service." *Journal of Electronic Resources Librarianship* 25 (4): 321–25. doi:10.1080/1941126X.2013.847694.

University of California Libraries. 2016. "Pay It Forward: Investigating a Sustainable Model of Open Access Article Processing Charges for Large North American Research Institutions." Mellon Foundation. http://icis.ucdavis.edu/wp-content/uploads/2016/07/UC-Pay-It-Forward-Final-Report.rev_.7.18.16.pdf.

Way, Doug. 2017. "Doubling Down on the Big Deal in Wisconsin." *Against the Grain* 29 (1): 23–24.

One Library's Story

*Creating and Sustaining a Hospital Library Consortium
for Purchasing Online Journals*

Kathleen Strube

The world was changing in the mid- to late 1990s. Journals had always been available in print. Now publishers were making them available online. It was an exciting time as librarians contemplated a new world. No matter where our customers were, they would be able to use their computers to find and print journal articles instead of having to come to the library or call the librarian. But librarians had a lot of questions. Would online access be reliable? Would all parts of the print journal be available? Could we fill interlibrary loan requests? Did the library have an intranet site to connect library customers to articles? And, perhaps most immediately, would we be able to afford these new online journals? University libraries were early adopters. Around 2000, hospital libraries wanted to be modern and provide easy access as well.

In early 2001, the director of the Aurora Health Care Libraries in Milwaukee, Wisconsin, worked with her Ovid sales representative on an idea to form a buying consortium to purchase access to the 140 Lippincott Williams & Wilkins journal titles. She wanted support from hospital administration for adding online journals and knew prices would be lower if she could offer a vendor many new customers, especially when it required only one negotiation and one contract. Consortial purchasing of electronic journal bundles was already popular for academic libraries and was just beginning to be explored for hospital libraries.

This new consortium would include large hospital libraries and the libraries for entire health care systems. Aurora Health Care, Inc., is a not-for-profit health care system in eastern Wisconsin that included ten hospitals at that time. The idea was to create a significant buying group of fifteen hospital or health system partners. Contacts were made, meetings were held, and the Ovid sales representative helped to find partners from Wisconsin, Illinois, and Michigan. The plan worked because hospital library buyers were a new market for Ovid Technologies at the time, and, therefore, it was possible to settle on low and reasonable prices. A contract was created that ensured that consortial members would be billed separately. A not-to-exceed yearly re-newal percentage was decided on. Archival rights were assured. Interlibrary loan by mail or fax (later by email) was allowed. The initial contract only allowed a certain number of concurrent users for the consortium as a whole, but later it became a site license. After the first year, the Michigan libraries split off to create their own consortium, but ten members from Wisconsin and Illinois continued, with a new member from Minnesota.

Once we had the framework, contract, and pricing for one publisher/vendor, it was easier to talk to other vendors about doing something similar. In subsequent years, we negotiated deals with the American Society for Clinical Oncology for *Journal of Clinical Oncology*, BMJ for journals, Clin-eguide, EBSCO for CINAHL, Elsevier for journals on the ScienceDirect platform, McGraw-Hill for AccessMedicine, Nature for journals, Springer for journals, and Wiley for journals. Our libraries soon became known for having quite a collection and our bosses appreciated the reasonable prices. The model was typically equal pricing for each consortial member or a set consortial price or percentage on top of what had been paid for print titles in the past. It was helpful to network at medical library conferences and view poster presentations to discover pricing models that had worked for other institutions. Yearly contracts eventually became multi-year deals.

Things have changed for hospital libraries since 2001, and the consortium has experienced some complications. The first complication arrived when hospitals and vendors decided they needed more formal contracts, and both sides wanted to review them. Earlier, it had been common for a librarian to sign vendor contracts, and professional library meetings offered training on what should be included. Later, hospitals and health care systems wanted their lawyers and contracts staff to review and sign the contracts. One of the benefits to the vendors of a consortial purchase was that they only had to negotiate once to create a contract for multiple institutions. This saved time, and therefore money, for the vendors. It was important to continue this for the consortium to work. It was decided that the Aurora Health Care librarian and legal team would create the contract for the group, and other members' institutions and legal teams would need to accept the contract without changes. The reward for members was that it was much better pricing than they could get on their own. This has generally worked but has not been easy for the non-Aurora member librarians to insist on. Aurora's legal team also wanted language in the contracts that clearly said that Aurora Health Care, Inc., was not responsible for the payment of any other member. Contract language had to be reworked to say that members were responsible for their own payments and compliance with the terms. Vendors grumbled a little but accepted this.

A recent trend and more difficult complicator is hospital mergers. Over the last few years, several of our consortial members have merged into larger hospital organizations. That process often takes several years, so consortial members needed contract language that stated that they could withdraw from the consortium at the yearly renewal time if their circumstances changed. The rest of us within the consortium needed language that assured us that we would not have to pick up the cost of losing a member. This was accepted by the vendors as they realized the practical reality of today's health care environment.

A result of mergers is that consortial members have sometimes added hospitals to the contract as their health system grew. This was a bonus for the member when it worked out, but vendors would not accept new hospitals being added for free if they had been subscribing to a product separately. Those members were required to continue with their previous contracts and payments, as vendors understandably did not want to lose money they were already earning. Some of our members have affiliated to greater or lesser extents with large national or regional health care systems. Adding those large systems to the consortial license was not feasible. So far, those members have been able to restrict access for the products to their original hospital sites; however, we may lose members in the future as full consolidations and information technology integrations are finalized. There has been incentive on the part of our members and their organizations to find a way to restrict access because our consortial pricing has been desirable.

Yet another trend in health care is hospitals having partner organizations, joint ownerships, minority ownerships, and affiliates of various sorts. These affiliated organizations may be given access to library resources. Publisher/vendor licensors and the hospital/health care system licensees may need to discuss authorized user language and pricing to accommodate entities that are affiliated with but not quite part of the original licensee.

Creating a hospital library consortium to purchase electronic book and journal packages has taken work and creativity, but the results have been worthwhile. Members of the WI-IL-MN Health Consortium feel lucky to have created good partnerships with many vendors, and both sides have prospered. Clinicians and, therefore, patients are benefiting from easy access to the latest evidence from the literature. Sustainability as hospitals continue to merge and health care systems grow even larger will be the challenge for the future, underscoring the need for the unique skills of hospital librarians who understand collection management, licensing terms, and how to work cooperatively with vendors and with each other. As long as consortial agreements continue to benefit both libraries and vendors, librarians will work to address and accommodate current and future changes.

Chapter Four

User-Oriented Collection Assessment

Linda A. Van Keuren

Twenty-first-century health sciences librarians have access to a vast amount of collection assessment data at their fingertips for decision making. The challenge that exists for librarians is how to keep patrons at the forefront of collection development decisions. Using collection data *alongside* user assessment data and professional knowledge, librarians can craft collections to successfully support their users and advance the mission of their larger organizations.

A library strategic marketing plan provides a good structure for a coherent approach to planning, evaluating, and implementing user-focused assessment activities. The concept of marketing originally comes from the corporate world and can be defined as "the process of determining the user communities' wants and needs, developing the products and services in response and encouraging users and potential users to take advantage of the products and services" (Johnson 2014). Note that the first step of marketing involves determining user needs, not developing or promoting products to users that they don't want or need. A realistic marketing plan not only promotes library services and resources to users but also can provide reassurance to library staff that the administration wants to actively plan for long-term library survival (Espe 2016). The four basic Ps of marketing—products, price, place, and promotion—can be adapted to be library focused (Bhardwaj and Jain 2016). The library's *products* are the collection, facilities, and services. The *price* is the cost and time invested in the resources for both the library and the users. *Place* considerations in the marketing plan include both physical and virtual access to the collections. And the final P is for *promotion*, the communication librarians have with their users about library resources. Implementing a marketing plan sends the message to both administration and library users that librarians are focused on being partners in the organizational mission.

COLLECTION ASSESSMENT USING LISTS AND BENCHMARKS

One of the earliest methods of assessing a library collection appeared in 1849 when a librarian at the Smithsonian Institution, Charles Jewett, used a checklist method for evaluation. This method involved comparing the collection against a published bibliography in an influential work (Gregory 2011, 116). Jewett's method continues to be useful today; for instance, health sciences librarians often look to lists like Doody's Core Titles to learn which books are considered "essential" for a collection. Books listing core resources in health sciences subject areas have also been published, such as *The Medical Library Association's Master Guide to Authoritative Information Resources in the Health Sciences* (Thompson et al. 2011). Subject-specific guides have been published by librarians, such as the Nursing and Allied Health Section of the Medical Library Association, which posts and updates their "Selected List of Nursing Journals" (NAHRS/MLA 2012). One method collection managers can use to evaluate journal collections is the Journal Citation Reports database from Clarivate Analytics (formerly from Thomson Reuters). Journal Citation Reports lists the top journals for various subject areas (such as Cell Biology, Pharmacology and Pharmacy, Pathology, or Surgery) by impact factor. While impact factors have been much maligned and questioned as to their validity for determining the importance of journals, and a backlash against them was announced by several publishers in 2016 (Callaway 2016), they remain a useful way to rank general importance of journals within their fields.

Sometimes librarians have found core lists for monographs or journals to be too general for analyzing a collection for coverage of a very specific subject area. In that case, it is possible to create a custom core list for a topic by analyzing the publishing in that area. Librarians at the health sciences library of the University of Wisconsin–Madison created their own core list of journals that cover the topic of drug resistance by analyzing the results of MEDLINE searches for the most productive journals for articles in that area (Bergen 1999).

Assessments of collection quality or completeness using lists or rankings of top monograph or journal titles have limitations because institutions have different needs. For this reason, some librarians try to assess their collections against peer or aspirational institutions. This is slightly more user focused than the use of lists because the comparison is with other institutions that presumably have similar user groups.

Many institutions will have compiled lists of their peer or aspirational institutions that can be used for benchmarking purposes, and librarians can find out about these peers from administrators. Peers can also be identified by an institutional research department within the organization or identified by searching for organizations with similar enrollments, missions, populations, or budgets. Academic libraries can use publicly available data from government organizations such as the National Center for Education Statistics (National Center for Education Statistics 2016) or data from library organizations like the Association of Academic Health Sciences Libraries (AAHSL) statistics, available online to members only and as a yearly published printed source (Squires 2016). Hospital statistical sources can help identify those with similar type, level of care, and numbers of beds (American Hospital Association 2016). Once peer institutions are identified, however, the challenge is to find library data that is available and meaningful to use as a benchmark, particularly for collections. The AAHSL annual statistics allow large academic health sciences libraries serving medical schools to compare physical collection size, circulation counts, and collections expenditures, and irregular AAHSL Resource and Services Surveys (available online to members only) allow a look at which libraries subscribe to which major databases (AAHSL 2016). But comparing physical collection size and circulations is irrelevant for many of the health sciences libraries that have switched to a mostly electronic collection, and library organizations are struggling with how to develop meaningful benchmarks for electronic collections. Comparing collection budgets, on the other hand, can be quite helpful for library directors or collection managers negotiating with their administrators, although budget numbers do not always tell the whole story about access to collections through consortia or other agreements. Modern health sciences libraries use benchmarks in conjunction with local user-oriented assessment data, as using both can be a more powerful practice than either one alone to demonstrate the library's usefulness and meaning within an organization.

EVIDENCE-BASED LIBRARIANSHIP

A culture of assessment permeates modern-day academia and the health care industry, as both are being required to run more like businesses than they have in the past. Librarians are smart to follow the lead of their institutions, and marketing plans that include user needs assessments can be valuable for that purpose. The notion that libraries collect a wide breadth of "just-in-case" collections for users is a goal for only the wealthiest of institutions, and collections evaluation needs to happen regularly for most libraries to stay relevant. Hospital libraries face shrinking budgets and closings due to perceptions that there is no added value to having information experts or a collection of information resources in house. Alongside this, however, the rise of evidence-based medicine (EBM) emphasizes decision making based on data, not just professional knowledge. The values of EBM have been translated into evidence-based librarianship (EBL) or evidence-based librarian and information practice (EBLIP). Similar to the way in which EBM processes shifted physicians' approaches to the practice of medicine, EBL has moved health sciences librarians to incorporate more evidence into their practice and has invigorated assessment research activities. Sentiment, professional experience, and even benchmarking are no longer enough to manage a collection. Evidence must be offered to administrators and patrons that the collections are locally meaningful, appropriate, used by the community the library serves, and produce outcomes that benefit the institution (Eldredge 2000).

EBL is a concept that was developed by Jonathan Eldredge (2000) to encourage sound decision making based on research and "enable health sciences librarians to practice the broad goal of continual, lifelong, self-directed learning while improving their practices." At the core of EBL is a process of creating an answerable research question, using appropriate methods to investigate the question, and acting upon the results. EBL brings sound research practices to user-focused assessment, driving librarians to produce reliable (i.e., repeatable) and valid (i.e., measuring what it states it is measuring) results. The five steps of EBL as outlined by Eldredge can be easily integrated as a part of a user-focused library marketing plan to assess use of the collection:

1. Formulate a clearly defined, answerable question that addresses an important issue in librarianship.
2. Search the published and unpublished literature, plus any other authoritative resources, for the best available evidence with relevance to the posed question.
3. Evaluate the validity (closeness to the truth) and relevance of the evidence.
4. Assess the relative value of expected benefits and costs of any decided-upon action plan.
5. Evaluate the effectiveness of the action plan. (Eldredge 2000)

Formulating a meaningful research question lives at the heart of the library strategic marketing plan, and some preparatory work may be needed prior to its creation. As part of writing the assessment plan and user-focused research question, general market research may be warranted to review the overall demographics of the institution served. Before launching into focus groups and other assessment techniques, both the twenty-year veteran and the new librarian can learn about their organizations with market surveys. Institutions are always changing, and librarian-held assumptions about a population should be verified and updated. Demographic data such as patron type or department affiliation can be mined from an integrated library system for review. Without exposing protected personal information, human resources or information technology departments can provide aggregate numbers and characteristics of the populations served. Mission and institutional strategic plans can be studied for indicators of the institutional goals. External library consortia or organizations can be consulted to find organizations with similar missions. This market research data can help crystallize a clearly defined EBL question and a target population for assessment. For example, once the raw institutional demographic numbers are available, librarians can consider whether it is beneficial to receive feedback from all library users, all non-library users, or some other specific demographic subset of the patron base. Health sciences libraries come in all shapes and sizes, serving a variety of user types with differing needs, and focusing on a specific characteristic or group of users can help keep the entire process manageable.

USER-FOCUSED ASSESSMENT IN DIFFERENT TYPES OF LIBRARIES

For libraries serving clinicians, market research can involve examining the characteristics of the health care institution, such as the number and type of employees, the departments with the highest number of employees, and characteristics such as educational level and job responsibilities. The Via Christi Regional Medical Center Libraries in 2007 undertook a large needs assessment to answer two questions: how could the libraries best serve their patrons, and, given limitations, how could the libraries best help the medical center improve patient care and outcomes. The survey results are dated now but showed demand by clinical professionals for "just-in-time" information at the point of care (Perley et al. 2007). Users in hospital libraries are short on time and are more likely to demand resources electronically, with an easy-to-use interface and a sophisticated searching mechanism that works well with tablets and other mobile devices.

Hospital librarians are in the unique situation to use the EBL process to demonstrate library impact on the quality of patient care and organizational costs. A survey was given to active library users by the librarians of Kaiser Permanente health care system to measure the influence of material and services provided by the librarians. The outcome of the survey successfully demonstrated the library's value, with many respondents reporting that library research avoided an adverse event, resulted in changes in practice, and contributed to a higher quality of care (Bayrer et al. 2014). Research results such as this can be a powerful statement to administrators when campaigning for library funds or staffing.

The advent of the Medicare and Medicaid EHR Incentive Program encouraging providers to use technology to improve patient outcomes (Centers for Medicare and Medicaid Services 2016) has created an opportunity for the integration of library resources into the electronic health record (EHR). As part of the market research process, information professionals serving clinical staff need to be aware of whether there is any meaningful use of information resources within the EHR. If librarians do not know the state of the EHR within the health care system, a marketing plan can be centered on learning more about that issue. If the EHR does not have an Infobutton (links between clinical information systems an online knowledge resources; Cimino 2007), the marketing plan could focus on involving librarians in creating that resource. Assessing users both pre- and post-Infobutton implementation to confirm that the best possible evidence is delivered to clinical staff in a way that does not impact their busy workflow could be very worthwhile.

On the other hand, academic medical libraries and large hospital libraries support research and teaching as well as clinical work. For academic libraries, conversations with the registrar and human resources staff or a review of data on their websites can reveal student and faculty population characteristics such as numbers of people by department, major, and location. For a library that supports a strong research community, the EBL research question may ask about user satisfaction with the depth and comprehensiveness of the collection. Research collection users may also have borrowing/use privileges at other research organizations, and libraries that are part of consortia will take those benefits into consideration as part of the marketing research, plan, assessment, and subsequent collection decisions. Assessment of the collection needs for teaching purposes could focus on both the instructors and students to see if there are differences in their needs and expectations, and assessment needs to focus on specific subsets of users rather than, for example, "students" in general. The needs of students in professional programs would be quite different from graduate students in research programs or undergraduate students. The introduction of a new academic program or degree can be viewed as an opportunity for user assessment of library collections and services from a student user point of view. When the University of Southern Indiana offered their first doctorate program in nursing, librarians used the occasion to launch a three-year research project assessing the ability of the library to meet the needs of this new student population. To answer their research question, librarians used a combination of usage data (from databases, interlibrary loan, and article delivery) with a user survey and citation analysis of student research papers to determine that the library was already mostly successful in meeting the needs of the doctoral students with some suggestions for additions to the collection (Whiting and Orr 2013).

Special libraries that support research and development in for-profit companies or government agencies have a highly focused user group for needs assessment. Human resources and a review of the organizational mission can help the librarian determine the scope of interests of patrons. The EBL research question for special libraries might ask whether the library collections and services enhance the company's mission and bottom line. An assessment completed by a special library serving the large constituency of the Minnesota Department of Health (MDH) used citation analyses to study information needs of the MDH user population by examining the publications of the MDH staff during a three-year time span. The study identified potential collection weaknesses as well as the use of the collections by type, age, and format (Rethlefsen 2007).

Libraries with consumer health information collections may need to do a different type of market research assessment than libraries, which only serve members of a closed institutional environment. In these cases, it is important for librarians first to define the community that they wish to serve, whether it is patients of a hospital or residents of an entire locale. Libraries that provide community health information to patients and families can discuss with an institutional public relations office the socioeconomic demographics of the community served or use data outside the institution from government information sources such as a national census or state, provincial, or city data sites. The EBL research question generated to assess user satisfaction with a consumer health collection asks about readability and accessibility of the information for the target user group. One consumer health user study, conducted by the University of Toronto, examined how women with mental health issues evaluated the quality of the information on mental health websites. Using a combination of online surveys, interviews, diary entries, and web activity tracking software, the authors learned the participants' key criteria for identifying quality information (Marton 2010). Much more inspiration for user assessment of consumer health collections can be found in *The Medical Library Association Guide to Providing Consumer and Patient Health Information* (Spatz 2014).

Finally, libraries with historical or special collections may find it more difficult to predict who will be using their collections and to develop a marketing plan to meet user needs. Such collections draw users from many different disciplines, such as history, social sciences, or art, and can draw traveling users from all over the world. Assessment in this case may focus more on the collection itself rather than the user, as condition of items, availability, and historical relevance are paramount. Because each special collection is, by definition, unique, benchmarks are also difficult. In the cases of historical collections, user assessment, with user surveys and usage data, may be completed after resources have been used. More about the special considerations of collection development for historical or special health sciences collections can be found in chapter 9.

The examples above demonstrate that, while the research questions appropriate for different institutions and kinds of libraries can vary, the techniques of user-centric collections assessment are similar. There are two broad categories of methods for assessing how well a collection meets local user needs. The first is to collect statistics behind the scenes. This requires work but does not require anything unusual of the users and can be easier to accomplish. The second category of techniques involves interactions between the library and the users in the form of surveys, focus groups, or the like. While it can be challenging to involve library users in the assessment of the collection, the strongest evidence is obtained when both types of assessment are implemented.

USER-ORIENTED ASSESSMENT WITH STATISTICS

Prior to health sciences collections becoming predominately electronic, assessment with usage statistics was difficult. Assessment occurred on an as-needed basis to support journal cancelations or other projects. With the development of almost immediate usage metrics for electronic resources, assessment can now be an integral and regular part of collection management decision making, whether for purchasing or for deselection. Circulation statistics have been available for a long time as indicators of monograph usage and are still useful. Circulation statistics are being used by many librarians engaging in downsizing projects and transfers of older materials to storage (see two such stories in this book). Even an inventory of stolen print items can indicate those subject areas where there is high interest and demand! Use of print journals is not as easy to assess. Manually noting the number of times journal volumes were reshelved involved extensive time and effort. Today, librarians have access to a tremendous amount of data about how patrons interact with the electronic resources, and use of journals and databases is very transparent. One common metric used is the COUNTER (Counting Online Usage of Networked Electronic Resources) statistics, developed to provide a consistent standard whereby usage is tracked (COUNTER 2016). Most large vendors use this standard, so COUNTER statistics have enabled librarians to compare usage of journals, databases, and e-book content across platforms and vendors, and improvements continue to be made to the standards and its implementation. Automated methods of collecting COUNTER statistics using the SUSHI (Standardized Usage Statistics Harvesting Initiative) protocol can make the usage data collection process relatively easy for librarians and leave more time for correlating to user feedback and other metrics. COUNTER data differentiates between searches on a platform and access/views of content on the platform, allows one to view usage by years or see monthly trends, and can be used to make decisions regarding renewal of electronic resources or concurrent user licenses needed. COUNTER statistics also provide turnaway information from content not subscribed to, another valuable tool for collection management librarians for future purchase planning. Circulation and electronic usage together are two of the most commonly consulted statistics by health sciences librarians as they move from benchmarks toward more data-driven collection management practices (Grigg et al. 2010).

For decades, librarians have been using citation studies to assess journal collections for supporting research. Such studies are much more time consuming than collecting simple usage statistics but indicate more about how parts of the collection are being used and can reveal important materials not owned by the library. One citation study using graduate theses in dentistry examined the types, ages, and current library subscription statuses of the sources cited to make collection management decisions about journal archive retention or subscription (Cox 2008).

Recently, librarians have been transforming the citation study into a tool to demonstrate institutional return on investment (ROI). These ROI studies provide a user-centered assessment of the collection, as the citation lists come from grant proposals created by researchers associated with the institution. Health sciences librarians from the University of Nebraska, University of Kansas, Creighton University, and Georgetown University compared the citations of funded grant proposals from their institutions to library holdings. Citation data was entered into a formula with the numbers and sizes of grants to determine the institutional ROI for library resource spending (Pisciotta et al. 2010; Varner et al. 2015). In today's environment, demonstrating that an investment in library resources is related to grant funding can be a very powerful message for administrators and funding agencies. Estimates of the ROI from those studies showed that for every dollar spent on the library, a range of $2.14 to $12.50 came back as grant funding (Pisciotta et al. 2010).

Some subscription tools are available to assist librarians in compiling and using metrics. Tools like InCites from Clarivate Analytics (which includes the former *Local Journal Utilization Report* from Thomson Reuters) generate custom analyses ranking journals that are most published in and most cited for any particular institution. Academic librarians and librarians at research institutions can use such analyses to see if their collections are supporting local needs as well as to justify collection expenditures to administrations.

Interlibrary loan (ILL) requests and purchase suggestions can both signal that the library may not be collecting as users need. Both represent users communicating to the library what it is they need to support their research, patient care, or studies. Purchase requests very directly provide guidance on new research or teaching areas that may not have been broadly announced, but not every user makes the effort or feels comfortable communicating with the library. Interlibrary loan statistics provide librarians with another way of learning what is needed, especially when there are multiple requests for a single title or specific area. Single requests may only indicate a single user doing one-time research, but longitudinal examinations of the subject areas borrowed via interlibrary loan may better indicate gaps in the collection. Many libraries use the interlibrary loan guidelines of the "rule of five" to determine what new periodicals will be under consideration for subscribing in the following year. The "rule of five" is derived from the National Commission on New Technological Uses of Copyrighted Works (CONTU) guidelines and applies to materials borrowed via interlibrary loan that are fewer than five years old. Its provisions state that a library may request up to five articles from a single periodical per year from issues published within the last five years before having to pay copyright fees (CONTU 2016). Both purchase requests and ILL requests provide the opportunity for librarians to start conversations with patrons about the resources and services provided.

Patron-driven acquisition (PDA) programs can be considered a form of user needs assessment since users, whether they know it or not, are directly making purchase recommendations for the collection. A PDA program for electronic materials, most often e-books, is one in which preselected, un-owned e-book records are added to the library online catalog and other finding aids. Patrons can find and use the content as needed. Purchase of the material is triggered when usage hits certain parameters previously arranged between the library and the vendor. The arrangements for purchase and titles of the e-book collections vary from vendor to vendor but ideally allow for a mix of librarian and patron decisions in the process.

An indirect collection assessment can be accomplished by comparing curricular, research, or hospital areas of excellence with the number of the library's books and journals classified in those subject areas in the library catalog. This type of study is broad as it involves matching a library's classification or subject-heading system with the areas of excellence, which may be difficult. Age and the amount of yearly publishing of various parts of the collection would also need to be taken into consideration. Further study can be done to demonstrate recent purchasing trends with recent enrollment or department trends to ensure that historical areas of collecting strength continue to be useful for the community and that the collection development policy is keeping pace with institutional changes (Bounds Wilson 2016). Performing similar studies on older content can help librarians make weeding decisions concerning removal of content that no longer aligns with user areas of interest. Evaluators may need to combine this data with other data such as publishing trends for that discipline and importance of historical works for study in that area.

Observational studies of in-person library activities provide insight on the use of physical collections and library-provided technologies used to access resources. Observation can reveal how library patrons naturally use library materials and provide a unique view that may not be revealed by hard usage numbers. For example, observing the use of print materials in the library can give librarians clues on user satisfaction with the physical arrangement of the collection and preference for print versus electronic. If print materials are observed in areas distant from where they are shelved, librarians may want to consider reorganizing the materials. Hospital librarians may be able to *carefully* use observation of dress (white coat length, scrub color, and other uniform clues) to get a very general idea of who comes into the library to use the collections and who does not. That type of observation would need to be very prudentially conducted as, of course, patrons may not always be dressed to fit their "category."

An online version of an observational study is the study of web or proxy transaction logs and logs of the search terms entered into databases. Web logs can trace the user through the library's website and demonstrate intriguing use statistics such as number of clicks and time needed to get to content. Logs serve as a good source for comparison about what users say they are doing and what they are actually doing. This time-stamped data can also be useful in determining user needs for library hours, physical resources, and levels of networking and Wi-Fi support (Gregory 2011). Transaction log analysis, originally used by programmers and network engineers to study system performance, can unobtrusively run in the background of a web interface and record every click and entry (a huge amount of data); the data extraction, anonymizing, and analysis, however, is time consuming and difficult (Troll Covey 2002). For those libraries that do not have in-house programming expertise, transaction log analysis may not be feasible. An alternative that librarians can discuss with their database vendors is the possibility of obtaining search entries from their logs. The texts of user-entered searches can be examined to identify usability of the resource, areas on which to focus library instruction, and subject areas of interest. Failed searches can indicate areas for further collection development or further instructional needs. These observational methods do not involve direct communication with users but can provide guidance on user needs that can aid in collection management decisions.

USER-ORIENTED ASSESSMENT INVOLVING PATRONS

User Surveys

Librarians undertaking user assessment involving their patrons for the first time should keep in mind sound research practices such as anonymizing user responses, removing obvious bias, and creating valid and reliable assessment tools. An investigation into best practices for research, such as those found in *Basic Research Methods for Librarians* (Connaway and Powell 2010), may prevent having to redo the survey, focus group, or other assessment technique due to sloppy data collection or irreproducible results. Institutional review boards or other organizational governing bodies may need to be approached for approval prior to undertaking any kind of assessment with users, particularly if librarians plan to publish or present the data at conferences.

One of the more commonly employed user assessments is the library survey, which provides direct feedback from users. Survey questions may center on a specific resource being considered for acquisition (ease of use, unique content, etc.), or around the general user experience and user expectations for their library. Surveys can be administered in a variety of ways: paper forms, emailed online surveys using such tools as SurveyMonkey, one-on-one discussions, or pop-up screens on the library's web page. Incentives, such as a raffled prize for survey participants, can be used to encourage user participation. Survey questions can be quantitative (e.g., how many times do you access the library's website in a week?) or qualitative and open ended (e.g., what would you like the library to provide in the future for your research?).

The National Library of Medicine Outreach Evaluation Resource Center has created a useful guide to help determine the appropriate methodology (Olney and Barnes 2013). Generally, if one is interested in trying to learn the *hows* of the collection (how many, how much, how often), quantitative research methods work best. If one is trying to learn the *whats* of the collection (what worked best, what didn't work), qualitative methods should be used.

Patron familiarity with the library collection needs to be considered when planning who will participate in the survey and how it will be delivered. One must determine ahead of time if the participants should be library users, nonusers, or both, as that determination can alter the methods of distributing and writing the survey. Non-library users will not physically be in the library or visit the library's web page, and a survey distribution plan for them should include using institutional communication channels such as emails or newsletters. Surveys can serve to promote the library resources to users by asking them to consider and comment on aspects of the collection that they may not have known about. Capturing data from users unfamiliar with the collection often leads to requests for material that the library already has, which can be another opportunity for promotion of resources.

As e-books replace many of the print books in library collections, a popular research question for librarians is to ask about user preferences by format. For this type of question, combining survey results with print and e-book usage statistics can address the same question from multiple angles. In a

Tulane University library survey, first- and third-year medical students and first-year residents were given a paper survey during their orientations asking them about their format preferences for reading. The authors suggested that, based upon their data, academic health sciences libraries should consider continuing to provide print copies of required textbooks for first- and second-year medical students. They noted that the preference for electronic resources increased as the students moved along in their curriculum, with electronic resources getting more preference with residents (Pickett 2016). If the authors had combined their survey data with usage statistics, they might have had an even fuller picture of their users' preferences.

Developing user surveys can be time consuming and difficult. Librarian bias can be hard to remove from questions, and users bring their own biases. There is temptation to include *all* the questions the library wants to ask, but keeping the research question focused within the library's marketing plan goals to avoid extraneous data collection is important. Surveys that are too long or detailed may result in less participation and survey fatigue. Too much data can also be hard for librarians to manage. Scope creep is a danger here as well, and keeping the survey focused and to the point is more likely to result in completion of the assessment project with actionable plans.

To help, some libraries look to outside entities to assist with the creation of user surveys, and these surveys have the benefit of combining a local user-centered view with comparison against other institutions. One such user survey and benchmarking tool, sponsored by the Association of Research Libraries, is LibQUAL+. LibQUAL+ surveys measure user perceptions of the library's services against expectations in three areas: helpfulness of staff, ease of finding information, and conduciveness of the physical environment for study. LibQUAL+ is web based and provides participants with prewritten, rigorously tested survey questions. While these surveys cover all aspects of the library, not just the collections, concerns and perceptions about the collections are included. Participating libraries can benchmark to peers to identify "industry" standards and practices (ARL 2016). Peer comparison can also provide guidance to libraries on areas to investigate further. LibQUAL+ questionnaires have been adapted for use at academic medical libraries by several members of the Association of Academic Health Sciences Libraries (Heath, Kyrillidou, and Askew 2014). Northwestern University's Galter Health Sciences Library was one of the first of these to use the LibQUAL+ data to highlight service and collection areas for further research, and they held focus groups with users for a "deep dive" into the areas of interest. Faculty were invited to discuss their impressions of the library's journal collection in focus groups, and the library learned much about their faculty's needs regarding format, depth, and accessibility of the collection (Shedlock and Walton 2004).

MINES (Measuring the Impact of Networked Electronic Services) for libraries is another prewritten survey assessment tool. MINES for libraries is an intercept survey that combines usage data collection with a web-based user survey to collect user demographics, location, and purpose. The benefit of an intercept survey is that it pops up on the screen to users after they have selected an electronic resource but before they are sent to the resource. This can link patron feedback directly to the resources used. One example of MINES use in a health sciences library is a study done by Plum and Franklin, who analyzed the use of over six thousand e-books in thirteen academic and health sciences libraries. In this implementation, print versions of the survey were also handed out to users walking into the library. Since the online survey interrupts patron research, the survey was kept to only four questions. Combining resource usage with patron demographics proved to be very useful and demonstrated that e-books were used for patient care, while e-journals or databases were used more for research (Plum and Franklin 2015, 93–121). For libraries with limited funding, benchmarking endeavors do not necessarily have to be undertaken via fee-based products such as LibQual+ or MINES. A thoughtful home-grown plan and methodology can work just as well. However, in both cases, it's important to keep in mind hidden costs such as staff time.

Focus Groups

Focus groups, either in conjunction with a survey or on their own, provide valuable opportunities to build relationships with user groups, do some user education, and gather information about users' priorities and impressions of the library's collections. Focus groups can consist of volunteers or invited groups of users. In addition to examining the recommendations of the book *Focus Groups: A Practical Guide for Applied Research* (Krueger and Casey 2015), librarians may want to consult with others in their institutions who have expertise in running focus groups (through a psychology, therapy, or similar department) for guidance on best practices for approaching potential participants and size, length of time, and types of questions. Some librarians may need to work with an institutional review board to ensure that the focus groups fall within institutional guidelines. Focus groups, even more than surveys, can provide meaningful data from non-library users if the library is able to encourage their participation. The more conversational tone of a focus group allows for non-library users to honestly state reasons for not using the library resources. These reasons may be ones that librarians would not have thought to include in a prescribed survey. Focus groups should be recorded to capture the conversation in the group. Afterward, this conversation should be de-identified and coded to gather the data for analysis. Qualitative data gathered from focus groups can be synthesized and used alongside quantitative usage data to give libraries a well-rounded view of users' impressions and needs for the collection. As part of a larger marketing plan to engage patrons and liaison librarians in the collection development process, the University of Southern California Health Sciences Libraries used focus groups of their pharmacy and medical students to determine student preferences for content, design, and navigation of e-book platforms. They combined this strategy with markers and flip charts placed around the library for a week to elicit student suggestions. Both methods provided valuable data for the librarians to make service and collection decisions.

Librarians need to be sure, once they have completed their assessments, to dedicate the time and resources needed to evaluate the data and form an action plan. A pitfall with assessment implementation is not thoughtfully interpreting and acting upon the data findings. Some decisions based on data do not require extensive evaluation—for instance, turnaway statistics may indicate a great need to get a new journal subscription. Interpretation of user surveys can be more difficult, as correlation of data does not necessarily indicate causation, and librarians need to beware of over interpreting their data. For example, users could respond that they are satisfied with library resource availability and that they have been published within the past year, but that does not necessarily mean that the collection is robust enough to increase the level of scholarly output of the institution. Reviewers of survey data need to be mindful that causation is very difficult to prove, even from the best written of surveys, as, to prove causation, all other possible explanations for a correlation must be accounted for. In the very general example above, researchers may have a high level of scholarly output and may be using resources outside of the library. It is possible for librarians to find that their selected assessment tools do not produce meaningful results. This can be considered part of the EBL process of self-directed learning, and librarians can take those lessons learned into the next assessment effort. Once data has been evaluated as objectively as possible, librarians can move on to making collection additions or changes and making sure that those decisions are communicated to library users or to administrators.

ROLE OF LIAISON LIBRARIANS IN ASSESSMENT AND MARKETING

Liaison librarians, even those that may not have specific job responsibilities for collections, should be active participants in the marketing plan implementation, the evidence-based librarianship research question creation, and crafting of a user-focused library culture and collection. Liaisons, with their frequent interaction with users, membership on institutional committees, and teaching encounters, can bring experiential knowledge to the marketing plan.

Liaison librarians' roles vary from institution to institution, but, at their core, they are the library ambassadors, working with patrons to ensure the collection and services are understood and needed, and communicating what they learn about patrons to collection managers. Liaisons can tell the persuasive library stories that are impactful when included in funding or resource requests to administration.

As liaisons develop personal relationships with patrons and talk to them, they gain unique insights into what users are hoping to get from the library, even if a formal assessment is not possible. Liaison librarians may have specialized degrees in biology, physiology, or other health sciences disciplines, in addition to their library or information science degrees, that make the conversation with patrons more meaningful. Liaisons often can suggest assessment participants, introduce the assessment tool to patrons, and explain the rationale behind the assessment. Liaisons can also help translate collection decisions for patrons by explaining the constraints and opportunities the library encounters in terms users can understand. Liaisons often have a pulse on the collection interests of library "champions" and can make sure that they are kept aware of library activities. Working with library "champions" creates strong partnerships and has positive political implications for the library. Many academic health sciences libraries are strengthening their liaison programs and dedicating more librarians to these roles. New York University Health Sciences Library developed their liaison system with very specific goals in mind to strengthen the connection between high-priority users and the library to better understand what information was needed and what access barriers existed. Understanding that today's world of electronic communication can seem impersonal, their liaison program allowed for more opportunities for the librarians to engage with users and support their research needs (Williams et al. 2014).

CONCLUSION

More about promotion of the collection and enhancing user discovery of the collection is discussed in chapter 6. Assessment and promotion are *both* part of an effective marketing plan for the user-centric library, and one informs the other to increase community support and build the relationship between users and the library. In 2013, the University of Tennessee Health Sciences Library wanted to better demonstrate to users the library value and engaged in a systematic marketing plan to gather user feedback, adjust collection purchases, demonstrate library values, and better align collections to campus priorities. They surveyed the literature, defined goals, used collection and user data to reshape their collection, and, finally, publicized the new resources to campus. The librarians involved determined that using a systematic marketing plan was effective and planned to continue to fine-tune it in future years (Fought, Gahn, and Mills 2014). Marketing plans are, at their essence, an orderly strategy for communication between the library and its patrons, and librarians should be aware of the best ways to communicate with their library users or potential users.

The user-focused assessment process must be evaluated and refined regularly. Librarians that use the EBL structure to focus their research questions and thoughtfully schedule their user assessment activities into the institutional schedule will likely find that their libraries have more user engagement. It is important to note that all assessment methods are imperfect and that better results will be obtained when librarians compile the results of more than one assessment method, combining the quantitative with the qualitative. Simply looking at raw usage statistics can give a sense of resource popularity but cause librarians to discount important usage of smaller but more focused resources. On the other hand, focus groups and surveys can sometimes allow a few loud voices to unduly influence decisions. Libraries often have a great deal of data going unused, and combining collection data with user data when possible provides a more comprehensive view of library user collection needs. Ideally, collection managers have time to focus on assessment efforts alongside all of their other duties.

Although the value of information is understood in the information economy, library value and return on institutional investment must be made self-evident to those that make budgeting and administrative decisions. Busy administrators today may be approached by information product vendors directly, bypassing collection development librarians for purchase and management of traditionally library-managed materials. Performing user-focused assessment endeavors is worth the time and effort it takes to ensure that administrators consider the library collections and librarians a vital part of the institution.

REFERENCES

American Hospital Association. 2016. "American Hospital Directory." American Hospital Association. Last modified October 10. https://www.ahd.com/.

Association of Academic Health Sciences Libraries (AAHSL). 2016. *Annual Statistics of Medical School Libraries in the United States and Canada, Services and Resources Surveys.* Association of Academic Health Sciences Libraries. Accessed October 11. http://www.aahsl.org/annual-statistics.

Association of Research Libraries (ARL). 2016. "LibQUAL+ : General Information." Association of Research Libraries. Accessed October 8. http://www.libqual.org/home.

Bayrer, Rebecca, Suzanne Beattie, Elizabeth Lucas, Dawn Melberg, and Eve Melton. 2014. "What Have We Done for You Lately? Measuring Hospital Libraries' Contribution to Care Quality." *Journal of Hospital Librarianship* 14 (3): 243–49. doi:10.1080/15323269.2014.888514.

Bergen, Phillip L. 1999. "An Assessment of Collections at the University of Wisconsin–Madison Health Sciences Libraries: Drug Resistance." *Bulletin of the Medical Library Association* 87 (1): 37–42.

Bhardwaj, R. K., and P. K. Jain. 2016. "Marketing of Library Resources and Services: A Structured Literature Review." *DESIDOC Journal of Library & Information Technology* 36 (3): 119–25. doi:10.14429/djlit.36.3.10027.

Bounds Wilson, Jamie. 2016. "Assessing Collection Development and Acquisitions at the Millsaps-Wilson Library, Millsaps College." *Mississippi Libraries* 79 (1): 4–7.

Callaway, Ewen. 2016. "Beat It, Impact Factor! Publishing Elite Turns against Controversial Metric." *Nature* 535 (7611): 210–11. doi:10.1038/nature.2016.20224.

Centers for Medicare and Medicaid Services. 2016. "Electronic Health Records (EHR) Incentive Programs." Centers for Medicare and Medicaid Services. Last modified November 22. https://www.cms.gov/Regulations-and-Guidance/Legislation/EHRIncentivePrograms/.

Cimino, James J. 2007. "An Integrated Approach to Computer-Based Decision Support at the Point of Care." *Transactions of the American Clinical and Climatological Association* 118: 273–88. http://www.ncbi.nlm.nih.gov/pmc/articles/PMC1863602/.

Connaway, L. S., and R. R. Powell. 2010. *Basic Research Methods for Librarians*. Santa Barbara, CA: Libraries Unlimited.

COUNTER. 2016. "About COUNTER." COUNTER. Accessed December 5. https://www.projectcounter.org/about/.

Cox, Janice E. 2008. "Citation Analysis of Graduate Dental Theses References: Implications for Collection Development." *Collection Management* 33 (3): 219–34. doi:10.1080/01462670802045558.

Eldredge, Jonathan. October 2000. "Evidence-Based Librarianship: An Overview." *Bulletin of the Medical Library Association* 88 (4): 289.

Espe, Sue. 2016. "Health Sciences Librarians Off the Radar." *Journal of the Medical Library Association* 104 (3): 236. doi:10.3163/1536-5050.104.3.012.

Fought, Rick L., Paul Gahn, and Yvonne Mills. 2014. "Promoting the Library through the Collection Development Policy: A Case Study." *Journal of Electronic Resources in Medical Libraries* 11 (4): 169–78. doi:10.1080/15424065.2014.969031.

Gregory, Vicki L. 2011. *Collection Development and Management for 21st Century Library Collections: An Introduction*. New York: Neal-Schuman Publishers.

Grigg, Karen S., Bethany A. Koestner, Richard A. Peterson, and Patricia L. Thibodeau. 2010. "Data-Driven Collection Management: Through Crisis Emerge Opportunities." *Journal of Electronic Resources in Medical Libraries* 7 (1): 1–12. doi:10.1080/15424060903585685.

Heath, Fred M., Martha Kyrillidou, and Consuella Askew, eds. 2014. *Libraries Act on their LibQUAL+ Findings : From Data to Action*. Hoboken: Taylor & Francis.

Johnson, Peggy. 2014. *Fundamentals of Collection Development and Management*. Chicago, IL: American Library Association.

Krueger, R. A., and M. A. Casey. 2015. *Focus Groups: A Practical Guide for Applied Research*. 5th ed. Thousand Oaks, CA: SAGE Publications, Inc.

Marton, Christine. 2010. "How Women with Mental Health Conditions Evaluate the Quality of Information on Mental Health Web Sites: A Qualitative Approach." *Journal of Hospital Librarianship* 10 (3): 235–50. doi:10.1080/15323269.2010.491422.

National Center for Education Statistics. 2016. "Library Statistics Program." Institute of Education Sciences, U.S. Department of Education. Accessed December 9. https://nces.ed.gov/surveys/libraries/.

National Commission on New Technology Uses of Copyrighted Works (CONTU). 2016. "CONTU Guidelines on Photocopying under Interlibrary Loan Arrangements." Coalition for Networked Information. Accessed December 9. http://old.cni.org/docs/infopols/CONTU.html.

Nursing and Allied Health Resources Section of the Medical Library Association (NAHRS/MLA). Research Committee Journal Project Team. 2012. "NAHRS 2012 Selected List of Nursing Journals." Medical Library Association. http://nahrs.mlanet.org/home/images/activity/nahrs2012selectedlistnursing.pdf.

Olney, Cynthia A., and Susan J. Barnes. 2013. *Collecting and Analyzing Evaluation Data.* . 2nd ed. Planning and Evaluating Health Information Outreach Projects, booklet 3. Seattle, WA: National Network of Libraries of Medicine, Outreach Evaluation Resource Center. https://nnlm.gov/neo/guides/bookletThree508.

Perley, Cathy M., Camillia A. Gentry, A. Sue Fleming, and Kristin M. Sen. 2007. "Conducting a User-Centered Information Needs Assessment: The Via Christi Libraries' Experience." *Journal of the Medical Library Association* 95 (2): 173. doi:10.3163/1536-5050.95.2.173.

Pickett, Keith M. 2016. "Resource Format Preferences across the Medical Curriculum." *Journal of the Medical Library Association* 104 (3): 193. doi:10.3163/1536-5050.104.3.003.

Pisciotta, Robert A., Crystal Cameron-Vedros, Deborah Carman, Nancy Woelfl, and James Bothmer. 2010. "ROI! Return on Investment Studies in Libraries." Midcontinental Chapter of the Medical Library Association. http://mcmla.org/resources/Express/2010/roi.pdf.

Plum, Terry, and Brinley Franklin. 2015. "What Is Different about E-Books? A MINES for Libraries Analysis of Academic and Health Sciences Research Libraries' E-Book Usage." *Portal: Libraries and the Academy* 15 (1): 93–121. doi:10.1353/pla.2015.0007.

Rethlefsen, Melissa. 2007. "Citation Analysis of Minnesota Department of Health Official Publications and Journal Articles: A Needs Assessment for the RN Barr Library." *Journal of the Medical Library Association* 95 (3): 260. doi:10.3163/1536-5050.95.3.260.

Shedlock, James, and Linda Walton. 2004. "An Academic Medical Library using LibQUAL+: the Experience of the Galter Health Sciences Library, Northwestern University." *Journal of Library Administration* 40 (3–4): 99–110. doi:10.1300/j111v40n03_08.

Spatz, Michele. 2014. *The Medical Library Association Guide to Providing Consumer and Patient Health Information.* Lanham: Rowman & Littlefield.

Squires, Steven J., ed. 2016. *Annual Statistics of Medical School Libraries in the United States and Canada.* 38th ed. Seattle, WA: Association of Academic Health Sciences Libraries.

Thompson, Laurie L., Mori Lou Higa, Esther Carrigan, and Rajia Tobia. 2011. *The Medical Library Association's Master Guide to Authoritative Information Resources in the Health Sciences/Authoritative Information Resources in the Health Sciences.* New York: Neal-Schuman Publishers.

Troll Covey, Denise. 2002. "Usage Studies of Electronic Resources." In *Usage and Usability Assessment: Library Practices and Concerns.* Washington, DC: Council on Library and Information Resources. https://www.clir.org/pubs/reports/pub105/pub105.pdf.

Varner, Douglas L., Jennifer C. Kluge, Nancy N. Woelfl, Jett McCann, Linda A. Van Keuren, and Grant Connors. 2015. "Library Return-on-Investment: Collaborating with Research Administration to Develop of Model for the Health Sciences Library in Support of Research." Medical Library Association Conference 2015. https://georgetown.box.com/s/8cjzhzswh2hzg4057matm23dglil045y.

Whiting, Peter, and Philip Orr. 2013. "Evaluating Library Support for a New Graduate Program: Finding Harmony with a Mixed Method Approach." *The Serials Librarian* 64 (1–4): 88–98. doi:10.1080/0361526x.2013.760329.

Williams, Jeff, Aileen McCrillis, Richard McGowan, Joey Nicholson, Alisa Surkis, Holly Thompson, and Dorice Vieira. 2014. "Leveraging Technology and Staffing in Developing a New Liaison Program." *Medical Reference Services Quarterly* 33 (2): 157–66. doi:10.1080/02763869.2014.897515.

One Library's Story

*All or Nothing: The University of California Walks
Away from ClinicalKey*

Sarah McClung, Rikke Sarah Ogawa,
and Bruce Abbott

The University of California (UC) system consists of ten campuses, of which seven have health sciences programs. Five are medical centers with medical and health professional schools, one is a stand-alone medical school without a medical center, and one offers health sciences programs without a medical school or center. Together, these seven campuses have multiple hospitals and an array of health professional schools in dentistry, medicine, nursing, optometry, pharmacy, public health, and veterinary medicine. Because the UC libraries have a history of negotiating consortially for desirable licensing terms and pricing, librarians identified as health sciences selectors across the UC campuses frequently work together to license medical resources.

Through 2014, six of the UC libraries consortially licensed MDConsult, a clinical database procured by Elsevier from Harcourt in 2002. The UC subscription to MDConsult consisted of a small collection of journals and e-books, as well as patient care handouts and a drug reference. Elsevier discontinued MDConsult in December 2014 and replaced it with ClinicalKey, a clinical search engine that contains over a thousand books and six hundred journals, including the previous MDConsult resources. While MDConsult had various customizable subscription options allowing libraries to add books to the collection on an à la carte basis, ClinicalKey was marketed as the comprehensive suite of Elsevier's medical content to be subscribed to as a unit. Before MDConsult's end, the UC libraries were faced with assessing what value ClinicalKey would add to its suite of medical content and clinical decision-making tools and whether or not the libraries should migrate to this new database.

The UC campuses began discussions with Elsevier's ClinicalKey representatives in 2013, shortly after the database was released. The UC health sciences selectors spent the next two years negotiating with ClinicalKey representatives, evaluating pricing proposals and content options, and assessing data concerning MDConsult and ClinicalKey in order to make an informed decision about the product's utility. With the distinct possibility of the ClinicalKey proposal falling through, each campus also prepared a contingency plan that included strategies for filling in collection gaps through consortial journal subscriptions and local book purchasing, as well as communication with campus stakeholders.

Our main concerns regarding subscribing to ClinicalKey were the substantial cost, inflexible content model, and lack of perpetual access. The UC Libraries had purposefully managed the content and cost of MDConsult to make it an affordable resource that supported the educational mission of our medical programs; however, ClinicalKey's pricing and content models were based on it being a comprehensive clinical search engine. After several rounds of negotiations, UC's final quote was an increase of nearly 95 percent over what we had paid in 2014 for MDConsult. At a time when most of the UC libraries had faced years of either reduced or flat budgets, finding additional funds to pay for ClinicalKey would have required sacrificing other content we were not willing or able to cancel. While it makes sense for Elsevier to charge more for a product that has more content than MDConsult, the UC libraries had not previously acquired all comparable content of ClinicalKey and did not intend to. ClinicalKey's bundled content model did not align well with the UC libraries' preference for package flexibility. The lack of ability to exercise our expertise in selecting and providing access to specific, relevant content to the institution's needs troubled the health sciences selectors. Furthermore, while ClinicalKey does offer subject-based collections as an alternative to their whole database, we were informed by our representatives that, due to our size, the UC libraries would wind up spending more if we subscribed to these smaller subsets of content.

Among a more foundational set of concerns for the UC libraries is that of subscription-based book collections. Whenever possible, we believe that libraries should own the content for which they have paid. To further this goal and other goals related to the access and collecting of e-books, the UC Libraries Collection Development Committee created a document titled the "UC Libraries E-book Value Statement," which is posted on the California Digital Library website (http://libraries.universityofcalifornia.edu/groups/files/cdc/docs/UC_Libraries_E-Book_Value_Statement.pdf). The value statement addresses five areas of concern, one of which is that e-books should have a sustainable and fair business model. One aspect of a sustainable model is that perpetual access and archival rights be guaranteed for purchased online content. This mirrors the perpetual access that libraries have always had with print clinical textbooks and journals even after cancelation. The model proposed by ClinicalKey at the time of negotiation did not guarantee future access in the case of cancelation, effectively making the annual subscription cost a content rental fee.

In addition to the information provided to us about ClinicalKey, the UC librarians collected and assessed many other types of data while making our decision. We evaluated online usage reports for MDConsult and the print circulation statistics of the books on both the MDConsult and ClinicalKey platforms and discovered that the bulk of the usage was concentrated on a small number of titles. We reviewed lists of required textbooks for our health sciences programs, course reserve titles, and past patron requests to see how many titles were clinical Elsevier imprints. While many foundational texts were included in both databases, most titles that were required reading for the UC's undergraduate medical education programs were, surprisingly, not published by Elsevier.

In December 2014, after careful consideration and analysis, the UC campuses decided not to subscribe to ClinicalKey. Because the untenable subscription cost and unfavorable content model were particularly egregious given our stated principles and fiscal reality, the UC libraries also decided not to move forward with local subscriptions to ClinicalKey. The campus contingency plans were put into place to make our previously identified changes to the collection and communicate with users.

Access to journals was handled consortially, while the clinical texts were handled at the campus level. Because the journals were available on the ScienceDirect platform, and the UC libraries already had a consortial license with Elsevier for many journals on ScienceDirect, we were able to transfer access to this existing contract and eliminate some duplication of content. For niche subject-area journals, the UC health sciences selectors evaluated usage and their campus-specific importance to determine whether or not they were added. Together, the health sciences selectors established a cost model that enabled us to add system-wide journal subscriptions for less than our previous MDConsult campus cost shares.

MDConsult e-books were not available for à la carte purchase on ScienceDirect. Some titles were available on third-party platforms with a wide variety of pricing and access models. No simple consortial option existed to address all of the UC libraries' budgets and concerns, so each campus took a different approach in replacing the e-book content, using our shared licensing value statement as a guide. Purchasing decisions were further complicated by Elsevier's announcement that subsequent e-book editions would only be available on ClinicalKey. Regardless, many campuses, including UC Los Angeles and UC Davis, purchased e-books on one or more third-party platforms. Titles purchased were based on the evaluation of usage reports and patron requests. One campus, UC San Francisco, purchased only print copies to replace the e-books after deciding the e-books on the third-party platforms were cost prohibitive and that purchasing them would only be a stopgap measure. Again, usage and patron requests, as well as required text lists, influenced which print books were ordered.

Each library communicated to its users the UC system's choice not to subscribe to ClinicalKey and how this decision affected access to previous MDConsult resources. Most campuses directly emailed key stakeholders, including medical faculty members, student representatives, deans, and residency coordinators, as well as posted news items on their library websites and in newsletters. UC Davis also created a LibGuide to outline the changes.

Regardless of the methods used on the campus level to replace MDConsult content, the UC libraries received remarkably few requests and complaints as a result of losing a top clinical resource. While some campus medical centers have expressed interest in subsets of ClinicalKey content, the UC librarians are diligent to explain the rationale for our decision. Overall, the UC libraries consider this experience a success in exercising fiscal responsibility and asserting our values without causing extensive inconvenience to our primary clientele. This situation highlights how e-book subscriptions tend to be more problematic than e-book package purchases, how it takes extra time and effort to work consortially to make decisions, and how it is challenging to provide a consistent user experience with multiple electronic platforms. Our largely positive experience unsubscribing from a large, well-known medical content database is encouraging as we continue to analyze and evaluate existing and future resources in order to be good stewards of funds, meet user needs, and uphold professional standards. UC libraries' undertaking demonstrates both the benefits and the complications of a collaborative approach to licensing a core clinical and educational information resource.

Chapter Five

Collaborative Collection Management

Esther E. Carrigan, Nancy G. Burford, and Ana G. Ugaz

Cooperation and collaboration have a long-established history in libraries, and that history is well documented in the literature. The two terms are used interchangeably. The *Oxford English Dictionary* (OED) defines them in similar terms: cooperation is "the action of working together towards the same end" (OED Online 2017a); collaboration is "united labor" (OED Online 2017b). Libraries of all types have formed consortia, defined by OED as a partnership or association, to formalize cooperative efforts across various library activities. In the health sciences library world, the National Library of Medicine (NLM) and its National Network of Libraries of Medicine (NN/LM) can be considered a kind of national consortium. Begun over fifty years ago, that network of medical libraries, in effect, laid the groundwork and created the infrastructure for many of the cooperative programs that have developed across health sciences libraries.

Collaboration can be and has been applied to any activity or service within libraries. Libraries share collection resources through interlibrary lending; share human resources and expertise through cooperative cataloging and virtual reference services; and share electronic licensing buying and negotiating power through consortia such as the Greater Western Library Alliance (GWLA). From a collection perspective, collaboration typically involves a cooperation or coordination of collection activities to achieve common goals.

Collaborative collection management might take place between different types of libraries, across libraries within a defined geographic region, such as the eight regions of the NN/LM, or among libraries with narrowly defined subject areas, such as hospital, veterinary medicine, or pharmacy. Johnson defines collaborative collection management as "the sharing of responsibilities among two or more libraries for the process of acquiring materials, developing collections, and managing the growth and maintenance of collections in a user-beneficial and cost-beneficial way" (Johnson 2004, 236). Burgett, Haar, and Phillips define it as "multiple libraries coordinating the development and management of their collections with the goal of building broader, more useful combined collections than any library in the group could build individually" (Burgett, Haar, and Phillips 2004, 4). These definitions are useful in establishing some of the parameters and expectations for collaborative collection management ventures.

The overarching goal for any collaborative collection initiative is to increase access to resources for the library user, but there are often many more focused, specific objectives factored into the collection collaboration decision. From a collection development perspective, these include increasing the effectiveness of the collection budget and reducing unnecessary overlap or duplication, using the formal collaborative plan to coordinate individual library collection responsibilities. From a collection management perspective, these include coordination of retention, deselection, storage, and preservation decisions (Richards and Eakin 1997).

The Medical Library Assistance Act of 1965 (MLAA) authorized "NLM to provide grants to improve medical library services and facilities and to create a regional medical library network to facilitate the sharing of collections" (DeBakey 1991). This network was later renamed the National Network of Libraries of Medicine (NN/LM), and it divides the United States into eight geographical regions. As technology advanced throughout the 1970s and 1980s, NLM not only provided access to its collections, but networks developed by NLM, such as MEDLINE and DOCLINE, facilitated resource sharing directly among all types of medical libraries, both within the NN/LM regions and across those regions (NLM 2011). These networks fueled the growth of health sciences library collaborations built on the foundation of a national system of Regional Medical Libraries (RMLs), one located within each of the NN/LM regions.

These RMLs are large academic medical libraries that, in addition to their regular staffing and services, complement house NLM employees who administer the regional office and coordinate NLM programs and collaboration within that region. In most regions, the RML establishes several resource libraries (RL), which are typically larger academic health sciences libraries that can address information and service requests from local hospital, community college, or other medical-related libraries (Bunting 1987). These resource libraries, along with the RML, develop or provide leadership for the collaborative programs within a region. The current mission of the NN/LM program, taken from the website, is to advance medical progress and improve public health by providing and improving access to biomedical information for both the health professional and the public. This broad goal has guided the NN/LM program since its inception. Librarians within a region provide training on the use of NLM-created biomedical information resources, work with a variety of libraries within the region to improve access to these resources through technology enhancements, and promote their use. NN/LM collaborative collection initiatives have long included not only coordinated collection development programs but also resource-sharing initiatives. Specific programs and initiatives vary across the regions and continue to evolve over time, but all support the overarching mission and goal of the NN/LM program.

GROWTH OF HEALTH SCIENCES LIBRARY CONSORTIA

Many health sciences libraries have been involved with one or more collaborative agreements, primarily to broaden their access to necessary literature. While the launch of MEDLINE in 1971 improved the retrieval of clinical and scientific literature, it was NLM's DOCLINE system that strengthened the links between libraries by providing a quicker, automated method of routing interlibrary loan (ILL) requests. To improve the efficiency of ILL between health sciences libraries, the Serial Records Section at NLM oversaw the creation of the SERHOLD database, completed in 1981, to provide the serials holdings information that would fuel DOCLINE routing (Willmering et al. 1988). DOCLINE and SERHOLD provided the infrastructure to support the effective resource sharing that is essential to the success of any collaborative collection management initiative.

In addition to the MLAA and the resource sharing and regional consortia it facilitated, NLM itself also directly supported the formation of consortia by launching its Resource Improvement Grant program in 1975 to provide funding for the planning and implementation of consortia. Applicants were expected to provide the rationale and objectives for the consortia development, such as establishing reciprocal borrowing privileges or centralized cataloging, increasing communication among members, establishing a mechanism for coordinating acquisitions, and developing continuing education and training programs (Kabler 1980). Although the twenty-first-century world of collections has changed dramatically, these are still valid and meaningful goals and objectives for consortia today.

Health sciences libraries, with journals as the heart of their collections, were especially hard hit by the collection cost inflation, and, in particular, journal inflation that plagued all library budgets beginning in the 1980s. This economic environment and the ongoing need to stretch collection dollars has made the potential benefits of collaborative collection initiatives well worth the inherent efforts and challenges and has made participation in consortia an attractive option for many libraries. While collaborative collection initiatives have changed over the years, they continue today, largely driven and shaped by economic incentives.

COLLABORATIVE PRINT PURCHASING AND RETENTION

Collaborative purchasing or collaborative collection-building activities are a logical extension of resource sharing. In fact, in the earliest years of the NLM regional network, a number of programs were developed by the RMLs to "share information resources and coordinate the development of regional collections" (Bunting 1987, 27). For example, the South Central Regional Medical Library Program (SCR) successfully set up duplicate exchange services and a union list of serials. The SCR resource libraries began their collaborative collection management efforts with a program (Hendricks 1976) in which each resource library agreed to retain certain serial subscriptions and a cooperative effort to complete backfiles for those institutional title commitments. In 1979 these same SCR resource libraries implemented a cooperative acquisition program for print monographs with objectives to increase the number of monographs available in the region, limit duplication, equitably distribute the purchasing responsibilities, increase the predictability of particular monographs being available in the region, and reduce subjectivity in acquisition responsibilities (Kronick 1979). Resource libraries were assigned particular publishers and committed to purchasing all of the monographs from the assigned publishers that matched agreed-upon profile parameters (Kronick 1979). A 1984 assessment found that the program was most successful with two of its five program objectives: increased coverage of the chosen publishers and reduction of overall duplication (Bowden, Comeaux, and Eakin 1984). Budget pressures across many of the participating libraries curtailed this program in the 1980s.

The Pacific Southwest RML focused on a cooperative acquisition plan for serial titles that were held by fewer than three libraries (Cooperative Serials Acquisitions Program), and the Greater Midwest RML initiated a project to coordinate collection development among member libraries using the Research Libraries Group Conspectus collection management tool. Collaborative purchasing initiatives varied by region but had the same goal of trying to extend collection budgets by reducing duplicate purchases of lesser-needed materials and distributing the acquisition of that material for sharing across the group. These early examples of collaborative print purchasing programs reveal the double-edged sword that economic pressures have been, and continue to be, to collaborative programs. On the one hand, reduced collection budgets encourage cooperative acquisitions by libraries attempting to stretch collection dollars. On the other hand, reduced collection budgets inevitably force libraries to focus on local collection needs and create an environment where external collaborations are challenging.

Health sciences libraries did find that distributing the responsibility for acquiring and maintaining print serials subscriptions offered some relief from the escalating costs of medical journals. Since one library's decision to cancel a journal would impact other libraries in a region, efforts to coordinate and share these decisions were logical. Collaborative initiatives to coordinate the purchase of print materials have been overshadowed in recent years by collaborative print weeding, retention, and preservation programs. The digital age has brought immense changes to libraries, especially health sciences libraries. The increased demand for user space combined with limited funding for building expansions has compelled many libraries to move collections out so that they can transform open stacks spaces into user spaces. Two stories of such projects are included in this book. As the education of health professionals changes, there is also increasing demand for conversion of library space to support changes in learning assignments, related student services, and other needs. Legacy print collections, both monograph and serial, are being reviewed by librarians to decide whether they should be moved into a storage facility or even whether they should be retained at all. Health sciences libraries that have been involved in collaborative collection-building programs often coordinate weeding, retention, and storage decisions with their collaboration partners. In one sense, these weeding, retention and storage decisions complete the cycle begun with consortial serials subscription management and monograph purchasing programs. Coordination of these decisions can include the development of shared print repositories. Collaborative print repositories and preservation initiatives will be covered in more depth at the end of this chapter.

CURRENT CONCERNS AND THE FUTURE FOR PRINT COLLECTION COLLABORATIONS

Challenges often cited with the sorts of purchasing and retention commitment collection projects described above are fundamentally tied to the loss of autonomy and the issue of who drives local collection decisions, especially when budgets are tight. Questions inevitably arise about whether a library should spend local funds on the acquisition of materials used by patrons at other libraries, whether collaborating libraries will fulfill their commitments, whether the library will lend more than it borrows, and most certainly how to assess the benefits versus the costs (labor and materials) of collaborative projects (Burgett, Haar, and Phillips 2004). These political questions and thorny issues are present in any print collaborative purchasing or retention initiative.

The future of collaborative print acquisitions, both monograph and serial, has been scripted by the shift in the nature of health sciences collections and publishing, which reflect the user preference for electronic formats, the concomitant drop in the use of print resources, the rise of open access, and the speed at which information is needed and conveyed. The Association of Academic Health Sciences Libraries reported that the typical academic health sciences library in 2014–2015 was spending over 97 percent of its collection budget on electronic resources (mean value reported of $2,077,443), leaving little (mean value reported of $58,690) for print and other format purchases (Squires 2016). Those print purchases would most likely be driven solely by local needs. Most of the cooperative print collection programs are focused on retention and preservation, not collection building, and these programs heavily emphasize legacy serials. As libraries continue to collect fewer and fewer materials in print, there will be less print to retain and preserve. Current collaborative collection-building initiatives are largely for electronic resources, not print.

COLLABORATIVE PURCHASING LEADS TO CONSORTIAL LICENSING

Collaborative print-purchasing ventures among health sciences libraries and their academic colleagues accomplished their intended goal: libraries were able to provide access to more comprehensive print collections than any of them could provide alone. In the short term, these alliances increased the buying power of individual libraries, and, in the long term, they offered the tremendous potential of planned cooperative collection building and resource sharing (Landesman and van Reenen 2000). The successes experienced and the value derived from these cooperative collection ventures set the stage for the evolution of simple print purchasing into collaborative or consortial licensing. Peer-reviewed, online journals in the sciences made their appearance beginning with *The Online Journal of Current Clinical Trials (OJCCT)* in 1992 (Brahmi and Kaneshiro 1993). In many ways, this journal heralded a new era in collection development that would have profound effects on collaborative collection management.

Fueled by advances in technological innovation and networking infrastructure, including the Internet, electronic journal content exploded in the 1990s. By the end of the decade the major publishers of scientific, technical, and medical journals offered not only individual journal titles in electronic format but also package deals for their content that were available to both individual libraries and consortia. First libraries, and then publishers, recognized the advantages of licensing electronic resources through consortial agreements. The initial goal of collaborations in the print world, of providing their users with access to increased content, continued for libraries in the electronic realm and is seen by many libraries as the chief benefit of these collaborations (Turner 2014).

Each year the Association of Academic Health Sciences Libraries (AAHSL) gathers statistical data from libraries that serve medical schools in the United States and Canada about their collections, expenditures, personnel, services, and use. This management tool has been produced since 1974/1975 to provide comparative data from peer libraries. A survey committee discusses, tweaks, expands, simplifies, or eliminates some of the data points included in the survey in order to capture significant changes in the library environment. As a result, the annual survey is a revealing source for trends and significant changes in academic health sciences libraries and in health sciences libraries in general. This is especially true concerning collections, and the statistics chronicle milestones in the evolution of collaborative collection management within the health sciences community.

By the end of the 1990s, the AAHSL statistics indicated the growing importance of collaborative purchasing/licensing in the academic health sciences library community. The 1998–1999 survey added a new data point for expenditure on electronic resources via a consortia or shared arrangement (Shedlock 2000). The AAHSL survey from 2014 to 2015 reports that the typical academic health sciences library spends just under 28 percent of its electronic resource dollars on consortial purchases (Squires 2016). Clearly, collaborative licensing of electronic resources remains an important strategy for academic health sciences libraries in today's information resource marketplace.

LICENSING FUELS COLLABORATION ACROSS DIFFERENT TYPES OF LIBRARIES

Collaborative collection management in a print-based world has many more constraints than in the digital world. Participants in print-based collaborative ventures must give up the convenience of having all items in their local collection in exchange for the benefit of broadening the collaborative collection strength. Technology advances can mitigate some of the delays inherent in sharing across a print-based collaborative, but not eliminate them. Collaborative purchasing or licensing of electronic resources brings many benefits with few of the print-based limitations or drawbacks. It does not require many of the difficult collection policy decisions that are integral to the planning that underpins print-based collaborative initiatives. Libraries band together in varying degrees of formal arrangements to enhance their buying and negotiating power for electronic resources, usually to achieve a reduced subscription cost for those resources (Burgett, Haar, and Phillips 2004). The growth in collaborations to license electronic resources in many ways paralleled the explosive growth seen in the resources themselves, especially during the 1990s and early 2000s.

Obviously, licensing electronic resources removes any geographic limitations on possible collaborations that are inherent in a print collaborative world. It also makes collaborations more feasible across different types and sizes of libraries. The primary prerequisites for collaborative electronic licensing seem to be a desire to license the same resource, an agreement about who will handle the vendor negotiations, and a mutually agreed upon formula for sharing costs. For collaborative licensing to work, however, vendors must be able to see the benefits for themselves. Vendor restrictions can sometimes impact and hinder possible collaborations. Sometimes they are unwilling to allow libraries from different institutional categories, such as academic, clinical, hospital, or for-profit companies, to license materials together. Another vendor-driven impact on the number and variety of library collaborations has been the development and proliferation of the "Big Deal" or "all-you-can-eat" model. This model (which is described in chapters 1, 2, and 3) applied to a consortium typically involves the consortium licensing an aggregate of all the journal subscriptions from a particular publisher that the participating libraries had been subscribing to individually, or, alternatively, the consortium could simply license the full package of titles from a publisher. These comprehensive publisher packages or Big Deals accomplish the long-standing goal of most collaborative initiatives of providing access to a greater array of information resources (Streib and Blixrud 2014). The Big Deal scenario in collaborative licensing has been of great interest to the health sciences library community since the publishers involved in them include the primary science, technology, and medical publishers.

There are a variety of collaborative licensing possibilities and opportunities for health sciences libraries, especially under the expanded umbrella of possible partners and less cumbersome arrangements than in the print marketplace. One of the most obvious collaborations is between academic health sciences libraries and the university libraries or universities of which they are members. According to the periodic descriptive statistics included in the Association of Academic Health Sciences Libraries annual statistics, about a third of academic health sciences libraries in 2013 reported to either the university library or university administration, rather than directly to a medical school (Squires 2014). These libraries are logically positioned to take advantage of collaborative licensing with their institutional academic library counterparts. Disparate libraries across an entire university system can also successfully band together to license collection content. Health sciences libraries also participate in statewide electronic resource programs that encompass a broad spectrum of libraries and increase their access to non-core and peripheral subject areas, often including consumer health information and more general health resources. Collaborating to gain access to more peripheral content is one of the long-established objectives for libraries engaged in collaborative collection management. The South Central Academic Medical Library Consortium (SCAMeL), established in 1982 by resource library directors within the South Central Region of the National Network of Libraries of Medicine, built on the foundations of its programs for resource sharing to embark on a collaborative licensing initiative in 1999. Key incentives for this program were to expand access to electronic resources across the region, consolidate license negotiation, and lower the cost of licensing through consortial discounts. Those consortial licensing efforts continue today (Van Schaik and Moore 2011).

Hospital libraries within the regional medical library network have also been active in collaborative licensing initiatives. Some hospital libraries and libraries for hospital systems have created their own consortia, and one story of a successful hospital library consortium for purchasing is included in this book (see "One Library's Story" after chapter 3). Other hospital libraries have joined collaborations with their academic medical library institutional partners or broader groupings of health libraries to license electronic resources (Harris and Peterson 2003). California can boast about its Statewide California Electronic Library Consortium (SCELC) with over a hundred members that has partnered with the Pacific Southwest Region of the National Network of Libraries of Medicine to provide a program that gives hospital libraries the opportunity to purchase access to electronic resources at reduced rates (Prottsman 2011). In a 2012 survey of the Medical Library Association's Hospital Libraries Section, 55 percent of respondents purchased electronic resources as part of a consortium. Vendor packages were purchased by 64 percent of the respondents, and 79 percent felt they were overspending for e-journals (Roth 2013). Clearly there is interest, need, and opportunities for collaboration among hospital libraries.

LICENSING CHALLENGES TO COLLECTION COLLABORATIONS AND RESOURCE SHARING

While licensing of electronic resources brings immediate benefits to libraries and their users in the short term, it also creates some immediate and long-term challenges for resource sharing and collaborative collection management. Challenges to resource sharing most often come from publisher licenses with restrictive clauses that put constraints on the ability of libraries to share electronic content through interlibrary loan. It is essential that libraries continue to review license agreements from the perspective of any limitations placed on the ability and processes used to legally share that content with other libraries under the doctrine of fair use. Many libraries, particularly those that have agreed to be resource libraries for their regions, consider interlibrary loan restrictions a "deal-breaker" in a license for an electronic journal.

Licenses for electronic book content are even more restrictive than those for journals, with digital rights management software threatening to override fair use protection and the ability to share book content (Turner 2014). Publishers have been slow to allow interlibrary loan of electronic book content, and it is still not possible for health sciences libraries to lend whole electronic books rather than a chapter at a time. Some health sciences publishers do not even provide electronic book chapters in PDF because of a fear of books being posted illegally online. Interlibrary loan is hampered when book chapters are only available as HTML web pages, usually without page numbers corresponding to the printed book. Restrictions on the use of electronic book content also can impact their use in electronic course reserves and course management software.

Usage restrictions are an example of the potential benefit of collaborative licensing, where a single consortial entity, with consolidated licensing expertise and more leveraging power than an individual library, can negotiate for more favorable access provisions for members of the consortium. Meeting these resource-sharing challenges is becoming even more important as redundant print alternatives to digital content become the exception for most libraries.

There have been some successes in consortial electronic book licensing, chiefly among academic libraries and often "characterized by experimentation and pilot initiatives" (Machovec 2013). In one approach, libraries have purchased publisher-based collections, similar to the print monograph acquisitions programs in health sciences consortia. These deals are often based on historical publisher spending by consortial members but attempt to greatly expand the content available for that same price—or a little more. In this model, traditional resource sharing through interlibrary loan is replaced by all participating libraries getting direct access to the total publisher aggregate content. Another approach successfully used in consortial electronic book licensing has been to use the demand-driven acquisitions (DDA) model. The concept is the same as demand-driven arrangements for a single institution. The participants agree to offer and make discoverable a certain kind and number of titles (for example, a subject area or publisher) and collectively trigger the short-term loans and purchases of the titles. The number of short-term loans (minimal use of the content) allowed before a purchase is triggered, the pricing of the purchase, access limitations, and the way costs are apportioned across the group are negotiated and governed by the license. Some of the statewide consortia that have piloted these electronic book projects do contain academic medical libraries. Participants of one state system pilot project concluded that "a consortial e-book DDA program can be a cost-effective way of equitably increasing access to a greater number of resources" (Harrington and Douglas 2014). These examples of consortial electronic book licensing are creative ways to mitigate the resource-sharing limitations of e-book licenses. It is important to note that while these arrangements do solve the problem for members of the consortia, they do nothing for resource sharing across the broader library community.

A more fundamental challenge to resource sharing, both in the short and the long term, is the fact that licensing electronic books and journals, especially through publisher Big Deals, means that more of the collective library dollars are being spent by libraries to purchase the same, or nearly the same, content. This is the direct opposite of the results of collaborative collection management in the print world. It is also very likely that libraries will spend more of their collection budgets to pay for the licensed content of a few large publishers. Both situations can reduce a library's budget, ability, and flexibility to build the focused, local collection that can best meet local needs and be of value as a shared resource for a collaborating collection partner library. In other words, there is less money for a library to purchase different or unique content that is of value to local users and collection partners alike. When viewed in the longer term, this reduction in a library's ability to develop specialized local collections would undermine, or make impossible, the ability for a library to follow its collaborative collection management plan and obligations to its consortial partners. Too strong an emphasis on collaborative licensing of electronic resources could also make it less feasible for a library to enter into a collaborative collection management partnership. Ultimately, it could even begin to threaten the survival of primary source collections. While it is certainly a collaborative collection activity, the goal and result of collaborative licensing can be in direct conflict with the traditional goals of collaborative collection management.

RENEWED FOCUS ON SPECIAL AND UNIQUE COLLECTIONS AND ACCESS TO THEM

For over a decade, academic librarians, particularly those with interests in the humanities and similar subjects, have warned that so much money spent on collaborative purchasing of large packages is creating library collections that are homogeneous and do not have the variety or depth of earlier collection environments (Burgett, Haar, and Phillips 2004). It is unclear whether this applies to health sciences libraries in the same way, even to academic health sciences libraries. In addition to its annual survey, every few years AAHSL also gathers data from academic medical libraries to capture the landscape of current resources to which they subscribe. The survey specifically asks, of a list of named resources, whether libraries "plan to continue offering, plan to drop or have dropped, plan to add within the next 12 months, evaluated in the past 12 months, or are not currently considering." The categories and subject areas covered of the resources listed in that survey vary, and the overlapping nature of the publisher packages available make it difficult to do any deep analysis. However, it does appear that, in 2014, there were a few publisher e-book or e-journal packages that over 60 percent of the academic medical libraries surveyed subscribed to: McGraw-Hill's AccessMedicine, Elsevier's ClinicalKey, Lippincott Williams & Wilkins Total Access Collection, the *BMJ* journal package, *JAMA* journal package, Nature Publishing journal package, some kind of Elsevier journal package, and a Wiley Big Deal journal package (Squires 2015).

The mission and collection scope of health sciences libraries is different from that of general academic libraries, however. The packages listed above are from the top medical publishers and contain many of the most important books and journals that were listed as "core" back in the print era. One assumes these same libraries likely purchased or subscribed to many of these journals and books back then, too. Furthermore, although much is made of dwindling monograph budgets, it needs to be noted that many health sciences monograph purchases have merely been transformed into package subscriptions, a detail that is not always made clear in AAHSL data collecting. Hospital libraries, even more than academic, are focused on supporting clinical care with the best resources they can buy with limited budgets, and unique content is not a priority. Similarly, small academic libraries, such as those supporting new medical schools, are focused on access to top educational resources, not on building research collections. Health sciences librarians, particularly academic ones, shouldn't completely dismiss the concern about homogeneity and the fact of collection budgets being tied up in a few large packages. Collection managers that purchase outside of the mainstream clinical subjects—for instance, history of medicine, sociology of medicine, international public health information, veterinary medicine, and bioethics— or those that need to support focused, research-intensive programs, should carefully consider collection allocation and the need for collection strategies and balance. These managers can also work to develop collection policies or statements that specify and prioritize local needs, when appropriate, and they can become and stay engaged in consortial committees so that they are aware of consortial decisions (Kinner and Crosetto 2009).

ENSURING CONTINUING ACCESS
TO RESOURCES: PRESERVATION

Print and digital preservation pose many opportunities and challenges for a collaborative approach to collection management. Preservation of print items, both monograph and serials, encompasses both the preservation of the intellectual content and the preservation of the physical information container. Digitization and electronic preservation of what was originally print material tends to focus only on the intellectual content. Repositories of digitized monographs and serials, most initiated as collaborative ventures, are already having a significant impact on ensuring access to the scholarly record. Examples of these initiatives are HathiTrust, Internet Archive, Portico, and LOCK-SS/CLOCKSS. HathiTrust is a partnership of academic and research institutions offering a collection of millions of titles digitized from libraries around the world. The aim is to build a comprehensive archive of published literature and to develop shared strategies for managing and developing their digital and print holdings in a collaborative way (www.hathitrust.org). Internet Archive is a nonprofit library of millions of free books, movies, software, music, websites, and other content. Its stated mission is "universal access to all knowledge" (https://archive.org/). Portico is a digital preservation and archiving service, one of the largest community-supported digital archives in the world. Its purpose is stated as "Working with libraries and publishers, we preserve e-journals, e-books, and other electronic scholarly content to ensure researchers and students will have access to it in the future" (www.portico.org). Many libraries describe this dark archive as an insurance policy. The LOCKSS/CLOCKSS program, based at Stanford University Libraries, provides libraries and publishers with "open source digital preservation tools to preserve and provide access to persistent and authoritative digital content" (www.lockss.org). These are alliances that span across research libraries, academic medical libraries, nonprofit organizations, and commercial entities. While these are each unique organizations with differing missions and methods, they share many common goals for digitization and digital preservation to ensure continuing access to the intellectual content of both print and digital resources, whether monograph or serial.

University libraries and their constituent academic medical libraries, through formal consortia and other cooperative collection management programs, have also undertaken focused print-archiving initiatives such as regional shared print repositories. The Center for Research Libraries (CRL), an international consortium of university, college, and independent research libraries, is again taking a leadership role through the development of a searchable Print Archives Preservation Registry (PAPR). This registry, which is a massive database undertaking, is being developed in phases to gradually implement and enhance its functionality. PAPR already includes a searchable database, downloadable reports, and a consolidated display of titles and holdings from multiple print-archiving programs (Reilly 2013). The purpose of CRL is to support original research and teaching "by preserving and making available to scholars a wealth of rare and uncommon primary source materials from all world regions" (www.crl.edu). The work of CRL offers health sciences libraries and their users access to peripheral content, one of the chief goals of collaborative collection initiatives.

One of the more recent developments in cooperative collection management is the growth of shared remote storage facilities, with a goal of preserving access to the print physical artifact (Clement 2012). For health sciences libraries, this is a logical extension of early RML efforts to develop regional plans for serials retention, such as the Regional Coordination of Biomedical Information Resources Program, begun in the 1980s by the Medical Library Center of New York. Shared repositories are primarily focused on legacy print collections, "older" monographs and serials that are no longer used enough to justify their shelving in open collection spaces. Most interesting and exciting are those shared storage initiatives that facilitate and encourage the resource-in-common model, where libraries can claim a copy of a resource already ingested into the storage facility as a resource-in-common and discard their own copy. This has proved very successful in the University of Texas system–Texas A&M University system collaborative storage initiative that includes eight academic health sciences libraries. (The story of the development of this repository follows this chapter.)

Academic health sciences library use of collection storage is rising sharply. AAHSL first added a question in their annual survey about items shelved remotely with the 2004–2005 annual survey. At that time the total volumes held in storage for all the participating libraries was around 2 million (Shedlock and Byrd 2006). By the 2014/2015 annual survey, there were over 5 million total volumes in storage (Squires 2016), and by 2015/2016 the number was close to 6 million (Squires 2017). The National Library of Medicine and its National Network of Libraries of Medicine provided a strategic plan and coordinated program for a National Cooperative Medical Journals Print Retention Program, MedPrint, in 2011 (NLM 2016). By August 2016, various libraries had committed to retaining all but three journal titles from the 250 primarily *Abridged Index Medicus* titles in print and had agreed to make them accessible for resource sharing through September 2036.

Given the success of existing ventures, the common pressure across libraries for increased user space, and the trend cited above, a reasonable expectation is that a large percentage of existing health sciences library print collections, both monograph and serial, will move into coordinated or shared management facilities within the next several years (Dempsey, Malpas, and Lavoie 2014). A logical next step would be for these programs that preserve legacy print collections through shared print repositories to be integrated into current collaborative collection management activities through an organized plan that clarified which institution within this shared repository consortium would take responsibility for purchasing items in print while others within the consortium could purchase online only. Since many libraries have already gone online only with many subscriptions, however, this kind of plan may be challenging to implement.

THE FUTURE OF COLLABORATIVE COLLECTION MANAGEMENT

A consideration of the underlying potential of collaborative collection management helps to predict its future relevance. At its best, collaborative collection development can allow a library to optimize its financial resources, help to address increasing space pressures and storage needs, allow a library to focus on the development of unique materials to meet local needs, and build a foundation for other collaborative initiatives across libraries. Even a cursory review of the history of academic and health sciences library collaborations suggests that there is a bright future ahead. As the very nature of what is meant by the "collection" continues to evolve, collaborations will play an integral part. Health sciences libraries have a rich history of successful collaborations over more than a century, and the growth of the digital enterprise, interdisciplinary research, and translational science/medicine suggests that the collaborations between those libraries will be even more essential than in the past. Health sciences libraries will very likely work together in new ways to support the fundamental goal of collaborative collection management—increasing the information resources available to users.

There is much still to be done in the more traditional collaborative collection roles—to accomplish shared print and digital repositories, to strategically plan the digitization of primary scholarly resources, and to engage in a collaborative plan to develop and enhance local "special" and unique collections that can serve as a resource to the broader library and user community. There are also increasing opportunities for new roles in collaborative collection management that move far beyond the "buyer's club" role. Some of those expanded activities are already happening today: support and advocacy for developments in scholarly communication, involvement in data management plans and curation, and creation of collection management tools. As librarians hone their advocacy roles, there is potential to reshape the collections marketplace, perhaps even to make it a buyer's market rather than a seller's. As libraries and collections continue to evolve there will be countless opportunities to discover and define collaborative collection roles for the future (Landesman and van Reenen 2000).

REFERENCES

Bowden, Virginia M., Elizabeth A. Comeaux, and Dottie Eakin. 1984. "Evaluation of the TALON Cooperative Acquisitions Program for Monographs." *Bulletin of the Medical Library Association* 72(3): 241–50. http://www.ncbi.nlm.nih.gov/pmc/articles/PMC227455/.

Brahmi, Frances A., and Kellie Kaneshiro. 1993. "The Online Journal of Current Clinical Trials (OJCCT): A Closer Look." *Medical Reference Services Quarterly* 12(3): 29–43. doi:10.1300/J115V12N03_03.

Bunting, Allison. 1987. "The Nation's Health Information Network: History of the Regional Medical Library Program, 1965–1985." *Bulletin of the Medical Library Association* 75(3 Suppl.): 1–62. http://www.ncbi.nlm.nih.gov/pmc/articles/PMC280609/.

Burgett, James, John Haar, and Linda L. Phillips. 2004. *Collaborative Collection Development: A Practical Guide for Your Library.* Chicago: American Library Association.

Clement, Susanne K. 2012. "From Collaborative Purchasing toward Collaborative Discarding: The Evolution of the Shared Print Repository." *Collection Management* 37(3/4): 152–67. doi: 10.1080/01462679.2012.685413.

DeBakey, Michael E. 1991. "The National Library of Medicine: Evolution of a Premier Information Center." *JAMA: The Journal of the American Medical Association* 266(9): 1252–258.

Dempsey, Lorcan, Constance Malpas, and Brian Lavoie. 2014. "Collection Directions: The Evolution of Library Collections and Collecting." *portal: Libraries and the Academy* 14(3): 393–423. doi: 10.1353/pla.2014.0013.

Harrington, Eileen G., and C. Steven Douglas. 2014. "Collaborative Collection Building: Health Sciences Librarians and a Consortial Ebook DDA Program." http://www.doody.com/dct/PublicFeaturedArticle.asp?SiteContentID=206&SID=percent7B2FF62C78-D8FF-41A5-849E-C99479652177%20percent7D.

Harris, Lindsay, and Mary Peterson. 2003. "Sharing the Burden: A Model for Consortium Purchasing for Health Libraries." *Journal of the Medical Library Association* 91(3): 361–64. http://www.ncbi.nlm.nih.gov/pmc/articles/PMC164400/.

Hendricks, Donald D. 1976. "TALON—The First Five Years." *Bulletin of the Medical Library Association* 64(2): 203–11. http://www.ncbi.nlm.nih.gov/pmc/articles/PMC199001/.

Johnson, Peggy. 2004. *Fundamentals of Collection Development and Management.* Chicago: American Library Association.

Kabler, Anne W. 1980. "NLM's Medical Library Resource Improvement Grant for Consortia Development: A Proposed Outline to Simplify the Application Process." *Bulletin of the Medical Library Association* 68(1): 25–32. http://www.ncbi.nlm.nih.gov/pmc/articles/PMC226410/.

Kinner, Laura, and Alice Crosetto. 2009. "Balancing Act for the Future: How the Academic Library Engages in Collection Development at the Local and Consortial Levels." *Journal of Library Administration* 49(3): 419–37. doi: 10.1080/01930820902832561.

Kronick, David A. 1979. "A Regional Cooperative Acquisition Program for Monographs." *Bulletin of the Medical Library Association* 67(3): 297–301. http://www.ncbi.nlm.nih.gov/pmc/articles/PMC226933/.

Landesman, Margaret, and Johann van Reenen. 2000. "Consortia vs. Reform: Creating Congruence." *Journal of Electronic Publishing* 6(2). Retrieved August 18, 2016, from journal website: doi: 10.3998/3336451.0006.203.

Machovec, George. 2013. "Consortial Ebook Licensing for Academic Libraries." *Journal of Library Administration* 53(5–6): 390–99. doi: 10.1080/01930826.2013.876833

NLM (National Library of Medicine). 2011. "175 Years: Our Milestones." National Institutes of Health, United States Department of Health and Human Services. https://apps.nlm.nih.gov/175/milestones.cfm.

———. 2016. "MedPrint—Medical Serials Print Preservation Program." National Institutes of Health, United States Department of Health and Human Services. Last updated November 17. https://www.nlm.nih.gov/psd/printretentionmain.html.

OED Online (Oxford English Dictionary Online). 2017a. "collaboration, n [Def. 1]." Oxford University Press. Accessed May 2. http://www.oed.com/view/Entry/36197.

———. 2017b. "cooperation, n [Def. 1]." Oxford University Press. Accessed May 2. http://www.oed.com/view/Entry/41037.

Prottsman, Mary Fran. 2011. "Communication and Collaboration: Collection Development in Challenging Economic Times." *Journal of Electronic Resources in Medical Libraries* 8(2): 107–16. doi: 10.1080/15424065.2011.576585.

Reilly, Bernard F., Jr. 2013. "The Future of Cooperative Collections and Repositories." *Library Management* 34(4/5): 342–51. doi: 10.1108/01435121311328681.

Richards, Dan T., and Dottie Eakin. 1997. "Cooperative Collection Development." In *Collection Development and Assessment in Health Sciences Libraries*, 199–208. Lanham, MD: Medical Library Association and Scarecrow Press, Inc.

Roth, Karen L. 2013. "Shared Ownership: What's the Future?" *Medical Reference Services Quarterly* 32(2): 203–8. doi: 10.1080/02763869.2013.776905.

Shedlock, James, ed. 2000. *Annual Statistics of Medical School Libraries in the United States and Canada*. 22nd ed. 1998–1999. Seattle, WA: Association of Academic Health Sciences Libraries.

Shedlock, James, and Gary Byrd, eds. 2006. *Annual Statistics of Medical School Libraries in the United States and Canada*. 28th ed. 2004–2005. Seattle, WA: Association of Academic Health Sciences Libraries.

Squires, Steven J., ed. 2014. "Descriptive Statistics Tables, 2013." In *Annual Statistics of Medical School Libraries in the United States and Canada*. 36th ed. 2012–2013, 127–203. Seattle, WA: Association of Academic Health Sciences Libraries.

———. 2015. "Services and Resources Summary Tables, 2014." In *Annual Statistics of Medical School Libraries in the United States and Canada*. 37th ed. 2013–2014, 127–136. Seattle, WA: Association of Academic Health Sciences Libraries.

———. 2016. *Annual Statistics of Medical School Libraries in the United States and Canada*. 38th ed. 2014–2015. Seattle, WA: Association of Academic Health Sciences Libraries.

———. 2017. *Annual Statistics of Medical School Libraries in the United States and Canada*. 39th ed. 2015–2016. Seattle, WA: Association of Academic Health Sciences Libraries.

Streib, Karla L., and Julia C. Blixrud. 2014. "Unwrapping the Bundle: An Examination of Research Libraries and the 'Big Deal.'" *portal: Libraries and the Academy* 14(4): 587–615. doi: 10.1353/pla.2014.0027.

Turner, Christine N. 2014. "E-Resources Acquisitions in Academic Library Consortia." *Library Resources & Technical Services* 58(1): 33–48.

Van Schaik, Joann, and Millie Moore. 2011. "Group Purchasing by a Regional Academic Medical Library Consortium: How SCAMeL Made It Work." *Journal of Electronic Resources in Medical Libraries* 8(4): 412–22. doi: 10.1080/15424065.2011.626353.

Willmering, William J., Martha R. Fishel, and Dianne E. McCutcheon. 1988. "SERHOLD: Evolution of the National Biomedical Serials Holdings Database." *Serials Review* 14(1/2): 7–13. doi: 10.1016/0098-7913(88)90004-4.

One Library's Story

Building a Texas-Sized Shared Print Repository

Esther E. Carrigan, Nancy G. Burford, and Ana G. Ugaz

The two largest and oldest public university systems in the state of Texas are Texas A&M University System (TAMU) and the University of Texas System (UT). Together they include twenty-one universities and seven health institutions. The flagship campuses of these systems, Texas A&M in College Station and the University of Texas in Austin, had a long-standing history of rivalry that included not only athletics but also academics, each vying to be "The University" for the state of Texas by exceeding the other in whatever national poll or ranking was currently being published. That rivalry is part of the institutional past and traditions, but it is now "history." The flagship campuses and the systems they represent are collaborating on an impressive array of initiatives, including shared print repositories. The question of what triggered the increased willingness and desire to collaborate, rather than compete, remains the subject of speculation. Some believe the paradigm shift occurred after the 1999 bonfire collapse in which twelve students died. (The bonfire tradition was tied to football rivalry.) Certainly the move of Texas A&M from the Big 12 athletic conference and into the Southeastern Conference (SEC) in 2012 ended the conference rivalry between them and all that it fueled. Other individuals, whose perspective extends beyond football, believe it was simply the realization by the leadership at both campuses and systems that they could accomplish more to educate and advocate for higher education within the political arena by joining forces and working together. Regardless of the exact causes, the result has been an era of collaborative initiatives.

The libraries within the A&M and UT systems have a combined print collection of over 26 million volumes. Each of the seven health institutions within the UT system has its own medical library. Our library, the Medical Sciences Library (MSL), is one of the campus libraries at Texas A&M, College Station, and the only academic medical library in the A&M system. Between MSL and the libraries of the seven health institutions of the UT system, the full gamut of health professional schools are supported: medicine, nursing, pharmacy, dentistry, public health, veterinary medicine, and various allied health professions. The medical libraries of both systems, due primarily to their roles as resource libraries within the National Library of Medicine National Network of Libraries of Medicine (NN/LM) South Central Region, have decades of experience working together in many areas, especially in resource sharing and collaborative collection initiatives. These collaborations began with coordinated print collection management initiatives and developed into consortial licensing with the arrival of electronic journals. All the libraries within each system have a history of collaborative collection management, primarily through system-level licensing of electronic resources and managing the Texas Digital Library.

Growing demands for increased user spaces at both the UT Austin and A&M College Station libraries led to joint discussions of collection storage possibilities. UT Austin had already converted an older building on their local research campus into a preservation quality storage facility. In 2009, A&M College Station Libraries signed an agreement with UT Austin Libraries for space in that storage facility. However, the location in urban Austin allows little room for future expansion. The success of the shared storage in Austin between the two flagship libraries led the two systems to plan for a new shared storage facility on less-developed land that would allow expansion for future storage modules closer to College Station.

In May 2013, a collaborative project began that was cooperatively funded by both the UT system and the Texas A&M system. The project was to open a high-density storage facility, the Joint Library Facility (JLF), about ten miles north of the main Texas A&M campus. The first module was designed to hold 1 million volumes of low-use print materials from the libraries of both university systems. Construction costs for the facility were shared; Texas A&M agreed to cover all operational and maintenance costs and to provide all staff for JLF. The impetus for this project came from a couple directions: the ever-increasing demands for user space in all system libraries and limits to funding for additional campus libraries. We decided to use committees made up of representatives from numerous campus libraries to create the operational and governance policies and processes for JLF. They decided to operate JLF on the Resource In Common (RIC) model. Each title/volume would be placed into JLF as a potential RIC, which means that any participating library that owns that title/volume may claim it as a RIC and withdraw its local copy, while JLF adds that library's symbol to the JLF record.

Space pressures of varying kinds made the academic health sciences libraries of participating institutions in JLF eager to send their collections to storage. Serious weeding of some medical library collections in Texas had already begun, even before JLF was a reality. The earliest medical library participants either wanted to convert space that was housing little-used collection materials into user space, or were under generalized space pressure from parent institutions that were looking for additional campus space for expanding student services. Those eager to participate were developing workflows to review their collections and submit lists of what they wanted to ship to JLF. The JLF director was busy accepting lists, prioritizing shipments, and making orderly plans. Then the cruel hand of fate struck and wreaked havoc on this orderly process! One medical library was suddenly ordered by its parent institution to clear out most of its collection within a few months so the space could be repurposed for student learning spaces. Other medical libraries already in the JLF queue stepped aside to let this library go to the head of the line. About a year later it was déjà vu with another medical library in another Texas city. Had JLF not been an option for these libraries, they would have been forced to discard materials. As a result of these crises, around half of the initial half million volumes processed for JLF came from academic medical collections. Some of the most comprehensive medical collections in Texas were transferred to JLF, making the shared JLF medical collection quite extensive, and, with the RIC model in place, each volume was unique. By 2017 the six medical library participants had transferred nearly 280,000 volumes to JLF and claimed almost an additional 200,000 volumes as RIC—clearly an efficient, effective, collaborative storage model. Librarians used several standard collection management tools for deciding which volumes to send to JLF and for the ingestion process, including individual library holding lists, centralized lists of intended deposits, and an online catalog of all holdings within JLF. Each library created its own policies about what to keep and what to send to storage, but most decisions were based on similar factors: age; circulation history, and whether the library had electronic equivalents. The single consistent requirement for the materials of all libraries sent to JLF was that the material met the Resource In Common requirements. Our library (MSL) used this set of criteria to choose monographic storage candidates:

- older than ten years and not used in the last five years or
- older than five years and never used, and
- not in a pre-identified protected classification (e.g., veterinary medicine).

Logistics and staging of shipments was one of the greatest challenges, especially with the extreme time pressures on some of the medical libraries to clear their stacks. It took a lot of teamwork from both the JLF staff and the medical libraries to accomplish these collection transfers. The solid foundation of collaboration built among the medical libraries of Texas as resource libraries in the south central region was an important factor in the overwhelming success of this project.

Near the end of 2015, a progress update from the JLF director made it apparent that JLF was becoming the shared print repository for medical collections in Texas. It did not take long for the idea of JLF becoming a MedPrint participant to take hold. MedPrint is a program of the National Network of Libraries of Medicine (NN/LM) and the National Library of Medicine (NLM) to ensure the preservation of and continued access to the biomedical literature through a national cooperative medical serials print retention program. In consultation with the Regional Medical Libraries (RML), NLM initially identified approximately 250 Abridged Index Medicus (AIM)/PubMed Central (PMC) journals as the primary set of materials to preserve in print. Libraries participating in the MedPrint program make commitments to have a volume run of a particular journal title that is at least 95 percent complete, retain that title for twenty-five years, and share the MedPrint collection through active lending.

Other libraries have helped fill in missing volumes, and JLF is anticipated to become a complete MedPrint repository by the end of 2017. It will be the first regional comprehensive node in the MedPrint network, able to not only preserve key biomedical journals but actively share them within Texas, the south central region, and across the United States. We have put a priority on rapid filling of requests and can report a DOCLINE fill rate of 89 percent and an average turn-around time of four hours.

The success of the MedPrint initiative within the UT and TAMU system libraries and the willing collaboration of other regional libraries have been encouraging. Buoyed by the MedPrint success, librarians are now setting their sights for JLF on a VetPrint project, an initiative among academic veterinary librarians that parallels the MedPrint initiative, intended to preserve the important 123 veterinary journal titles included in the "Basic List of Veterinary Medical Serials," third edition. The veterinary library community is very small compared with other health sciences library communities, so the project is nationwide rather than regional. Informal work to identify holdings in various veterinary libraries is already underway.

The chief lessons we learned from this shared print repository project were to never underestimate the power of collaboration and to make collaboration a habit within a group. The medical libraries involved naturally came to the aid of each other and worked together to solve their collection and space pressures as a result of their history of successful collaborations. Not only were participating JLF libraries eager to contribute, but other libraries, hearing about the increasing success of this ambitious project, wanted to find a way to contribute and participate as well. JLF with its shared collection, a stellar example of collaborative collection management, is succeeding beyond our wildest expectations.

Chapter Six

Discovery of the Health Sciences Collection

Susan K. Kendall

When librarians building health sciences collections are making purchasing decisions, they have to imagine how new resources will fit into their existing collections and how they will be found. No one wants to buy materials that get no use, and budget and space constraints make it imperative that selectors buy materials that will get significant usage. It is impossible to accurately predict which materials will get use and which will not, which is why collection managers are constantly evaluating their collections and gathering usage data to help them make decisions. Librarians sometimes forget, however, that they have the power to influence and drive usage. Decisions they make both prior to and after purchasing have a significant impact on how easily users can find and use the resources.

For health sciences libraries these days, the library websites are more important presences than their physical footprints. Downsizing space is a trend for health sciences libraries in hospitals and academic medical centers (Freiburger 2010). Some have maintained their space but repurposed much of it away from collections toward other needs. Libraries have traditionally used their physical spaces to highlight parts of their collection or advertise new materials. Without a physical space as a place to promote resources, librarians will want to invest quite a bit of time and energy into their websites as the most powerful tools for promoting use of the collection. In smaller organizations, there may be one librarian wearing many hats as collection management librarian, cataloger, website developer and maintainer, and outreach librarian. In larger organizations, the collection management librarian might work with a team of librarians from different departments: acquisitions, cataloging, website maintenance, and outreach to promote collections on the website. Some of these departments might not be in the health sciences library but might be shared with other subject areas across a whole university library system. In those cases, the health sciences collection librarian might have more of a challenge because decisions about what is promoted on the website will allow for a large range of needs. Knowing how a resource might appear to users on the website should affect collections decisions, and being able to work with librarians in these other departments to ensure the best discoverability of the health sciences collection will benefit the health sciences collection librarian.

Librarians are often disappointed to find that studies of information-seeking behavior reveal that potential health sciences library users are unaware of what their library has to offer, tend not to explore offerings outside their few favorite known resources, and prefer to use Google rather than the library website to find and access resources (De Groote, Shultz, and Blecic 2014; Haines et al. 2010). Rather than lament this, librarians should take note of how their users are finding resources and use that information to make their collections easier to discover. Warnings that librarians ignore marketing at their own peril are plentiful, from a series of articles about a 2012 *Library Journal* survey of public libraries to articles encouraging academic libraries to develop a marketing orientation (Almquist 2014; Delawska-Elliott, Grinstead, and Martin 2015; Dowd 2013). A marketing orientation, discussed in more depth in chapter 4, is more than just providing publicity for collections and services; it is a long-term approach of identifying user needs and working to meet those needs. One recurring need underlying information-seeking behavior studies is for library users to be able to find things without having to think like a librarian, know beforehand what resources are available, use advanced searching techniques, and navigate complicated library websites and catalogs. Unfortunately, collection management librarians know that the landscape of their collections *is* complicated, although it is not their fault. There is overlapping content on multiple platforms, there are separate individual and institutional versions of electronic books (e-books), and, of course, not everything is "free on the internet." While librarians have the freedom to design their services to directly meet user needs they have identified, they do not quite have the same level of control over the resources they purchase. Users want to seamlessly move among resources without regard to publisher, platform, firewalls, copyright restrictions, or subscription limitations. Vendors and publishers, on the other hand, naturally want to protect their intellectual property from theft and promote their own resources rather than other publishers' resources. Their goals can be at odds with user goals. Librarians are caught in the middle trying to meet user expectations within limits. One of the biggest challenges for them in the primarily electronic environment of current collections is that the resources they are purchasing come from multiple publishers and vendors. In the printed world, books and journals from multiple publishers interacted very nicely. They used the same paper and print technology—they even came in standardized sizes—and could sit side-by-side on the shelf in any configuration or classification the librarian chose. Records for items in the library catalog or in an indexing service were the same from resource to resource and publisher to publisher. There was no difference between how well books and journals "worked," whether they were from small publishers or large publishers. On the other hand, in the electronic environment, books and journals from multiple publishers are not "housed" together; they are on completely separate platforms. Books and journals from one publisher may have completely different functionality than books and journals from another publisher. More and more librarians must make collections decisions and present their holdings to users based on the publisher or platform rather than the content, resulting in the dreaded "silos" of information that are uniformly disparaged. Interaction of electronic resources across publishers is a "holy grail" sought by librarians and being worked on by some vendors, but that ideal has yet to be realized. Health sciences collection management librarians often find themselves forced to purchase products for the sake of the content despite serious functionality problems, or they must decide between two products, each of which has both good and bad aspects. Whenever possible, however, collection management librarians can use their power of purchasing to choose products designed for better functionality and interaction and thereby reward publishers and vendors who adhere to new industry standards for interoperability. A good knowledge of finding tools for resources and the discoverability of resources should be an important piece of the collection management librarian's evaluation process for new materials.

LEVELS OF ACCESS

Libraries have always been about searching for and discovering information, and they have employed multiple means of putting users in touch with resources. Cataloging and indexing have been primary tools for collating similar materials and employing the use of controlled vocabulary to aid the finding process. Because librarians know that the best, most relevant content for any particular search comes from a variety of sources and publishers, they have tended to emphasize the use of publisher-neutral library catalogs and literature indexes such as PubMed. Unfortunately, library users tend to find these methods clumsy and confusing for getting into full-text content. Lately, the landscape of access points for library resources has opened up tremendously. Someone might access any given journal article, for instance, by following links from a Google search, the library list of e-journals, the journal in the library catalog, PubMed or another index, the references list of an e-book chapter or another article, a LibGuide, the electronic health record, or a course management system. A lot of the time users have no idea how they got into a specific resource and aren't even sure if they are in a book, a journal article, or something else. More access points mean more opportunities for the collection to be discovered and used, which is a good thing. People will use different methods at different times. Librarians do have a challenge, though, in that they have control over the presentation of some of these access points and no control over others.

At the point of electronic resource purchase, the collection management librarian will want to think about three potential levels of access to the product: the whole resource/database level, the individual book or journal title level, or the article and chapter level. Different finding tools will take the user to different levels. The first thing the librarian might think about would be at which of these levels, or some combination of these, the resource is able to be linked or accessed. Second, the librarian would want to decide the level of access that best meets their library users' needs. Third, the librarian would need to put the answers to the above questions in context of their limitations in tools or staff time needed to provide the chosen level of access. If a librarian is trying to decide between two good products, but one allows the librarian to provide better access for less effort than the other, that may be the deciding factor about which one to purchase.

PROVIDING RESOURCE-LEVEL ACCESS

Resource-level access is the easiest and most straightforward and works well for certain types of resources and certain types of libraries. A link to a database on the library website or in the library catalog is an example. For some very small libraries, resource-level listing is the only access they are reasonably able to provide for most things, and that will influence their collections decisions. For them, purchasing the most content in the simplest packages makes sense. Librarians might seek out self-contained, full-text e-book packages from one publisher or subscribe to an aggregating service, such as Ovid or EBSCO, which provides access to books and journals from multiple publishers through one portal. Because they only have a few resources, small libraries can easily direct users to their collections, and users will quickly get familiar with what is available.

Larger hospital and academic health sciences libraries will also want to provide resource-level access for some of their collections. The types of databases for which simple resource-level access makes the most sense are point-of-care tools, drug information databases, indexes to the literature, and data sets. All of these operate as stand-alone portals without individual journals or books that need to be found as separate entities. Services have recently become available to help libraries track databases at the resource level, and larger academic libraries trying to manage many subjects, including the health sciences, are taking advantage of these services to streamline the way they provide access on their websites. Springshare is partnering with Pro-Quest Serial Solutions to enable libraries to create A–Z and subject-classified database lists for library websites, and the subject groupings of databases can be customized for a particular library's needs.

Vendors tend to focus on access to their products at the resource level. Many invest a lot of time into creating information portals for searching across multiple types of content that they produce. The unstated assumption of some of them is that their content should be sufficient for users. Linking outside their own content is maybe only grudgingly enabled. Some of these are enormous, like Elsevier's ClinicalKey, which contains all of that company's medical content. Others are subject-specific, like McGraw-Hill's Access products and Lippincott Williams & Wilkins's Health Libraries. Still others, like EBSCO, Ovid, and Rittenhouse, aggregate content like e-books or journals from multiple publishers onto one platform. While users do sometimes get used to one of these portals as a favorite place to visit when they need information on a topic, there are other times in which simple portal access is less useful. Librarians know that no one publisher has a monopoly on all the important information and that they need to provide a way for people to get into books and journals by title without regard to the portal or platform.

PROVIDING TITLE-LEVEL ACCESS

Compared with resource-level access, providing title-level access is a much bigger challenge but very necessary. Larger libraries are purchasing resources from a wide range of sources and publishers, some small and some large, and these resources can often include multiple parts and material types, such as journals, books, and videos. Providing access to the individual titles within large databases is the key to preventing users from having to guess which database contains the book they want. Despite promoting their web portals for keyword searching of content, the vast majority of publishers do provide title-level access with stable links to individual books or journals housed on their platforms if asked. Providing access to the titles of journals and books can happen through a library catalog, the library website, or both. A study from 2006 looked at the websites of libraries for the top-twenty-ranked research-oriented medical schools to determine how they were providing access to their collections of medical textbooks, particularly the Brandon-Hill listed medical textbooks, a set of books still thought to be some of the most important for each medical subject area (MacCall 2006). Almost every library provided access in at least two different ways—through a catalog and through a list. These lists were alphabetical, subject classified, or both. This is an example of libraries maximizing the options for users, allowing searching or browsing by topic or by title, and indicates that librarians find their users to be looking for e-books, for instance, just as they looked for physical books. Because the research for the study was done purely by inspection of publicly available websites, there was no evaluation or discussion of exactly how librarians were creating the access to e-books by title on their web pages and how much time was involved in cataloging or creating the lists.

The study noted above is now over ten years old and has not been updated, but, anecdotally, it appears that much remains the same for e-book access. A perusal of health sciences library websites from both large and small institutions shows that many are still presenting e-book title lists (alphabetically or by subject) as well as title access through a catalog. While there were a lot of e-books in 2006, there are so many more now that the organization and presentation of e-books on health sciences library pages is increasingly a challenge. A 2012 post on the Krafty Librarian blog about organizing e-books generated much discussion among health sciences librarians about how difficult it is to present them in a way that makes sense for library users (Kraft 2012). Most agreed that patrons do not like to use a library catalog, but most also agreed that the catalog is still one of the best, most comprehensive ways for librarians to keep track of their e-book holdings. Quite a few indicated that they created manual lists of e-books on their library websites despite the time-consuming nature of that activity and the burgeoning number of e-book titles—in one library's case, over six thousand of them. Many used a service like EBSCO A-to-Z or ProQuest Serial Solutions to track their e-books, automatically add MARC records and links to their catalogs, and automatically generate A–Z subject lists of e-books for the website. Using services like these is essential for most libraries and removes the need for a lot of manual link updating in catalogs or on websites. They allow a library to maintain a list of the e-book packages or individual e-books they subscribe to or have purchased individually in a knowledge base. In turn, that knowledge base is continually updated by publishers with stable URLs at the title level. Libraries can regularly receive MARC records based on the knowledge base and librarians can upload these into their catalogs. Title lists can be generated for library web pages by subject area or by title, although it appears that many health sciences libraries have given up on lists of e-books due to the sheer numbers of them. Collection management librarians expect when purchasing e-book packages that they will be able to track the titles using one of these services, and, very occasionally, they might come across a small (often society) publisher that is not familiar with working with a third-party e-book tracking service. The number of publishers like that should diminish over time, and librarians should pressure publishers to keep up with industry standards. Finally, some health sciences libraries have combined several approaches to tracking and presenting their e-books to library users. They list e-book packages at the resource level for users looking for databases by name; they encourage users to search their catalogs for access to the complete collection of e-books by title or subject; and they have created manual lists of important e-books because users still love and demand lists even if they are impractical and incomplete. Librarians may believe that a manual list is worth the work because it promotes their collection in ways that the catalog can never do.

Compared with e-books, organizing and providing title-level access to electronic journal collections is much easier. The services mentioned above from EBSCO or ProQuest have existed even longer for managing serials than they have for e-books, and libraries have been using them to upload MARC records for journals into their catalogs and create A–Z and subject lists of journals for their library websites. While libraries differ on whether they provide title lists of e-books, most libraries seem to provide title lists for journals, and these title lists are often favored by health sciences library users over the catalog for finding and accessing journals (De Groote, Shultz, and Blecic 2014). It should be noted that libraries do not have control over the subject categorization of journals within these services and they cannot customize the lists; nevertheless, they seem to do a good enough job. A newer method of providing access to journals at the title level, and one that may serve to showcase the collection even better, is through a service that pulls library-subscribed journals into a uniform platform like BrowZine, which is available for library subscription. BrowZine's web and app versions allow users to create easily accessible, browsable bookshelves of favorite library-subscribed journals for which current issues can be accessed in full text with authentication through the library (Swogger and Linares 2016). The web service allows librarians to create subject lists of electronic journals on their websites. The advantage of BrowZine's lists over subject lists created by the EBSCO or Serial Solutions services mentioned above is visual. BrowZine shows thumbnail images of journal covers and provides a consistent platform for reading journals from different publishers. The disadvantage of BrowZine is that not all journals are available through that service, and the lists will not be comprehensive. Users also lose any special features that would be available on the publishers' websites. There are a few free app competitors to BrowZine for the physician audience, such as Docwise or QxMD's Read, and it will be interesting to follow their reach into the market. QxMD's Read may, for instance, work better for hospitals. It is likely that these types of resources will continue to be developed as vendors see the need libraries have for promoting their collections in more visually accessible ways.

PROVIDING ARTICLE-LEVEL ACCESS

Moving up another level of complexity, librarians will want to think about access to information sources at the article or chapter level. Traditionally this has been done using indexes, which, for the health sciences, have been primarily for the journal literature, but also for some monographic series and other types of resources. Even in the age of Google and Google Scholar, PubMed, CINAHL, and Embase, among many other indexes, remain important means of article-level finding and access of the literature, particularly for researchers. Librarians may use indexing in one of these databases as reassurance that a resource will be findable and more likely to be used. But librarians must assume their library users are coming into articles from a variety of online portals and search engines. The end goal for users is the full text of the article or book chapter, not just an abstract, and link resolvers using the OpenURL standard make that possible. Librarians are familiar with link resolvers by now, and they are a crucial tool that allows linking across platforms, between resources from different publishers, and between indexes and full-text articles. Several vendors have their versions, and libraries generally choose a link resolver as part of a package for resource management along with an integrated library system, a serials management system, and possibly a discovery system (see below). For academic health sciences libraries, many of these decisions are made at the whole university library level. The health sciences collection management librarian may not have a final say in which product is chosen but should remain informed and understand how it will affect the presentation of the collection. While link resolvers can lead to dead ends and errors more than one would like, collection management librarians still want to make sure that subscribed databases allow this kind of linking and that the resources they purchase are in the knowledge bases of these systems. The more links and opportunities for users to move around from one resource to another, the more likely patrons are to actually use library resources online, so the key is maximum interoperability among systems. Fortunately, standards in that area are constantly being evaluated and updated as systems become more and more complex (Lagace, Kaplan, and Leffler 2015).

A recent trend for libraries is the addition of a web-scale discovery layer on top of the library's catalog and other resources. These discovery layers are designed to provide users the ease of a "Google-like" one-box search interface for navigating all of the library's collections at once, from print holdings to electronic articles and book chapters from multiple publishers and platforms, combining the functionality of a library catalog, article indexes, and full-text databases all in one (Hoy 2012). The idea is that users will not have to think about what resources are available from which publishers or figure out which index would be more appropriate to use. Search results can be refined after the fact, allowing users to tell the system whether they want to limit by date, material type, subject, or other customizable facets.

Such discovery systems dig down to search the full text of articles and can drive user access toward resources that may have remained more hidden in the traditional access modes of the library catalog and indexes. Implementation of these discovery layers is not an easy or quick task. Whole books have been written for academic libraries on the topic of evaluating different discovery layers and implementing them (Popp and Dallis 2012). How well the discovery tool works with the library's existing resources is a consideration since each tool is designed to work maximally with that company's own products, such as link resolvers, electronic resource management systems, and indexes and databases. During implementation, librarians must make decisions such as how many databases and resources to include in the discovery search, how many facets to show for search refinement, and how to display results. They have to balance the desire for a comprehensive search with concerns about users being frustrated with irrelevant results. Collection management librarians are ideally involved at many points of these decisions, as they will affect which resources will get used and future purchasing decisions.

Sommer Browning from the University of Colorado points out the necessity for collection management librarians to consider discovery of content as one of the collection development criteria (Browning 2015). At her institution, two collaborative teams of librarians were created once their discovery layer had been implemented: one to maintain and oversee the discovery layer and one to troubleshoot problems. Collection development librarians were included in both teams, working alongside technical services and electronic access librarians to keep the discovery layer working well and to bring information back to other librarians in the collection development department. A new electronic resources trial workflow was established to test how any proposed new purchase might work with the discovery layer, an idea that other libraries may also want to adopt. It's clear that collection development librarians bring an important voice to institutional discussions about and maintenance of discovery layers, and collaboration and communication between them and technical services, public services, and access services librarians should be promoted.

But how well do discovery layers work for health sciences libraries? A lot of the articles on web-scale discovery systems discuss implementation across a whole university library system. Health sciences libraries are sometimes part of a larger university system but sometimes completely separate. In either case, health sciences libraries have begun investigating the pros and cons of implementing such a system for their own user groups. Discovery layers are not yet the norm for health sciences libraries. A 2014 visual survey of the websites of 144 libraries affiliated with the Association of Academic

Health Sciences Libraries revealed that less than 40 percent had implemented a discovery tool, and even those that had one tended not to emphasize it (Kronenfeld and Bright 2015). Some had chosen not to employ the discovery tool that their own university library had implemented for other subject areas.

Kronenfeld and Bright suggest that perhaps health sciences librarians have found that the way their university libraries have customized the tool for other types of users does not work well for health sciences users. For instance, they note that the tools do not do a good job of answering clinical questions. The more different types of databases that are searched by a discovery tool, the higher the likelihood of health topic searches picking up results from magazines, newspaper articles, and general databases geared toward a non-health professional user. Even results from scholarly journals or textbooks can be much more information than a clinician needs. This is the opposite of the goal of dedicated point-of-care tools, which are set up to provide a fast, best, fairly short answer for a busy clinician, not comprehensive search results from multiple platforms and databases.

Possibly web-scale discovery systems work better for health sciences research and education than for clinical questions. Ketterman and Inman at East Carolina University compared one of the discovery tools, ProQuest's Summon Discovery Service, with PubMed for searches on "health information management," "medical information," and "electronic health records" (Ketterman and Inman 2014). They were pleased with the results from the discovery layer search and recommended it, at least for students, as a supplement to PubMed. They liked the fact that it reached deeper into the collection by finding book chapters and searching the full text of articles.

A 2016 article compared three popular web-scale discovery systems for health sciences research and found they were all similarly effective in returning relevant results for searches in the disciplines of applied health sciences, dentistry, medicine, nursing, public health, and pharmacy (Hanneke and O'Brien 2016). They limited their results to scholarly journal articles, which likely was important for focusing the search to professional health sciences literature. The value of the discovery layer search for health sciences researchers was that a significant amount of literature was found that was not picked up by a similar PubMed search. This highlights the value of a discovery layer for being able to search full text at the article level, similar to Google Scholar.

Health sciences libraries that have the ability to set up a discovery layer on their own to meet the needs of their unique users can build a system that is more focused. Two papers discuss the implementation of EBSCO's Discovery Service in academic health sciences libraries and their decisions about which databases to include in the search (Pinkas et al. 2014; Thompson, Obrig, and Abate 2013). Unlike some others, EBSCO's Discovery Service allows one to provide an option for the user to try the same search they have just run in the discovery search directly in other individual databases. This gives health sciences librarians the best of both worlds: a one-box search plus the option to point users to a list of specialized databases like PubMed, CINAHL, Micromedex, ClinicalKey, or whatever is deemed useful for that library's clientele. Discovery services can be quite expensive, but even hospital libraries have begun to experiment with them as their budgets allow. Some have found that none of them yet really meet their needs, but others have taken the plunge of implementation (Brigham et al. 2016; Magnan, Duffy, and Mackes 2015). Most seem to promote searching of point-of-care databases separately on their web pages.

The landscape of discovery services is rapidly changing, and it will be important for collection management librarians to reevaluate their decisions regarding them as time goes along. Librarians should work with vendors to let them know how discovery tools can be optimized and developed for different user groups and to encourage metadata sharing among vendors, an important key to allowing databases to work with each other and with discovery systems. Perhaps a tool focused on health care professionals will develop over time. As discovery systems mature, more health sciences libraries may find that they are able to customize them to meet their needs and that they are worth promoting on their websites. What is certain is that whether a resource will be effectively searched through the discovery layer will be an important consideration for collection managers.

PUBLICIZING THE COLLECTION

After choosing resources for the collection, taking into account the level of access the library will be able to provide and ensuring the resource is listed on the website and discoverable through a library search engine or catalog, the health sciences collection management librarian's work is not necessarily done. Highly motivated library users, like researchers looking for access to their favorite journals, will manage to find the library website and perhaps the resource they were looking for (although they could probably benefit from learning about unfamiliar resources as well).

Other groups of users may need to be led to appropriate library resources: undergraduates who may only have experience using Google to find information, professional school students still unfamiliar with resources in their field, students in online programs not even aware they have access to a library, and busy clinicians needing fast access to information who may find the library website too time consuming to navigate. For these users, the library can best compete with easy, ubiquitous, freely accessible, but possibly lower-quality resources by putting the quality resources in front of the users' eyes in spaces that are targeted for them. Collection management librarians have to start thinking like advertisers for their collections, creating portals that are attractive because the resources are easy to find and use and targeted to a specific need. Collaborating with outreach, liaison, and instruction librarians will help with this.

A library's website offers multiple opportunities for advertising the collection. Many libraries employ features spaces to highlight new larger purchases, but this more traditional advertising technique is necessarily limited to promotion of a few new databases. Creating subject-specific guides for specific user groups, using a product like Springshare's LibGuides, is very popular and a way for librarians to create spaces on the web targeted for specific users. Libraries of all types—from community colleges to large academic libraries to hospital libraries—are using LibGuides to organize and promote their resources. Some choose to organize resources into subject categories, creating guides to highlight resources for dentistry, nursing, global health, drug information, genetics, or orthopedics. Others have created guides targeted to the needs of users in specific programs or classes, such as a guide for surgery residents or a guide for students in the "Nursing 480" class.

Essentially, librarians are acknowledging that, for many of their users, the collection is overwhelming. By curating subcollections of resources around a topic or for specific needs, librarians make the collection more manageable and understandable. These guides act as alternative portals for users, as tools for self-guided instruction, or as reinforcement after an in-person instructional session on finding resources (Gerberi, Hawthorne, and Larsen 2012; Neves and Dooley 2011).

Collection development librarians who are also liaisons to their users are in a strong position to promote library resources and guides to resources in day-to-day interactions, instruction sessions, orientations, or the like. Many health sciences libraries, however, do not necessarily follow this model. Health sciences librarian position postings have shown a trend for hiring embedded librarians, informationists, and other librarians doing liaison or instruction work without also being responsible for a collection (Cooper and Crum 2013). This makes sense, as there is a push to get librarians out of libraries and more directly involved in curriculum, research, and clinical care. All of these new activities leave little room for multiple librarians doing collection management. Communication between the collection development librarian and librarians in these other positions is crucial, however, to developing a collection that is marketed to the users by identifying and meeting their needs. There are many ways in which liaisons can help promote resources to users, from one-on-one interactions to group communication. Liaisons should be familiar with current awareness tools and be able to help users set themselves up with electronic table of contents delivery, alerts, or RSS feeds, all of which are usually available directly from journal websites (Kramer et al. 2011).

A study in 2012 showed that most health sciences journals had RSS and other social media features and a large number had social bookmarking tools to allow users to share and promote content to their friends (De Groote 2012). Of course, users will typically promote and request current awareness alerts from resources they already know about, so strategic input from librarians can help users learn about unfamiliar resources. Librarians can communicate with library users as a group using email, blog posts, or various types of social media. Being engaged on social media and using it to the best advantage to advertise collections and services requires a time commitment.

It is easy for librarians to become excited about new methods of communication, but if there is not enough time to keep up a blog, for instance, it is better not to have one at all. There are ways to save time by automatically sending out the same information on multiple social media platforms, but these efforts will probably be less successful than if librarians put in the time and effort to optimize their content for each platform, such as using hashtags to best advantage in Twitter (Cuddy, Graham, and Morton-Owens 2010). Twitter and Facebook require interested users to "follow" the library to get the information that is posted, so these may end up reaching only those that already have a strong interest.

The collection management librarian will need to thoughtfully consider which modes of communication make sense for which users and types of information. A 2012 study looked at academic health sciences libraries on Facebook. Only a few provided library resource links, such as links to recent articles in the *New England Journal of Medicine*. Most often the content on Facebook tended to promote library events rather than collections. There was a direct correlation between library popularity (in numbers of fans) and the presence of photo and video content (Garcia-Milian, Norton, and Tennant 2012). Only a few of these libraries had more than two hundred Facebook fans.

The Lister Hill Library of the Health Sciences set out to try multiple social media platforms and evaluate which ones worked the best for them. They created a presence on Facebook, Twitter, Pinterest, and YouTube, and they had six active library blogs. Facebook was their major outlet but was used primarily to promote events. Blogs were more often used to promote library resources and were linked to emails that liaison librarians sent. A YouTube channel contained videos about using such resources as PubMed, CINAHL, and the Cochrane Library, and users were directed to these videos through LibGuides or in virtual reference encounters.

These librarians noted that the number of users reached through Facebook had begun to decline slightly in the fall of 2012. At that point they created a Pinterest account to advertise resources and made a more concerted effort to incorporate hashtags in their use of Twitter (Vucovich et al. 2013). Their conclusion was that each social media platform reached a different set of users and served a different purpose and that they reached enough people that it was worth their time investment. The ever-changing landscape of social media means that librarians wanting to reach their users will need to be nimble and keep up with the platforms as they wax and wane in popularity.

EMBEDDING THE COLLECTION

While publicizing the collection has the goal of getting users to come to the library website, or some portion of it, and discover the wealth of resources there, the next logical step to meeting user needs is delivering the collection to them at their point of need where they already are on the web. Decentralization of library functions is already taking place in the form of embedded librarians in departments and research and clinical teams. Librarians should also think about embedding collections. This can be especially crucial when trying to reach users that are physically distant from the library. Even though everyone may be primarily using the library online, distance students and remote users especially tend to forget that they have access to a library online.

Since most courses, at community colleges and all the way up to medical schools, involve at least some online delivery, many libraries have moved reference and instruction services into the course management system with instructional modules and "ask a librarian" widgets. Information resources from the collection similarly have been embedded in course management systems as direct links or links in guides so students stumble across them when accessing lecture or assignment materials (Blevins and Inman 2014).

Calls for educational reform have proposed the "flipped classroom" approach that is now currently being implemented in many undergraduate, graduate, and health professional programs. Unfortunately, the discussion taking place about these changes in professional, non-library literature never mentions the role the librarians can play in this educational approach, despite the fact that librarians would be able to help identify and purchase online instructional materials and deal with copyright considerations (Critz and Knight 2013; McLaughlin et al. 2014; Prober and Khan 2013). Interestingly, discussion in the library literature also seems focused on flipped information literacy instruction as a method and tends not to mention collection issues (Youngkin 2014).

Similarly, in the clinical environment, librarians are embedding resources into electronic health records to be available at the point of need for health care professionals. For both of these embedded examples, librarians must carefully select the most appropriate resources to promote, or they lose the value of the opportunity. In 2009 the Association of Academic Health Sciences Libraries convened a symposium on "Electronic Health Records

(EHR) and Knowledge-Based Information: State-of-the-Art and Roles for Libraries in Health Information Technology," and papers from that symposium were published in the July 2010 issue of *Journal of the Medical Library Association* (Curtis 2010).

Some library directors cautioned librarians against simply embedding a library toolbar or a tab for library resources, encouraging librarians to consider their clinicians' needs for fast point-of-care information. One library created a custom clinical information tool that used several licensed library databases in subject search tabs covering diagnosis, diseases, drugs, evidence-based medicine, and patient education (Epstein et al. 2010).

Similar to the process of implementing and customizing a discovery layer for a library's users, customizing this clinical information tool for searching multiple databases at once was very time consuming. Other libraries have also reported that a lot of time and effort are needed to choose appropriate resources and customize them where possible to successfully integrate decision support systems into electronic health records. Simple implementation of basic diagnostic tools tended to give diagnoses that were too broad and not useful. Physicians appreciated when the tools were set up to generate automatic searches of multiple databases based on their own diagnoses and keywords (Fowler et al. 2014).

When health sciences librarians have been invited to collaborate with physicians, hospital administration, and information technologists on these projects, the outcome is usually more satisfying than cases where the hospital administration chooses to integrate one resource into the electronic health record without consulting the library. On the other hand, librarians will have the challenge of deciding how much staff time they devote to such projects because they are so much more involved than the strategy of just putting "the library" in front of the users.

While electronic health record integration of information resources at the point of need for physicians and nurses is still being developed, it is far ahead of such information integration for practitioners in other health sciences fields such as veterinary medicine or public health (Alpi et al. 2011; Revere et al. 2007). Infrastructure development and interoperability of different kinds of resources is something librarians in these fields can push vendors to work on.

Embedding collections is in the early stages. Library administrations already struggle with the scalability of embedded librarians, as the ratio of librarians to students, clinicians, research faculty, or whatever user group is being served is usually very small (Guillot, Stahr, and Meeker 2010). The concept of embedded collections—for instance, in the electronic health record example above—can similarly involve a whole new workflow and workload that some libraries may not be able to handle. But the idea is worth exploring. It makes sense that embedded collections accompany embedded librarians. Academic library managers have discussed sustainability primarily in the context of embedding librarians (and presumably collections, too) into course management systems, posing such questions as how many courses one librarian can realistically be involved in at one time (Burke and Tumbleson 2013).

Wu and Mi present a five-level working model for embedded librarianship, demonstrating that librarians can approach the concept of embedding themselves at different levels of depth as staff time allows (Wu and Mi 2013). At many of the levels they describe, embedded librarians are creating curated subcollections to support the users they are working with. At the highest level of embedding (level 5), librarians collaborate with users in decision making and reaching strategic goals such as helping to develop a curriculum for a program rather than merely supporting existing curricula.

An SLA-funded research project on embedded librarians recommended that librarians move toward strategic engagement (similar to Wu and Mi's level 5) for the best chance of long-term success (Shumaker and Makins 2012). How would the collection management librarian who is not necessarily the one who is embedded fit into this picture? Wu and Mi place the "resource purchaser," developing the collection to support a course or curriculum, at level 1 on their scale of embedded librarianship. However, the collection development librarian who collaborates closely with faculty to help shape a curriculum by choosing and integrating resources is actually operating at a higher level of embedded librarianship and is taking a strategic proactive approach to collection development rather than a reactive one. Collection management librarians, like embedded librarians, may need to get out of the library and become more involved with their users.

CONCLUSION

If health sciences libraries are truly to be user-centric, librarians have to meet the needs of those users with collections that not only have the content users want but also the functionality, interoperability, and discoverability that bring that content to the users' attention where and when they need it. Collection management librarians will find themselves needing to keep informed about many other areas of librarianship, from technical services and web systems to instructional needs and social media. It can be daunting but exciting to be involved in promoting access and usage of the collection at all these different levels, and, far from acting solely in the background, collection management librarians may find themselves front and center in their libraries, helping to develop and improve systems of access for users or embedding content in user spaces. All the knowledge they get from being involved in these projects will come back to inform their choices and creativity in collection building, bringing the story full circle.

REFERENCES

Almquist, Arne J. 2014. "The Innovative Academic Library: Implementing a Marketing Orientation to Better Address User Needs and Improve Communication." *Journal of Library Innovation* 5 (1): 43–54.

Alpi, Kristine M., Heidi A. Burnett, Sheila J. Bryant, and Katherine M. Anderson. 2011. "Connecting Knowledge Resources to the Veterinary Electronic Health Record: Opportunities for Learning at Point of Care." *Journal of Veterinary Medical Education* 38 (2): 110–22. doi:10.3138/jvme.38.2.110.

Blevins, Amy E., and Megan B. Inman. 2014. "Integrating Health Sciences Library Resources into Course Management Systems." *Medical Reference Services Quarterly* 33 (4): 357–66. doi:10.1080/02763869.2014.957071.

Brigham, Tara J., Ann M. Farrell, Leah C. Osterhaus Trzasko, Carol Ann Attwood, Mark W. Wentz, and Kelly A. Arp. 2016. "Web-Scale Discovery Service: Is It Right for Your Library? Mayo Clinic Libraries Experience." *Journal of Hospital Librarianship* 16 (1): 25–39. doi:10.1080/15323269.2016.1118280.

Browning, Sommer. 2015. "The Discovery–Collection Librarian Connection: Cultivating Collaboration for Better Discovery." *Collection Management* 40 (4): 197–206. doi:10.1080/01462679.2015.1093985.

Burke, John J., and Beth E. Tumbleson. 2013. "The Sustainability and Scalability of Embedded Librarianship." In *Embedded Librarianship: What Every Academic Librarian Should Know*, edited by Alice L Daugherty and Michael F Russo. Santa Barbara, CA: Libraries Unlimited.

Cooper, I. Diane, and Janet A. Crum. 2013. "New Activities and Changing Roles of Health Sciences Librarians: A Systematic Review, 1990–2012." *Journal of the Medical Library Association* 101 (4): 268–77. doi:10.3163/1536-5050.101.4.008.

Critz, Catharine M., and Diane Knight. 2013. "Using the Flipped Classroom in Graduate Nursing Education." *Nurse Educator* 38 (5): 210–13. doi:10.1097/NNE.0b013e3182a0e56a.

Cuddy, Colleen, Jamie Graham, and Emily G. Morton-Owens. 2010. "Implementing Twitter in a Health Sciences Library." *Medical Reference Services Quarterly* 29 (4): 320–30. doi:10.1080/02763869.2010.518915.

Curtis, James A. 2010. "Introduction: The Association of Academic Health Sciences Libraries Symposium: 'Electronic Health Records and Knowledge-Based Information: State-of-the-Art and Roles for Libraries in Health Information Technology.'" *Journal of the Medical Library Association* 98 (3): 204–5. doi:10.3163/1536-5050.98.3.004.

De Groote, Sandra L. 2012. "Promoting Health Sciences Journal Content with Web 2.0: A Snapshot in Time." *First Monday* 17 (8). doi:10.5210/fm.v17i8.4103.

De Groote, Sandra L., Mary Shultz, and Deborah D. Blecic. 2014. "Information-Seeking Behavior and the Use of Online Resources: A Snapshot of Current Health Sciences Faculty." *Journal of the Medical Library Association* 102 (3): 169–76. doi:10.3163/1536-5050.102.3.006.

Delawska-Elliott, B., C. Grinstead, and H. J. Martin. 2015. "Developing a Marketing Orientation in Hospital Library Services: A Case Report." *Medical Reference Services Quarterly* 34 (4): 481–89. doi:10.1080/02763869.2015.1082390.

Dowd, Nancy. 2013. "The Results Are In and They Aren't Good." *Library Journal*. http://lj.libraryjournal.com/2013/02/marketing/the-results-are-in-and-they-arent-good-library-marketing/.

Epstein, Barbara A., Nancy H. Tannery, Charles B. Wessel, Frances Yarger, John LaDue, and Anthony B. Fiorillo. 2010. "Development of a Clinical Information Tool for the Electronic Medical Record: A Case Study." *Journal of the Medical Library Association* 98 (3): 223–37. doi:10.3163/1536-5050.98.3.010.

Fowler, Susan A., Lauren H. Yaeger, Feliciano Yu, Dwight Doerhoff, Paul Schoening, and Betsy Kelly. 2014. "Electronic Health Record: Integrating Evidence-Based Information at the Point of Clinical Decision Making." *Journal of the Medical Library Association* 102 (1): 52–55. doi:10.3163/1536-5050.102.1.010.

Freiburger, Gary. 2010. "Introduction: Be Prepared. Loss of Space for Medical Libraries." *Journal of the Medical Library Association* 98 (1): 24. doi:10.3163/1536-5050.98.1.009.

Garcia-Milian, Rolando, Hannah F. Norton, and Michele R. Tennant. 2012. "The Presence of Academic Health Sciences Libraries on Facebook: The Relationship between Content and Library Popularity." *Medical Reference Services Quarterly* 31 (2): 171–87. doi:10.1080/02763869.2012.670588.

Gerberi, Dana, Dottie M. Hawthorne, and Karen E. Larsen. 2012. "Rethinking Responsible Literature Searching Using LibGuides." *Medical Reference Services Quarterly* 31 (4): 355–71. doi:10.1080/02763869.2012.723981.

Guillot, Ladonna, Beth Stahr, and Bonnie Juvé Meeker. 2010. "Nursing Faculty Collaborate with Embedded Librarians to Serve Online Graduate Students in a Consortium Setting." *Journal of Library & Information Services in Distance Learning* 4 (1–2): 53–62. doi:10.1080/15332901003666951.

Haines, Laura L., Jeanene Light, Donna O'Malley, and Frances A. Delwiche. 2010. "Information-Seeking Behavior of Basic Science Researchers: Implications for Library Services." *Journal of the Medical Library Association* 98 (1): 73–81. doi:10.3163/1536-5050.98.1.019.

Hanneke, Rosie, and Kelly K. O'Brien. 2016. "Comparison of Three Web-Scale Discovery Services for Health Sciences Research." *Journal of the Medical Library Association* 104 (2): 109–17.

Hoy, Matthew B. 2012. "An Introduction to Web Scale Discovery Systems." *Medical Reference Services Quarterly* 31 (3): 323–29. doi:10.1080/02763869.2012.698186.

Ketterman, Elizabeth, and Megan E. Inman. 2014. "Discovery Tool vs. PubMed: A Health Sciences Literature Comparison Analysis." *Journal of Electronic Resources in Medical Libraries* 11 (3): 115–23. doi:10.1080/15424065.2014.938999.

Kraft, Michelle. 2012. "Organizing eBooks." *Krafty Librarian* (blog), August 22. http://www.kraftylibrarian.com/organizing-ebooks/.

Kramer, Sandra S., Jennifer R. Martin, Joan B. Schlimgen, Marion K. Slack, and Jim Martin. 2011. "Effectiveness of a Liaison Program in Meeting Information Needs of College of Pharmacy Faculty." *Medical Reference Services Quarterly* 30 (1): 31–41. doi:10.1080/02763869.2011.540210.

Kronenfeld, Michael R., and H. S. Bright IV. 2015. "Library Resource Discovery." *Journal of the Medical Library Association* 103 (4): 210–13. doi:10.3163/1536-5050.103.4.011.

Lagace, Nettie, Laurie Kaplan, and Jennifer J. Leffler. 2015. "Actions and Updates on the Standards and Best Practices Front." *The Serials Librarian* 68 (1–4): 191–96. doi:10.1080/0361526X.2015.1017420.

MacCall, Steven L. 2006. "Online Medical Books: Their Availability and an Assessment of How Health Sciences Libraries Provide Access on Their Public Websites." *Journal of the Medical Library Association* 94 (1): 75–80.

Magnan, Deborah, Christopher Duffy, and Robert T. Mackes. 2015. "Implementing a Discovery Tool in a Hospital Library: A Tale of Two Success Stories." *Journal of Hospital Librarianship* 15 (4): 435–43. doi:10.1080/15323269.2015.1079767.

McLaughlin, Jacqueline E., Mary T. Roth, Dylan M. Glatt, Nastaran Gharkholonarehe, Christopher A. Davidson, LaToya M. Griffin, Denise A. Esserman, and Russell J. Mumper. 2014. "The Flipped Classroom: A Course Redesign to Foster Learning and Engagement in a Health Professions School." *Academic Medicine* 89 (2): 236–43. doi:10.1097/acm.0000000000000086.

Neves, Karen, and Sarah Jane Dooley. 2011. "Using LibGuides to Offer Library Service to Undergraduate Medical Students Based on the Case-Oriented Problem Solving Curriculum Model." *Journal of the Medical Library Association* 99 (1): 94–97. doi:10.3163/1536-5050.99.1.017.

Pinkas, María M., Megan Del Baglivo, Ilene Robin Klein, Everly Brown, Ryan Harris, and Brad Gerhart. 2014. "Selecting and Implementing a Discovery Tool: The University of

Maryland Health Sciences and Human Services Library Experience." *Journal of Electronic Resources in Medical Libraries* 11 (1): 1–12. doi:10.1080/15424065.2013.876574.

Popp, Mary Pagliero, and Diane Dallis, eds. 2012. *Advances in Library and Information Science: Planning and Implementing Resource Discovery Tools in Academic Libraries*. Hershey, PA: IGI Global.

Prober, Charles G., and Salman Khan. 2013. "Medical Education Reimagined: A Call to Action." *Academic Medicine* 88 (10): 1407–10. doi:10.1097/ACM.0b013e3182a368bd.

Revere, Debra, Anne M. Turner, Ann Madhavan, Neil Rambo, Paul F. Bugni, AnnMarie Kimball, and Sherrilynne S. Fuller. 2007. "Understanding the Information Needs of Public Health Practitioners: A Literature Review to Inform Design of an Interactive Digital Knowledge Management System." *Journal of Biomedical Informatics* 40 (4): 410–21. doi:10.1016/j.jbi.2006.12.008.

Shumaker, David, and Alison Makins. 2012. "Lessons from Successful Embedded Librarians." *Information Outlook* 16 (3): 10–12.

Swogger, Susan E., and Brenda M. Linares. 2016. "BrowZine: A Method for Managing a Personalized Collection of Journals." *Medical Reference Services Quarterly* 35 (1): 83–93. doi:10.1080/02763869.2016.1117292.

Thompson, JoLinda L., Kathe S. Obrig, and Laura E. Abate. 2013. "Web-Scale Discovery in an Academic Health Sciences Library: Development and Implementation of the EBSCO Discovery Service." *Medical Reference Services Quarterly* 32 (1): 26–41. doi:10.1080/02763869.2013.749111.

Vucovich, Lee A., Valerie S. Gordon, Nicole Mitchell, and Lisa A. Ennis. 2013. "Is the Time and Effort Worth It? One Library's Evaluation of Using Social Networking Tools for Outreach." *Medical Reference Services Quarterly* 32 (1): 12–25. doi:10.1080/02763869.2013.749107.

Wu, Lin, and Misa Mi. 2013. "Sustaining Librarian Vitality: Embedded Librarianship Model for Health Sciences Libraries." *Medical Reference Services Quarterly* 32 (3): 257–65. doi:10.1080/02763869.2013.806860.

Youngkin, C. Andrew. 2014. "The Flipped Classroom: Practices and Opportunities for Health Sciences Librarians." *Medical Reference Services Quarterly* 33 (4): 367–74. doi:10.1080/02763869.2014.957073.

One Library's Story

Supporting a Reimagined Medical School Curriculum with Targeted Library Collections and Licenses

Iris Kovar-Gough

Michigan State University's College of Human Medicine is a community-based medical school with an enrollment of eight hundred students across a four-year curriculum. Students complete their first two preclinical years at one of two campuses in Michigan, East Lansing or Grand Rapids, and their final two years in clinical clerkships at one of seven sites across the state. The Michigan State University Libraries supports this medical school with a physical collection located on the East Lansing campus and an extensive online collection.

For decades, medical school faculty were quick to request that the library subscribe to materials to support research but overlooked us as a partner in medical education. The curriculum was based on a traditional Flexnerian model that emphasized basic science courses for the first two years followed later by clinically oriented courses. Faculty relied heavily on printed texts and coursepacks for teaching. They worked directly with a course materials support unit on campus to produce the coursepacks, which consisted of curated text written by professors, images from multiple third-party sources, and PowerPoint slides containing lecture materials. Inclusion of many of the images involved labor-intensive permissions seeking by the course materials unit. Sometimes individual faculty worked with publishers directly to license image use for coursepacks on a semester-by-semester basis with the adoption of a required textbook. None of these interactions involved librarians or the library collection. While this approach made more sense before the advent of electronic books, it became clear that it was inefficient and expensive for faculty to continue to incur copyright fees by reproducing images from printed books and working out deals directly with the same publishers for which the libraries already had subscriptions. But finding an optimal intervention point was challenging.

In the fall of 2016, the College of Human Medicine began to implement a new competency-based and patient-centered curriculum with clinical experience integrated throughout the four years of medical school. The new curriculum uses online educational modules to deliver content with reflective student learning occurring in small and large discussion groups, labs, clinic hours, and learning societies and is a departure from the college's usual methodologies of in-person or recorded lectures and coursepacks. The new curriculum offered an ideal opportunity for us to engage with the college in new ways. With an emphasis on online materials and a move away from printed texts and coursepacks, the library's liaison to the college was able to reinvigorate our relationship with faculty, have a voice in curriculum development, and consequently alter our collection development and practices.

The goal of our project was to encourage college collaboration with librarians to facilitate use of library resources (particularly licensed image content) in the new curriculum. This would have several benefits: it would position the library as a partner in medical education, ensure faculty could easily find high-quality materials for course content, and, finally, save money in copyright fees that had previously been passed down to students in the cost of coursepacks. We wanted to empower faculty with skills and knowledge to make informed decisions about where to find curricular content outside of using the books on their desks or the results of Google image searches. The reduction in costs for medical students was also a goal of the university at the level of the office of the provost.

To carry out the project we employed three main strategies. First, we engaged in outreach efforts and relationship building. We attended curriculum meetings and carefully increased our participation to engage faculty in discussions about the materials they used to build curricula and the gaps in available resources. We also met with individual stakeholders to demonstrate librarian value and interest in medical education. Eventually, we were invited to participate in curriculum design workgroups and developed more meaningful collaborations with key players that exposed avenues for engagement and embedding of library resources and expertise. Second, we bought new products requested by faculty or that we thought would be useful. Third, when we purchased these new products or renewed existing subscriptions, we contacted vendors to request and amend license language to allow for more flexible online use of resources, particularly images and figures from textbooks.

To move the project forward quickly and effectively we focused on our library licenses for major products and vendors. Fortunately, most of the textbooks of interest to faculty were from the top three medical publishers. We contacted and met with representatives from Elsevier's ClinicalKey, McGraw-Hill Education, and Wolters Kluwer Health to check terms of use and amend licenses where needed to allow for embedding textbook images within curriculum online behind institutional firewalls. We found these vendors to be cooperative and supportive, although legal departments could be slow in approving language. We added subscriptions to new resources from other vendors that would increase our sources for images, such as the Thieme Teaching Assistants and VisualDx. We also purchased the Lippincott Williams & Wilkins Health Library–Clerkship Collection, which contained electronic books frequently requested by faculty. Requesting license changes for brand-new subscriptions was even more efficient than for existing subscriptions since vendors were eager to make a new sale. Next we created a LibGuide highlighting "approved" sources for images from the library subscriptions that would not require extra requests and fees for permissions. Being able to present the faculty with a curated list of sources for image content removed stakeholder-perceived barriers of access to library resources and anxiety about copyright issues.

There were many positive outcomes from this project. The college uses more library content than before, particularly high-quality anatomy images from Thieme and links to online textbooks like Lawrence's *Essentials of General Surgery*, which had previously been unavailable to us in electronic form. With more faculty–liaison librarian engagement at a curriculum design level, we can better scope our collection to meet their needs and drive collection development toward products with license terms and technical specifications that support online medical education. Finally, faculty perception of librarian expertise and range of job duties has expanded and led to more fulfilling relationships between the college and the library. Key faculty members on the curriculum revision committee made comments that the liaison librarian's expertise and input had been integral to the committee's success and had helped design the curriculum with the most efficient and effective long-term use in mind.

There have been a few challenges. There is still a small contingent of faculty who continue to use older content whose online use is not covered by the new licenses, and improved librarian-led outreach and education is needed to help them explore new resources. At the start of our project, some faculty envisioned offering course modules containing library-licensed resources on the open web. This was not realistic, but through targeted educational interventions and working with college programmers to find technological solutions to perceived barriers of access that underlay this altruistic vision, we came to acceptable compromises. The differences between copyright law and library licenses are also difficult for faculty to understand. We are creating materials for faculty to help make this distinction clear, and positioning ourselves as the "go to" people for questions about appropriate use of material in online environments.

We learned some interesting lessons during this project. In our discussions with content vendors like Elsevier and McGraw-Hill, we discovered that publishers' expectations about the terms of image use could often be more lenient than a conservative reading of our library licenses led us to believe. Some were surprised when we asked for explicit license terms to allow for putting textbook images online behind institutional firewalls and did not necessarily see the necessity of new license language. Initially we found it challenging to know exactly what to ask for in the requested addenda. Over time we realized that it was important to include terms allowing us to archive learning modules using the images, as faculty in the medical school wanted students not only to view the current semester's courses but also refer to past courses. Furthermore, we checked that the copyright information required by the vendors to accompany the images was easy to find and attach, since we knew that step needed to be simple if we expected faculty and staff compliance. Finally, we learned that, in order to develop our collection to meet college needs, we had to go outside our comfort zones and ask to be included in meetings and decision-making processes and, occasionally, tell faculty that their plans were not feasible while extending offers of help and viable solutions. By getting stakeholder input and buy-in, we have been successful in encouraging collaboration and embedding library materials in the new curriculum.

Chapter Seven

Usability and Accessibility for Health Sciences Collections

Jessica Shira Sender and Heidi M. Schroeder

Accessibility and usability are not new concepts in libraries, but there has been a renewed focus on what those terms mean in relation to collection development in the health sciences. In some respects, they are two of the most critical components of any collection. Both refer to how products are designed. Usability refers to the ease and effectiveness of use of those products, whether they are physical items, pieces of technology, or websites. Accessibility focuses on making sure that the design is not discriminatory for people with disabilities, impairments, or differences. Libraries can develop world-renowned collections, but if the resources contained within those collections are not usable or accessible, the collections do not serve their purpose. Libraries have always developed collections that are to be used rather than archived as museum pieces. Libraries also have a history of being inclusive and democratic institutions with a value of making information available to all kinds of users. A resource can be accessible, but if it is not usable, it is hard to justify the inclusion of it to the collection. Similarly, if a resource is designed with usability principles, but forgoes adhering to accessibility standards, it is not a true reflection of the best usability design. Keeping both concepts in mind ensures that all users are successfully able to use and leverage the resources that are a part of a library collection.

USABILITY CONSIDERATIONS FOR COLLECTIONS

Usability Principles

The growth of products, programs, and resources online has been beneficial to many, allowing more users to access more resources from anywhere, but this boom in online resources goes hand in hand with needing to understand and evaluate *how* users experience these resources. Print resources have usability considerations, but online resources offer a bigger variety of experiences. If a user is unable to use the resources provided or has a negative experience while using a website, database, or even physical collection, the user is unlikely to return to the library or its digital resources again. This is particularly apt for health sciences libraries and their users. Health sciences libraries and librarians often serve users who are in hospital or clinical settings, far from where a physical library or collection may be. Conducting usability testing on health sciences resources and employing sound usability principles when selecting resources and developing collections ensures that a health sciences collection is meeting the needs, however varied they may be, of the user. This chapter will largely focus on the usability of digital collections; however, many of the usability principles and user-testing methods discussed can and should be used to evaluate and assess physical collections, too.

Before delving into usability considerations for a health sciences collection, it is critical to understand what usability is. Jakob Nielsen is considered one of the founders of the modern concept of usability. Usability, as he defines it, is a "quality attribute that assesses how easy user interfaces are to use" (Nielsen 2012). He also says that usability refers to methods for improving ease of use during the design process (Nielsen 2012). Jakob Nielsen founded the Nielsen Normal Group, a research company that focuses on evidence-based user experience research, training, and consulting. They outline five major concepts that are critical to understanding usability. Those principles, listed on their website, are as follows:

- Learnability—how easy is it for users to accomplish basic tasks the first time they encounter the design?
- Efficiency—once users have learned the design, how quickly can they perform the tasks?
- Memorability—when users return to the design after a period of not using it, how easily can they reestablish proficiency?
- Errors—how many errors do users make, how severe are these errors, and how easily can they recover from the errors?
- Satisfaction—how pleasant is it to use the design? (Nielsen 2012)

The Usability.gov website from the United States Department of Health and Human Services also outlines what usability is and includes a set of six factors to define usability:

- Intuitive design: a nearly effortless understanding of architecture and navigation of the site
- Ease of learning: how fast a user who has never seen the user interface before can accomplish basic tasks
- Efficiency of use: how fast an experienced user can accomplish tasks
- Memorability: after visiting the site, if a user can remember enough to use it effectively in future visits
- Error frequency and severity: how often users make errors while using the system, how serious the errors are, and how users recover from the errors
- Subject satisfaction: if the user likes using the system (United States Department of Health and Human Services 2016)

There is significant overlap between these two sets of usability principles, which allows for a common foundational understanding of the important principles of usability. While usability is a term often applied when discussing how to design websites or products, usability principles and guidelines can be applied by librarians evaluating a variety of web resources for purchase or subscription. Much of what has been studied in relation to health sciences is the usability of health sciences websites, point-of-care tools, or health care technologies. This chapter will discuss the usability testing methods used in these studies and explore how they can be applied to evaluating and selecting resources for a health sciences collection.

Usability Testing Methods

Usability as a field of research originated from the human-computer interaction field, where a focus on how users interacted with programs, systems, digital resources, and even products shifted and began to inform research. The "user experience" (UX) initially referred to how companies designed new products, and it emerged into a field of study focused on why some products did well while others did not. Usability testing of products with representative users has become a critical component of product development in the corporate world. With the results of usability testing, companies can evaluate product marketability and user impact prior to releasing products to the general public.

As UX and usability testing have progressed in business and product development, they have become important components of the health care fields (Jonassaint et al. (2015). There has been substantial research conducted about usability on a variety of health technologies, such as electronic health records (EHRs), which have undergone rigorous usability testing as more clinical and hospital environments implement them (Ratwani 2017). There has been a rapid increase in the development and deployment of mobile fitness smartphone applications, which require usability testing at every stage of development and continual usability testing after release to the public (McKay et al. 2016). There has also been a growing increase in personal health-monitoring devices for dementia (Cho 2016), diabetes (Garcia-Zapirain et al. 2016), eating disorders (Nitsch et al. 2016), and a variety of other health concerns (Kortum and Peres 2015). These technologies require extensive usability testing to make sure that they will work for their intended users (Lyles, Sarkar, and Osborn 2014).

In contrast, there is a relative lack of literature or research about how usability principles can be applied to the types of resources in a health sciences library collection. Much of what has been studied in relation to health sciences libraries is the usability of library websites because they are products over which librarians have control. Collection management librarians are purchasing online products developed by companies that should be doing their own usability testing before bringing these products to market. For collection managers, then, understanding usability testing methods is not necessarily important because they will be doing extensive usability testing on each product they purchase, although they may be able to use some of the principles in their decision making. Primarily, it is important because understanding usability testing methods will allow them to understand what might go into product development and to be able to provide specific and targeted feedback to the vendors that are selling these products.

Baseline Usability Testing

As in any field, there are understood methods of conducting research. Baseline usability testing helps establish satisfaction with a website in order to direct future changes. Participants for such studies are chosen because they represent user groups for which a website is intended. A researcher observes these participants using the website to determine how they interact with the site, how they complete typical tasks associated with the site, and how satisfied they are with the experience. The researcher watches, takes notes, listens, and may ask questions. Sometimes users are asked to talk through what they are thinking as they are using the website. The data can inform the researcher about what resources are being used most often, what paths users take on the website to get to different resources, and what "pain points" may exist for users trying to find information. The study can be solely qualitative, or an attempt can be made to generate quantitative, measureable results as benchmarks against which the usability of future changes can also be measured.

Focus Groups

Another usability testing methods that requires more time and planning is the focus group. These have the potential to reap greater rewards with deeper insight than a simple observation. A focus group is a moderated discussion with a facilitator and about five to ten participants. Focus groups tend to be more discussion based and less structured than baseline usability tests. The goal of a focus group is to obtain information about the service, product, or resource in question but allow ample opportunity for wide-ranging discussion. While focus groups in a traditional corporate setting may be used to determine a direction for product development, in a health sciences library, focus groups can be used to help direct collection development by giving librarians a better understanding of the users' experiences and interactions with various library resources

Surveys

Another type of usability test is a survey, typically done online, although physical surveys may be an option. Surveys can vary in length and format, and the goal is to collect user feedback about a site, product, or issue of concern. Surveys not only offer flexibility of length, format, and anonymity, but can also provide a significant amount of quantitative data that can be analyzed. Additionally, surveys can be administered at any point or be continually ongoing, depending on the project and needed evaluation.

Surveys are perhaps the easiest way to conduct usability testing for health sciences collection development managers and other librarians. Since many of the users of health sciences collections are doctors, nurses, professors, and busy students, a survey that can be administered to a large group without needing the participants to spend a lot of time can be very beneficial. Additionally, since users may be spread across clinical sites, academic buildings, or statewide, an online survey is an easy way to reach those who might otherwise not be able to provide input face to face, something that both the baseline usability testing and focus group methods require.

Usability and user-centered collection assessment go hand in hand, and both survey and focus group methods can be used to gather data from users about many aspects of a website or product, not just usability. More on these methods for user-centered collection assessment is discussed in chapter 4.

Other Usability Testing Models

There are other common usability testing methods that are intended to be used for large information architecture projects, typically to develop a new site or redesign an aging website. These include card sorting, wireframing, and first-click testing. Card sorting is a method that involves users creating categories on index cards representing different services or resources that would be included on a website. This technique is usually used in the development phase of a website, as it gives structure to a site. A wireframe is an illustration of a website that shows the levels and connections of different subsites within the larger website. It displays the relationship between top, secondary, and lower-level pages. Both card sorting and wireframing show the website designer what users think is important to be able to find on the website. Lastly, first-click testing examines what a user would click on first when using a particular website to complete a given task. The test can be done either through a software installed on the computer that records the clicks, or observationally, as the researcher watches what the user does.

Typically, companies will employ several methods of usability testing, starting with baseline usability testing of an existing site or product to learn information that can be used when developing new products or creating the architecture of a redesign. Surveys and focus groups can fill in some of the qualitative details that may be missing. Many large vendors of databases with which librarians are familiar employ outside companies to do usability testing for them. Other, smaller vendors may have very little budget for usability testing, and librarians may find that the products they purchase reflect that difference. In both these cases, however, librarians should feel that they can also provide feedback to these companies based on any kind of usability testing they may be able to do with their own library users.

Usability and Libraries

As users and their experiences have become central to product development, site redesign, or system creation in the corporate business and health care world, libraries have begun to adopt the same usability principles. The core principles of usability design have a natural overlap with libraries, and libraries have actually been doing informal usability testing and responding to user needs for years. Libraries have a large web presence, with multiple access points to resources and information. The principles of usability, particularly learnability, efficiency, and memorability, are critical to the success of a library website. As an outward-facing, often first, point of contact for users, the library website needs to be easy to use and understand, efficient for users and their goals, and memorable to encourage their return.

Many libraries or institutions have already begun to do user experience research on their physical locations, spaces within the library, or websites. Health sciences librarians can leverage already existing data about their users and their needs by partnering with a user experience department or researcher at their institutions. The health sciences library at New York Medical College conducted both a survey and baseline usability testing to inform their understanding of how their users interacted with their website (Ascher, Lougee-

Heimer, and Cunningham 2007). From the results, they determined that users had a general approval of the website, but that navigation of the pages was difficult. Novice users were confused about how to carry out basic tasks, and the posttest interviews revealed that there was a steep learning curve in navigating the library's website. Participants in the study recommended making the site more task oriented. Keeping in mind usability principles and applying usability testing methods, this health sciences library was able to redesign their site in a way that better served their users. The same health sciences library later used usability studies to redesign their mobile site (Rosario, Ascher, and Cunningham 2012).

Usability testing could also help health sciences librarians determine what parts of the collection are and are not being used and why. In many library collections, the vast majority of resources goes unused and undiscoverable (Schwartz 2004). By conducting usability testing on different databases, e-book platforms, point-of-care tools (Howe 2011; Shurtz and Foster 2011) and resources, and even on the catalog itself, health sciences librarians could gain some insight into how users are interacting with their resources, and where there is confusion or barriers to use (Yeh and Fontenelle 2012). Additionally, health sciences librarians face the challenge that many of their library users are accessing library content using mobile devices. This means that the usability of any given resource should be tested on multiple sizes of devices and operating systems. Anything that librarians can learn about how usable these resources are and how different platforms affect the functionality of a resource can inform resource allocation, promotion of collections or newly acquired resources, and outreach to constituents.

Renowned user experience and usability researcher Steven Bell stresses that a user-centered library experience does not force users to interact with a website in a specific and potentially limited way dictated by the designer but allows them to encounter and interact with the resource in a way with which they are already familiar (Bell 2014). Ideally, collection managers can and should be evaluating the web platforms and mobile platforms of all of the electronic resources to which the library subscribes and the experience users have with the physical library collection. In reality, collection managers have many considerations when deciding on purchases and subscriptions, and usability can often take a back seat to content, price, demand, and other immediate concerns. Additionally, much of the content purchased by librarians is only available on one platform. Even if the interface is less than ideal, librarians still feel pressure to purchase or subscribe because the content is so valuable. Both librarians and library users can find this situation frustrating, and some publishers with valuable content may not make usability a priority. But there are some opportunities for librarians to make choices based on usability. When an e-book is available on multiple platforms, such as an aggregator platform like EBSCO or Rittenhouse's R2, as well as on a publisher's own website, there is an opportunity for usability testing to determine which platform may work better for library users. If there is no time or opportunity to do usability testing with multiple participants, collection management librarians can use their understanding of good usability principles in their own evaluation of resources during a trial period. Consultation of review sources such as *The Charleston Advisor* can also be valuable, as database reviews in the publication include an in-depth analysis and ranking of the user interface.

Collection management librarians should also take advantage of liaison relationships that they have developed with users or partnerships with liaison librarians. In the health sciences particularly, where the content is unique and targeted to a very specific type of user (nurse, physician, pharmacist), learning about and understanding the needs and experiences of these professionals can help librarians think more like them when they must do their own tests of usability.

The principles of usability and good usability testing can help inform sound collection development decisions. They can also provide librarians a better understanding of what users of all backgrounds and abilities want from both the physical and digital resources that make up the collection. As the focus on the user experience expands and shapes libraries, there has been an increase in webinars, programming, and resources available to librarians on how to conduct usability testing. Seeking out some of this programming for a better understanding of the field can be helpful for librarians even when there is not time, staffing, or the resources to do full-scale usability testing. Usability testing can be done one on one, from a distance, or even with small groups; librarians can keep this valuable feedback for themselves or share it with product vendors. Collection managers that keep usability in mind along with all the other considerations they have when making decisions ensure that users of all backgrounds will be able to successfully use and navigate their collections.

ACCESSIBILITY CONSIDERATIONS FOR COLLECTIONS

In an increasingly diverse world, libraries, including health sciences libraries, are striving to best meet the service and collections needs of *all* patrons. Following usability principles is a good first step, but accessibility goes a step further to address concerns that a product may be designed in a way that discriminates against users with disabilities. Although considering accessibility for persons with disabilities is not new to librarians, academic libraries, including academic health sciences librarians, may notice there has been more momentum surrounding the topic of accessibility on their campuses in recent years. This is probably due to proactive efforts to be more inclusive and, in the United States, also to Department of Justice and Department of Education lawsuits and complaints over inaccessible electronic resources at colleges and universities.

The accessibility of libraries' electronic resources and digital collections has been mentioned in these lawsuits and complaints and has been addressed in resolutions such as the resolution agreement between the University of Montana and the U.S. Department of Education (OCR 2014). The accessibility of library collections is not just a legal issue, it is also an ethical one. Libraries overwhelmingly take pride in promoting and providing their collections to the widest audience they can. Acquiring inaccessible e-resources and collections causes libraries to fall short of this goal, as users with disabilities are either completely unable to use certain library resources or the accessibility barriers are so great that their experiences are unequal with those of other library users.

The focus of this section will be on the accessibility of electronic resources and collections, not print, since print collections in most cases require remediation using assistive technologies. Electronic resources, however, if created and built with accessibility in mind from their inception or improved by those committed to accessibility, have the promising potential to be immediately accessible to all, regardless of ability. Also, the prevalence of—and often preference for—electronic collections in libraries, especially health sciences libraries, cannot be denied or ignored. Finally, the complicated and varied nature of e-resources presents unique accessibility challenges. There are numerous electronic resource types (e-books, databases, e-journals, streaming video, digital images, etc.), file formats (PDF, HTML, ePUB, JPEG, etc.), and vendors creating and disseminating these e-resources.

Accessibility Definitions, Laws, Standards, Testing, and Typical Barriers

When considering the accessibility of library and health sciences library electronic collections, librarians first need to understand the meaning of accessibility, accessibility laws and policies, accessibility standards, and typical accessibility issues and problems that exist in libraries' electronic collections. There are numerous definitions of accessibility, but many definitions refer to all people, regardless of ability or disability, being able to use and access things in their environment (Be. Accessible 2017; BBC 2014). Accessible electronic and information technology (EIT) is "technology that can be used by people with a wide range of abilities and disabilities (Accessible-Tech.org 2017). The Americans with Disabilities Act (ADA) in the United States defines people with disabilities as having "a physical or mental impairment that substantially limits one or more major life activities" (United States Department of Justice Civil Rights Division 2017).

Two pieces of accessibility legislation relevant to libraries in the United States are the Rehabilitation Act of 1973 and the Americans with Disabilities Act (ADA) of 1990. In a 2015 article, Kirsten Ostergaard provides an overview of the sections of the ADA and Rehabilitation Act as they relate to higher education (Ostergaard 2015, 160). The U.S. Department of Justice and the U.S. Department of Education's Office of Civil Rights enforce the ADA and the Rehabilitation Act and have increasingly been referring to Section 508 of the Rehabilitation Act's accessibility standards for EIT in complaints and lawsuits against academic institutions, even though Section 508 is only required for federal agencies (Ostergaard 2015). Many countries have some legislation that makes it illegal to discriminate against people with disabilities, such as the Equality Act 2010 in the United Kingdom, the Disability Discrimination Act of 1992 in Australia, and the Human Rights Act of 1977 in Canada. The laws generally don't specify technical standards for web accessibility, which change quickly, so many countries are using the Web Content Accessibility Guidelines (WCAG) 2.0, developed by the World Wide Web Consortium (Henry 2017).

In the United States, Section 508 has not been updated since 2000, and some feel the "checkpoints show their age" (McHale 2011, 156). Consequently, many institutions and libraries are using WCAG 2.0 guidelines instead. WCAG 2.0 has twelve guidelines organized into four principles: *perceivable*, *operable*, *understandable*, and *robust*. Each of the twelve guidelines are divided into testable success criteria for the graded levels of WCAG 2.0 compliance: A, AA, and AAA (Abou-Zahra 2012). Although it was published several years ago, an article published in the *Journal of Web Librarianship* provides a thorough overview of and more information about these two standards (McHale 2011).

Typical accessibility issues that exist for electronic resources and collections are the same problems found in other EIT. Users with various disabilities will encounter different barriers or experience accessibility issues differently. Common problems experienced by those with auditory, cognitive/neurological, physical, speech, and visual disabilities include, but are not limited to, audio content without captions and/or transcripts, audio without adjustable volume or that cannot be turned off, page content that cannot be resized or zoomed in and out, images and controls lacking alternative text, insufficient color contrast, sites that do not provide full keyboard support or do not allow users to only use the keyboard, inconsistent and complex navigation, content and tables without structure and headings, inaccessible forms or form fields, and no alternative formats or files provided for inaccessible content. Many people with disabilities use assistive technologies like screen readers, screen magnifiers, assistive listening devices, voice recognition, trackballs, and touch pads. In order for these assistive technologies to work well, it is critical that electronic resources are free of the barriers described above. The W3C's Web Accessibility Initiative provides an extensive list of barriers experienced by people with various disabilities (Abou-Zahra 2012).

Vendors sometimes make the argument that concerns about the accessibility of health sciences library products are irrelevant because health professionals and health professional students do not have disabilities. This is a misconception. Laws such as the ADA and the Rehabilitation Act in the United States bar schools from discriminating against students with disabilities. Recent court rulings, in fact, have ruled in favor of students with disabilities against medical schools, affirming that assistive technologies in many instances can be used and that medical schools must accommodate them (New 2014). Furthermore, many cognitive and learning disabilities are deemed "invisible disabilities," and other disabilities can be temporary. Medical students, for instance, may have dyslexia or ADHD and use assistive technologies like screen readers or text-to-speech, and they are not required to disclose these disabilities to their schools. And anyone could suddenly break an arm or wrist, becoming temporarily unable to use a mouse or keyboard and requiring assistive technology to access and read course or research materials. While many medical schools, for example, have a very low percentage of students with disabilities and do need to do much better at providing accommodations for students with disabilities, it has been suggested that training more doctors with disabilities will result in better care for patients with disabilities and that medical schools need to take more seriously this aspect of diversity (Zazove et al. 2016). Resources have been published to assist health professional schools in accomplishing this goal (Meeks and Jain 2016). Health sciences libraries, especially those supporting education, have an opportunity to show leadership in this area at their institutions.

Accessibility and Collections

There is not an overabundance of literature on the accessibility of library collections and library e-resources, which indicates more research and investigation in this area is needed. In a content analysis of disability and accessibility in the library and information science literature, Heather Hill found that, of 198 articles from 2000 to 2010, 25 percent examined accessibility as it related to electronic resources, but only 3 percent of the articles were focused on the general theme of "collections." These articles included recommendations for selection and building of accessible collections (Hill 2013).

A few studies have examined the accessibility of e-resources. In one, twelve vendors answered a survey about the accessibility of their databases, Section 508 compliance, and whether their companies conduct accessibility/ usability testing (Byerley, Chambers, and Thohira 2007). While all indicated they followed accessibility guidelines, and eleven out of twelve rated their resources at a four out of five for accessibility, the authors found that the majority of vendors reported they were not fully compliant with various 508 standards, only five of the twelve vendors indicated they had users with disabilities test their products, and none of the vendors addressed accessibility in their marketing efforts. In a 2010 study examining the accessibility of thirty-two library databases (including health sciences databases like PubMed, CINAHL, and CANCERLIT), authors found that twenty-five of thirty-two, or 78 percent, were "marginally accessible" or "completely inaccessible" when compared against an accessibility checklist (Tatomir and Durrance 2010). Another study, in 2011, had ten students use screen readers to complete basic tasks in three library databases, and authors found that, when students were unable to complete a task, nearly one-third of the time it was due to accessibility problems (Dermody and Majekodunmi 2011). Finally, in 2015, the accessibility of the PDFs from four journal publishers was examined against eleven standard PDF accessibility criteria, and significant and prevalent accessibility issues were found. None had consistent heading structure, none displayed titles when a PDF document was open, none had a tab order that followed the document structure, only 3 percent featured images with alternative text (a word or phrase that describes the contents of an image or visual element), and only 4.5 percent were tagged (Nganji 2015).

The news about the accessibility of library resources may seem grim, but libraries have begun to be more proactive about insisting that vendors work on the accessibility of their products. Many libraries have been or are beginning to request Voluntary Product Accessibility Templates (VPATs) from vendors and publishers in order to determine how compliant an e-resource may be with Section 508. A library vendor VPAT repository is available through the Libraries for Universal Accessibility (LUA) website (Libraries for Universal Accessibility 2017). Although VPATs provide vendors with an opportunity to accurately describe and disclose where their products are or are not meeting Section 508 criteria, it is well known in the accessibility community that VPATs are often inaccurate. One study examined 189 line items from seventeen vendor VPATs by comparing what the vendors reported to the findings of an automated accessibility scanner. Many common accessibility barriers were identified. In thirty-seven instances where vendors stated "not applicable" or "fully compliant," the scanner found compliance issues, indicating an inaccuracy rate of 19.6 percent (Delancey 2015). Nine of seventeen vendors stated they were fully compliant with alternative text, but the scanner found problems with fourteen of them.

Libraries interested in best practices and practical tips for building accessible collections have a few good resources and examples to consult. In a broader chapter on adaptive design and assistive technology in libraries, Tatomir and Tatomir suggest using an accessibility checklist during purchasing, requiring library vendors to submit VPATs, ensuring library website navigation to e-resources meets usability and accessibility standards, checking metasearch tools like federated searches and discovery layers for accessibility, and possibly creating or pointing to mobile apps that are more accessible (Tatomir and Tatomir 2012). Kirsten Ostergaard from Montana State University provides five strategies to help academic libraries acquire accessible electronic information resources (Ostergaard 2015). These include connecting with university administration and disability service offices to learn about accessibility on campus, modifying collection development policies to include accessibility language (or creating a general library accessibility statement that addresses collections), communicating and negotiating with vendors about accessibility, documenting communication from vendors regarding accessibility, and designating a library liaison to one's institutional disability services office. A detailed description of the Michigan State University Libraries' implementation of accessibility purchasing procedures for library e-resources and collections is described in the story following this chapter.

CONCLUSION

Many librarians have only just begun to think about the issues of usability and accessibility of their collections, and, with collections made up of so many resources from so many different vendors, they can find it daunting to know where to begin. Health sciences librarians wishing to understand more about the usability of their collections may need to "start small," conducting some testing as time and resources allow, and partnering with user experience librarians and others at their institutions with such specialties. Health sciences librarians wishing to investigate and improve the accessibility of their collections are encouraged not to let the "perfect be the enemy of the good" but to start by looking over the resources in the literature and resources available to them such as their institution's disability services offices. Being mindful of library values and the great impact libraries can have can help librarians continue to strive for resources and collections that are usable and accessible to all library patrons.

REFERENCES

Abou-Zahra, Shadi. 2012. "How People with Disabilities Use the Web: Diversity of Web Users (draft)." W3C Web Accessibility Initiative. Last Modified August 1, 2012. https://www.w3.org/WAI/intro/people-use-web/diversity.

AccessibleTech.org. 2017. "What Is Accessible Electronic and Information Technology?" ADA National Network. Accessed March 13. http://accessibletech.org/access_articles/general/whatIsAccessibleEIT.php.

Ascher, Marie T., Haldor Lougee-Heimer, and Diana J. Cunningham. 2007. "Approaching Usability: A Study of an Academic Health Sciences Library Web Site." *Medical Reference Services Quarterly* 26 (2): 37–52. doi:10.1300/J115v26n02_04.

BBC (British Broadcasting Corporation). 2014. "My Web My Way: What Is Accessibility?" British Broadcasting Corporation. http://www.bbc.co.uk/accessibility/best_practice/what_is.shtml.

Be. Accessible. 2017. "What Is Accessibility?" Be. Accessible. Accessed March 13. http://www.beaccessible.org.nz/the-movement/what-is-accessibility.

Bell, Steven J. 2014. "Staying True to the Core: Designing the Future Academic Library Experience." *portal: Libraries and the Academy* 14 (3): 369–82. doi:10.1353/pla.2014.0021.

Byerley, Suzanne L., Mary Beth Chambers, and Mariyam Thohira. 2007. "Accessibility of Web-Based Library Databases: The Vendors' Perspectives in 2007." *Library Hi Tech* 25 (4): 509–27. doi:10.1108/07378830710840473.

Cho, S., Je Hyeok, L., Il Kon, K., Min Gyu, K., Kim Young, S., & Eunjoo, L. (2016). The educational and supportive mobile application for caregivers of dementia people. *Studies In Health Technology & Informatics*, 2251045-1046. doi:10.3233/978-1-61499-658-3-1045

Delancey, Laura. 2015. "Assessing the Accuracy of Vendor-Supplied Accessibility Documentation." *Library Hi Tech* 33 (1): 103–13. doi:10.1108/LHT-08-2014-0077.

Dermody, Kelly, and Norda Majekodunmi. 2011. "Online Databases and the Research Experience for University Students with Print Disabilities." *Library Hi Tech* 29 (1): 149–60. doi:10.1108/07378831111116976.

Garcia-Zapirain, Begona, Isabel de la Torre Diez, Beatriz Sainz de Abajo, and Miguel Lopez-Coronado. 2016. "Development, Technical, and User Evaluation of a Web Mobile Application for Self-Control of Diabetes." *Telemedicine Journal and e-Health: The Official Journal of the American Telemedicine Association* 22 (9): 778–85. doi:10.1089/tmj.2015.0233.

Henry, Shawn Lawton. 2017. "Web Content Accessibility Guidelines (WCAG) Overview." W3C Web Accessibility Initiative. Last Modified March 10. https://www.w3.org/WAI/intro/wcag.php.

Hill, Heather. 2013. "Disability and Accessibility in the Library and Information Science Literature: A Content Analysis." *Library & Information Science Research* 35 (2) :137–42. doi:10.1016/j.lisr.2012.11.002.

Howe, Carol D. 2011. "Point-of-Care Healthcare Databases Are an Overall Asset to Clinicians, but Different Databases May Vary in Usefulness Based on Personal Preferences." *Evidence Based Library & Information Practice* 6 (4): 152–54.

Jonassaint, Charles R., Nirmish Shah, Jude Jonassaint, and Laura De Castro. 2015. "Usability and Feasibility of an mHealth Intervention for Monitoring and Managing Pain Symptoms in Sickle Cell Disease: The Sickle Cell Disease Mobile Application to Record Symptoms via Technology (SMART)." *Hemoglobin* 39 (3): 162–68. doi:10.3109/03630269.2015.1025141.

Kortum, Philip, and S. Camille Peres. 2015. "Evaluation of Home Health Care Devices: Remote Usability Assessment." *JMIR Human Factors* 2 (1): e10. doi:10.2196/humanfactors.4570.

Libraries for Universal Accessibility. 2017. "VPAT Repository." Libraries for Universal Accessibility. Accessed March 13. http://uniaccessig.org/lua/vpat-repository/.

Lyles, C. R., U. Sarkar, and C. Y. Osborn. 2014. "Getting a Technology-Based Diabetes Intervention Ready for Prime Time: A Review of Usability Testing Studies." *Current Diabetes Reports* 14 (10): 534–39. doi:10.1007/s11892-014-0534-9.

McHale, Nina. 2011. "An Introduction to Web Accessibility, Web Standards, and Web Standards Makers." *Journal of Web Librarianship* 5 (2): 152–60. doi:10.1080/19322909.2011.572434.

McKay, Fiona H., Christina Cheng, Annemarie Wright, Jane Shill, Hugh Stephens, and Mary Uccellini. 2016. "Evaluating Mobile Phone Applications for Health Behaviour Change: A Systematic Review." *Journal of Telemedicine and Telecare*. doi:10.1177/1357633x16673538.

Meeks, Lisa M., and Neera R. Jain, eds. 2016. *The Guide to Assisting Students with Disabilities: Equal Access in Health Sciences and Professional Education.* New York: Springer Publishing Company.

New, Jake. 2014. "Fighting Their Way into Medical School." *Inside Higher Ed*, July 28. https://www.insidehighered.com/news/2014/07/28/judge-orders-medical-college-accommodate-deaf-student.

Nganji, Julius T. 2015. "The Portable Document Format (PDF) Accessibility Practice of Four Journal Publishers." *Library & Information Science Research* 37 (3): 254–62. doi:10.1016/j.lisr.2015.02.002.

Nielsen, Jakob. 2012. "Usability 101: Introduction to Usability." Nielsen Norman Group. https://www.nngroup.com/articles/usability-101-introduction-to-usability/.

Nitsch, M., C. N. Dimopoulos, E. Flaschberger, K. Saffran, J. F. Kruger, L. Garlock, D. E. Wilfley, C. B. Taylor, and M. Jones. 2016. "A Guided Online and Mobile Self-Help Program for Individuals with Eating Disorders: An Iterative Engagement and Usability Study." *Journal of Medical Internet Research* 18 (1): e7. doi:10.2196/jmir.4972.

Office for Civil Rights (OCR). 2014. "Resolution Agreement." U. S. Department of Education Office for Civil Rights. http://umt.edu/accessibility/docs/FinalResolutionAgreement.pdf.

Ostergaard, Kirsten. 2015. "Accessibility from Scratch: One Library's Journey to Prioritize the Accessibility of Electronic Information Resources." *Serials Librarian* 69 (2): 155–68. doi:10.1080/0361526X.2015.1069777.

Ratwani, Raj M., A. Zachary Hettinger, and Rollin J. Fairbanks. 2017. "Barriers to comparing the usability of electronic health records." *Journal of the American Medical Informatics Association* 24 (e1): e191-e193 doi:10.1093/jamia/ocw117.

Rosario, Jovy-Anne , Marie T. Ascher, and Diana J. Cunningham. 2012. "A Study in Usability: Redesigning a Health Sciences Library's Mobile Site." *Medical Reference Services Quarterly* 31 (1): 1–13. doi:10.1080/02763869.2012.641481.

Schwartz, Ezra. 2004. "The Iceberg Problem—Is the Investment in Our Collections Visible to Patrons?" *Against the Grain* 16 (6): 28–32. doi:10.7771/2380-176X.4436.

Shurtz, Suzanne, and Margaret J. Foster. 2011. "Developing and Using a Rubric for Evaluating Evidence-Based Medicine Point-of-Care Tools." *Journal of the Medical Library Association* 99 (3): 247–54.

Tatomir, Jennifer, and Joan C. Durrance. 2010. "Overcoming the Information Gap: Measuring the Accessibility of Library Databases to Adaptive Technology Users." *Library Hi Tech* 28 (4): 577–94. doi:10.1108/07378831011096240.

Tatomir, Jennifer N., and Joanna C. Tatomir. 2012. "Collection Accessibility: A Best Practices Guide for Libraries and Librarians." *Library Technology Reports* 48 (7): 36–42.

United States Department of Health and Human Services. 2016. "Usability Evaluation Basics." U.S. Department of Health and Human Services. Accessed October 14. https://www.usability.gov/what-and-why/usability-evaluation.html.

United States Department of Justice Civil Rights Division. 2017. "Introduction to the ADA." United States Department of Justice. Accessed March 13. https://www.ada.gov/ada_intro.htm.

Yeh, Shea-Tinn, and Cathalina Fontenelle. 2012. "Usability Study of a Mobile Website: The Health Sciences Library, University of Colorado Anschutz Medical Campus, Experience." *Journal of the Medical Library Association* 100 (1): 64–68. doi:10.3163/1536-5050.100.1.012.

Zazove, Philip, Benjamin Case, Christopher Moreland, Melissa A. Plegue, Anne Hoekstra, Alicia Ouellette, Ananda Sen, and Michael D. Fetters. 2016. "U.S. Medical Schools' Compliance with the Americans with Disabilities Act: Findings from a National Study." *Academic Medicine* 91 (7): 979–86. doi:10.1097/ACM.0000000000001087.

One Library's Story

Developing Accessibility Purchasing Procedures for
Electronic Resources at the
Michigan State University Libraries

Heidi M. Schroeder

The Michigan State University Libraries consist primarily of a main library and one business branch library located on the campus in East Lansing, Michigan, and serve the entire university, including two medical schools, a veterinary school, a nursing school, public health program, biomedical research programs, and allied health programs. One result of consolidating almost all the collections, services, and librarians into one building is that policies and procedures for decision making about collections, for instance, are easily implemented across all subject areas uniformly. In 2008, Michigan State University implemented a web accessibility policy, and, in 2015, it incorporated accessibility into its electronic information technology (EIT) purchasing procedures. It became clear to librarians that the accessibility of library materials was an important aspect of this university-wide effort, and that we needed to be better informed about the accessibility of the online materials we were purchasing. Buying inaccessible library e-resources puts our institution at risk for lawsuits and complaints, results in acquiring resources we know users with disabilities cannot use, and, for those of us testing and remediating inaccessible e-resources, costs us time, money, and resources. Because we decided that trying to improve the accessibility of our electronic collections is not only the right thing to do but also fits with the libraries' mission and accessibility statement, we began to take the accessibility of our collections very seriously. In the fall of 2015 a librarian was assigned to be the accessibility coordinator for the library to develop accessibility purchasing procedures for electronic resources that closely align with the university's central accessibility policies and culture. We intended for these procedures to be implemented immediately for all new e-resources and implemented over the span of five years for existing e-resources. Because it would be impossible to tackle this project with thousands of vendors at one time, we decided to prioritize the largest vendors, such as Elsevier, EBSCO, and Wiley, because content from them affects the widest variety of our library users. In later years, we will focus efforts on smaller vendors. The procedures we have developed are divided into five steps.

Our first step was to ask vendors for accessibility contacts. By getting the names of accessibility staff, if they exist, we know who the best person/team is to contact if we have questions or want to provide feedback. This question also gives us insight into how dedicated to and knowledgeable about accessibility a vendor might be. For example, if companies have staff dedicated to accessibility, we interpret this to mean they might already be working on and addressing accessibility. In most cases, vendors have referred us to generic technical or customer support email addresses. A few vendors have referred us to their user experience teams, and even fewer have referred us to specific accessibility staff. Some of these contacts and teams have been more knowledgeable and proactive about accessibility than others.

Our second step was to request accessibility documentation. Specifically, we started asking vendors for Voluntary Product Accessibility Templates (VPATs), which document compliance against Section 508 of the Rehabilitation Act, and WCAG 2.0 documentation since MSU as an institution is striving for WCAG 2.0 AA compliance (for more information on this standard, see chapter 7). We have found that asking for this documentation is a good first step in starting accessibility conversations with vendors. We are also looking at and documenting public-facing accessibility web pages and sections of FAQs. Vendors who have this information readily available are indicating at least a minimal awareness of accessibility, which is encouraging. So far, it has been our experience that most major vendors have VPATs; fewer have WCAG 2.0 documentation. We are also evaluating some aspects of vendor VPATs in house, as it is common knowledge in the accessibility community that VPATs are often filled out incorrectly or inaccurately.

Thirdly, we began requesting that vendors insert accessibility language into or as an addendum to our licenses. To draft our proposed language, we used model language from the Center for Research Libraries, Association for Research Libraries, and other libraries that already had accessibility license language. We also received feedback from our university's general counsel. Our proposed language, which is the same as what the Big Ten Academic Alliance has adopted (www.btaa.org/docs/default-source/library/clistandar dizedagreementlanguage.pdf?sfvrsn=32), specifically mentions WCAG 2.0 AA and VPATs/Section 508. It also includes a sentence that attempts to make the vendor, not the library, responsible for timely remediation of inaccessible materials.

Fourthly, we have developed several methods for testing the accessibility of our electronic resources, including databases, e-books, and electronic journals. The library has been able to partner with another unit on our campus called Usability/Accessibility Research and Consulting (UARC) that provides, among other services, preliminary accessibility reports against WCAG 2.0 AA. We pay for these reviews, and the funding for these comes out of the collection budget, but the preliminary reports are ours to send to vendors. The libraries' accessibility coordinator and student accessibility employees also do some informal internal testing, although we do not have the robust training and knowledge that UARC's staff has. Finally, MSU has a central Accessibility Review Committee, which has completed accessibility testing of some of the major e-resources that go through central purchasing (our integrated library system from Innovative, LibGuides, and our interlibrary loan system, ILLIad). While the results of all of our testing have varied widely, all of our resources have had some accessibility problems like poor color contrast, lack or improper use of headings, problems with reading order, inaccessible image-based PDFs, images without alternative text, and the inability to tab through content. For several library e-resources, issues with PDF and image files, as opposed to interfaces, have been more serious and prevalent, especially for resources that contain historical content.

Finally, we are starting to carefully document information gathered from the previous steps and provide feedback to vendors. Communicating problems that we find with vendors is a very important step to encourage them to improve accessibility. Most of these conversations have been positive, although some vendors have been unresponsive to our inquiries or confused about our feedback and the topic of accessibility in general. UARC reports have been especially useful to pass along to vendors. They are purely factual (comparing the platform and content against WCAG 2.0 AA) and are coming from a "third party," which feels more objective.

Applying these procedures has been challenging and time consuming. We have found that while most vendors we have talked with are familiar with accessibility and also say that it is important, many do not seem to be putting adequate resources toward making sure their products comply with standards, nor are they incorporating accessibility concerns into discussions when they acquire third-party content. If this is the case for the large publishers and vendors we have started with, we suspect we will find smaller vendors, like society publishers, even less prepared for these discussions when we get to them. While we have high standards, we also have realistic expectations and must continue purchasing materials that are not yet fully accessible, especially if they are important for teaching, research, and learning. We have occasionally delayed purchasing e-resources to put some pressure on vendors to either improve accessibility or communicate how they plan to address issues in the future. We have also committed to the possibility of not purchasing some resources that have serious accessibility problems and to re-evaluating our standing orders with vendors that have not followed through on promises to fix problems. We have not yet canceled existing resources that have accessibility issues, but we might take such action in the future if vendors do not improve or help us remediate inaccessible content. We do not think our library is unique in having a wish list that is longer than the list of things we can afford, and we would like to reward vendors that create access-ible content.

While we coordinate accessibility testing, licensing modifications, and communication with vendors on a library-wide basis, we have also tried to keep individual subject specialists and collection managers apprised of our progress and our timeline with regular informational sessions. Most selectors will not be able to learn about every aspect of accessibility, but everyone has been able to learn about some basics so that they can be partners in the process. For instance, when looking at a new platform for streaming video content, selectors now know to check whether videos are closed captioned and have transcripts available. Since most new e-resource purchases are go-ing through our procedures, selectors have been concerned about delays or whether they would not be allowed to buy something that was needed. Com-munication has been key to making decisions cooperative and involving selectors in deciding when a delay or decision not to purchase makes sense.

We have seen in the past that it often takes many voices to convince vendors that a concern is important. We and others fought for archival, preservation, and interlibrary loan rights in our licenses and have largely been successful, at least with major publishers. Accessibility is more difficult because it requires vendors and publishers to make changes to their platforms and content, not just to their licenses. However, it is likely that we are on the cusp of accessibility becoming a much more common discussion, and that we will see many changes in the near future, making libraries' work in this area much easier, and, more importantly, resulting in e-resources that *all* of our library patrons can use.

Chapter Eight

Data in the Library

Considerations for Collection Development Policy and Practice

Lisa Federer

Libraries of the twenty-first century are often in the position to deal with problems and challenges that would have been unimaginable to librarians fifty, twenty, or even ten years ago. The increasingly rapid pace of technological advances has influenced the ways that people access, use, and interact with information in transformative ways. The influence of technology on information behaviors is especially evident in the sciences, where research practices have evolved substantively in the last several decades. As a result, the information needs of practicing researchers have changed, as have the learning outcomes and educational needs of students at all levels in these fields.

As information technology evolves, libraries must adapt their collection development policies and practices to ensure that they are acquiring materials that support their users' needs in terms of both subject matter and format. Many academic and research libraries have begun to think about how they will handle adding data resources to their collections. This chapter will discuss the rationale for developing a data collection development policy and explore existing data collection development policies at various institutions, as well as consider alternative methods for making data available to users.

TYPES OF DATA HEALTH SCIENCES LIBRARIES COLLECT

The term "data" can encompass many substantively different types of information. Philosopher of science Sabina Leonelli defines data as "a relational category applied to research outputs that are taken, at specific moments of inquiry, to provide evidence for knowledge claims of interest to the researchers involved" (Leonelli 2015). Given that research communities rely on many different types of evidence, what constitutes data may vary widely across disciplines and may include a broad range of topics and formats. Numeric data and statistics may come to mind most readily, but research data can also include texts, images, audio, video, and more.

Though the term "data" resists easy definition, many types of data fall within the scope of health sciences libraries' collections, including demographic and salary data on health practitioners, benchmarking data for universities or hospitals, scientific research data, public health data, and market research data. The types of data that different health sciences libraries collect will depend on their institution's mission and their users' interests and needs. In some cases, data are freely available, but in other cases, the data are proprietary and require one-time purchase or an ongoing subscription. Health sciences libraries supporting academic or research institutions may also host institutional repositories, collecting and preserving local data produced by researchers at the institution. In those cases, the library acts as both a publisher of the data and the repository of a unique collection, and special collection policies may govern the collection and preservation of that data.

Data have of course played an important role as the raw material of science since long before our current era of data-intensive science. However, researchers today can often make meaningful discoveries without ever having to gather their own data, simply by utilizing existing data resources. For example, using existing data, researchers have been able to discover new indications for previously developed drugs, thus potentially uncovering new disease treatments (Molineris et al. 2013; Sirota et al. 2011). Existing data sets also play an important role in developing algorithms and other methods that advance computational science. Machine-learning methods, for example, can help researchers uncover previously unnoticed patterns (Ashinsky et al. 2015) and make predictions (Hu et al. 2016), and some types of machine-learning algorithms rely on existing data to "train" the model and validate its performance (Alpaydin 2014).

Given the central role of data in the research enterprise, educators who are training the next generation of researchers must consider how to prepare students to work with data. Indeed, training in the effective use of data has come to be considered crucial across a variety of scientific fields (Grisham et al. 2016; Purawat et al. 2016; Westra et al. 2015). For librarian educators as well, data can play an important role in the training mission of the library. It has long been considered the purview of the librarian to teach information literacy, the set of skills needed to effectively locate and use information; likewise, many librarians have begun to extend this type of instruction to include data literacy (Schield 2004), sometimes termed data information literacy (Carlson et al. 2011).

DATA COLLECTION DEVELOPMENT POLICIES

A review of publicly available collection development policies reveals that libraries have a range of approaches for how they handle collecting data—if in fact they collect it at all. Some libraries, like Northern Illinois University Libraries, mention data and data sets in their overall collection development policy (2017). However, these general policies do not delineate practices or issues specific to the collection of data; rather, data are mentioned simply as a format that may be included in the collection. Other libraries do not mention data in their collection policies, perhaps because they do not consider data within the purview of their collection.

Even for libraries that do collect data, having a written collection development policy regarding data may not always be advantageous or even desirable. Some of the limitations of traditional collection development policies—their "inflexibility" and "unresponsiveness to changes that occur in the college or university"—are perhaps even more applicable with regard to data (Snow 1996, 192). However, in libraries that plan to collect data, having a clearly defined policy that specifies exactly what falls within the scope of the collection and what does not can help librarians determine what to acquire, exclude, and deselect. While libraries do not generally face limitations in terms of *physical* space they can devote to collecting data, items in digital collections still compete against each other for a limited set of resources and budget. Some data do not have adequate future value to merit retaining them on an ongoing basis (Kung and Campbell 2016), while other data may not be relevant to a specific library's collection. A successful collection development policy will give librarians specific guidelines about how to make this type of decision.

As of this writing, a handful of libraries have a publicly available collection development policy specific to data. The policies considered here come from several different types of academic libraries, from small liberal arts colleges to Ivy League research institutions:

- Brown University Library
- Columbia University Libraries
- Georgetown University Library
- James Madison University Libraries and Educational Technologies
- Laurence McKinley Gould Library (Carleton College)
- Michigan State University Libraries
- Penn State University Libraries

- University of California, Santa Barbara, Libraries
- University of Ontario Institute of Technology Library
- Yale University Library

The varying approaches these libraries take to collecting data reflect their diverse user populations and different priorities, but their policies include a number of common themes. While some of these libraries do not specifically serve the health sciences, considering their collection policies can still be instructive for health sciences librarians since some of the issues addressed in these policies apply universally to all types of data.

SCOPE AND FORMATS OF DATA COLLECTED

Many libraries' policies include a statement about the scope of data to be collected, which in many cases mirrors the scope considerations in a more traditional collection development statement, such as what subject areas will be collected. Some policies address language and geographical focus (Michigan State University Libraries 2014; Penn State University Libraries 2005; University of California, Santa Barbara, Library 2015; Yale University Library 2014), though making such determinations in terms of data may require different ways of thinking about scope. For example, rather than specify that resources must be in English, Yale's policy states that they should "generally be usable by English-language readers," which could include data that contain some "non-translated components" but contain "English-language labels" (Yale University Library 2014).

In terms of chronological focus, many policies specify that the library will collect not only current materials but also historic materials of relevance—provided they exist in a format that is still accessible using modern equipment (James Madison University Libraries and Educational Technologies 2011; Michigan State University Libraries 2014; Penn State University Libraries 2005; University of California, Santa Barbara, Library 2015; University of Ontario Institute of Technology Library 2016; Cornell University Library 2014). Perhaps a more meaningful way to talk about timeliness of data, at least regarding scientific and biomedical data, would be to address the data's currency, or its continuing relevance (University of Ontario Institute of Technology Library 2016). As scientific standards and technologies change, once-useful data can become out of date and insufficient for modern research purposes. For example, DNA-sequencing technologies have undergone dramatic advances over the last several decades (Heather and Chain 2016). Next-generation sequencing (NGS) technologies developed within the last ten years have made it possible to read longer sections of the genome and have facilitated better understanding of the complexity of the genome (Goodwin, McPherson, and McCombie 2016). As a result, data that were once considered state of the art may be completely irrelevant by today's more precise standards.

Data format is another pressing consideration of scope that many libraries address in their policies (Brown University Library 2010; Georgetown University Library 2016; Laurence McKinley Gould Library 2015; Michigan State University Libraries 2014; University of California, Santa Barbara, Library 2015; Yale University Library 2014). Some data are saved in file formats that require specific software to view or analyze; libraries may choose to exclude data saved in formats that are obscure or that cannot be opened using software that the institution can support. Some policies refer to formats that can be read by common statistical software packages (Georgetown University Library 2016; University of California, Santa Barbara, Library 2015) while the Michigan State University Library states a preference for "a proprietary-agnostic format" that can be opened by many different types of software, rather than being limited to a particular program (2014). Even for institutions that do have access to proprietary software, data saved in proprietary formats can be rendered unusable if that software becomes obsolete over time. Even if a program is still available, newer versions of the software may not be backward compatible, meaning that the new version might not be able to open an older file created with a previous version of the same software (Cornell University Library 2014). For example, newer versions of the popular statistical package SPSS are often not backward compatible for certain file types, so care must be taken to ensure that data sets are saved in the correct format or that the relevant version of the software is maintained, along with a computer running an operating system that is likewise compatible with this older software (IBM Support 2016).

Physical format can also be a concern worth addressing in a collection development policy, particularly regarding format obsolescence (Xie and Matusiak 2016). Though most policies considered here call for data to be made available via network or web access, some also refer to data saved on physical media that may be circulated to users or made available in person at the library (Columbia University Libraries 2016; Michigan State University Libraries 2014; Penn State University Libraries 2005; University of California, Santa Barbara, Library 2015; Yale University Library 2014). While the practice of referring to physical formats is common among the policies reviewed here, including this type of detail may necessitate more frequent updating of the policy as certain formats become obsolete. For example, several policies refer to data on CD-ROM, a physical format quickly approaching obsolescence (Columbia University Libraries 2016; Michigan State University Libraries 2014; University of California, Santa Barbara, Library 2015; Yale University Library 2014), and some even mention floppy discs (Columbia University Libraries 2016) and microfiche formats (Penn

State University Libraries 2005), which, by most accounts, are now obsolete. Libraries that do continue to collect and retain data in these formats should consider how to ensure ongoing access to the data after the physical media become obsolete. For example, laptop computers sold today often do not have a CD-ROM drive, so many users with newer computers would not be able to access a data set that circulates on a CD-ROM; Brown University's policy therefore specifies that it will keep computers with drives available for users who need to access these data (Brown University Library 2010).

DATA QUALITY AND DOCUMENTATION

Most of the policies make some reference to data quality, which in many cases refers to the character of the data, including their accuracy, level of documentation, and the like, but can also be understood to mean its integrity, such as whether the file is still readable or has become corrupted or otherwise inaccessible (James Madison University Libraries and Educational Technologies 2011; Michigan State University Libraries 2014; University of California, Santa Barbara, Library 2015; University of Ontario Institute of Technology Library 2016; Yale University Library 2014). In either definition, addressing data quality involves taking steps to ensure that users will have continuous access to authoritative, clearly understandable data.

The saying "garbage in, garbage out" applies to data-driven research and data reuse in its many forms; poor-quality data will invariably produce inaccurate or incomplete results. The *Bad Data Handbook* outlines "the four Cs of data quality analysis," a set of general criteria for assessing the quality of data: good data are Complete, Coherent, Correct, and aCcountable (McCallum 2012). These criteria can also serve as guidelines for assessing the quality of data for the purposes of collection decisions, and indeed, many of the policies considered here include these or similar criteria. Data sets that are *complete* include not only all data necessary to effectively make the data set suitable for use and analysis but also all documentation that would be needed to completely understand the data, including codebooks and metadata (Brown University Library 2010; Georgetown University Library 2016; Michigan State University Libraries 2014; University of California, Santa Barbara, Library 2015; University of Ontario Institute of Technology Library 2016; Yale University Library 2014). Assessing whether data are *coherent* involves considering whether a data set has internal consistency, and may be a task best suited to a subject matter expert or a librarian with expertise in evaluating data. Assuring that data are *correct*—or accurate, as is more frequently used in the policies considered here (Laurence McKinley Gould Library 2015; University of Ontario Institute of Technology Library 2016)— may also be a task best suited to a subject matter expert. Working with vendors or data producers who have a reputation for producing high-quality data sets can help libraries trust that data are accurate (Laurence McKinley Gould Library 2015; University of California, Santa Barbara, Library 2015; University of Ontario Institute of Technology Library 2016). Finally, an authoritative source should be *accountable* for a data set; in terms of library data collections, this accountability can mean that a vendor or data producer is available to provide support or respond to questions about the data set (James Madison University Libraries and Educational Technologies 2011; Laurence McKinley Gould Library 2015; University of Ontario Institute of Technology Library 2016).

Even with data that meet these criteria for quality, the problem of data integrity can raise serious ongoing concerns; after all, if libraries are going to invest in data, they should try to ensure that the collection remains accessible and in good condition. Though data are not subject to the same damage as physical items through overuse and simple wear and tear, data can suffer a similar fate in the form of data degradation, often called "data rot." Data are often stored on physical media like hard drives or other discs, which are subject to physical damage and deterioration over time. Even the best cared-for drives will eventually fail, though some media have a longer life span than others (Mike Wirth Art 2016). Fortunately, unlike their physical collection counterparts, data can generally be duplicated with ease (except when license terms prohibit doing so) and multiple copies stored on separate drives, so that data are not entirely lost in the event of catastrophic drive failure or damage. For example, Brown University Library's policy details how their Social Sciences Data Center maintains multiple copies of data in different locations, a good practice in general and even more important when the original data are stored on fragile media like floppy discs and CDs (2010).

CONFIDENTIALITY AND LICENSING RESTRICTIONS

Data that are considered sensitive may come with licensing requirements that detail how and where they are stored and may require that users apply for access; fulfilling these obligations may be difficult for libraries. Accordingly, some policies specify that the library will not collect data that are considered confidential or restricted (Columbia University Libraries 2016; University of California, Santa Barbara, Library 2015; Yale University Library 2014). Even when data are not considered sensitive or confidential, data providers sometimes set licensing restrictions that limit how many users may access the data or restrict use to a specific individual or department. Just as most libraries would likely not purchase a book if its use were to be restricted to just one researcher, many of the policies considered here exclude data with usage restrictions, specifying that the data must be available to all of the institution's students, staff, and faculty (Laurence McKinley Gould Library 2015; Michigan State University Libraries 2014; University of California, Santa Barbara, Library 2015; University of Ontario Institute of Technology Library 2016; Yale University Library 2014). Some policies also state a preference for data whose licensing terms allow not only in-person access but also networked, remote, or off-campus access for authorized users (Laurence McKinley Gould Library 2015; University of California, Santa Barbara, Library 2015; Yale University Library 2014).

OTHER CONSIDERATIONS

The issues discussed here cover a broad range of concerns that are common to many of the publicly available policies that address data, but this list of considerations is not necessarily exhaustive. Libraries may also wish to address other questions when making choices about acquiring a data set or, more broadly, creating a data collection policy:

- What costs are associated with acquiring and maintaining the data set? These costs may include both up-front costs, like licensing fees, and long-term costs, like those associated with maintenance and preservation.
- Are similar data sets available through free or open repositories?
- How relevant are the data to the teaching, research, or clinical activities of the larger institution?
- Who will be responsible for selecting data for acquisition—a subject specialist or liaison librarian, a data librarian, a committee, or someone else?
- What level of support, if any, will the library provide for users wishing to use the data?

ALTERNATIVE APPROACHES

While the policies and procedures described thus far have, to a large extent, mirrored those associated with more traditional collection development, alternative approaches may be more appropriate for some libraries and data types. Some libraries, for example, may lack the technological infrastructure to host and store data locally, funds to invest in purchasing expensive data sets, or staff with appropriate subject matter expertise. Fortunately, libraries do not necessarily have to maintain their own collections to provide access to important data or to facilitate discovery of data that may be freely available.

For libraries that do not wish to maintain their own local data collections, a consortial arrangement can be an effective way of providing access to data to their institution. The Inter-University Consortium for Political and Social

Research (ICPSR), which includes psychological, health care, and other health-related data, is a well-known example of a consortium that provides access to research data for member institutions (ICPSR 2016). By paying an annual fee, member institutions receive access to thousands of research data sets as well as tools for analysis and technical help on how to use the data. Joining a consortium or organization like ICPSR makes it possible for libraries to make authoritative, high-quality data available with minimal effort and little risk.

While many data sets do involve some sort of fee, a great deal of data is available for free through repositories and other open sources, including government agencies and other international organizations. While access to some of these data sets requires permission of the agency, many are easily and freely accessible on the web. A number of institutes within the National Institutes of Health (NIH) support specialized repositories (BMIC 2017), and the National Center for Biotechnology Information (NCBI) at the National Library of Medicine (NLM) also plays an important role in providing access to a wide array of health sciences-related data (NCBI 2016).

In many research disciplines, the last few years have seen a move toward increased acceptance and expectation of data sharing. For example, in their 2015 follow-up to their original 2011 study, Tenopir et al. found that respondents were significantly more willing to both share and reuse data than they had been in the baseline survey (Tenopir et al. 2011, 2015). Many journals, such as the *Nature* and *PLOS* journals, now require authors to share the data that support their findings (SpringerNature 2017; PLOS 2016). Funders have also begun instituting policies that require funded researchers to share their data. These policies do not yet universally apply to all NIH-funded researchers—a variety of policies apply to different types of funding and data (BMIC 2014)—but the general move toward requiring sharing means that more research data are freely available.

Despite the greater availability of freely available data, finding these data sets remains challenging for many researchers; in the absence of a federated search or data index, data can be difficult to locate unless researchers already know exactly where to look. Efforts are also underway to help facilitate data discovery, such as the ongoing development of an NIH-funded "data discovery index" (bioCADDIE 2016) and various other initiatives aimed at making data "FAIR": findable, accessible, interoperable, and reusable (Wilkinson et al. 2016). Even so, libraries can also play an important role in enhancing discoverability by helping to connect their users with data resources that they might otherwise have difficulty locating.

New York University's Health Sciences Library's (NYUHSL) approach provides a useful example of how libraries can connect researchers with data without having to heavily invest in a data collection. They have developed a data catalog that not only allows their users to find data of interest but also to connect with local experts who can provide assistance (Surkis and Read 2016). In addition to indexing publicly available data sets, the catalog also includes internal data sets created by NYU researchers and data sets that individual NYU departments have already licensed and that others can make use of, thus cutting down on duplicate licenses across multiple departments (NYU Health Sciences Library 2016). By adding information on local experts at NYU for many of the indexed data sets, the data catalog also helps facilitate collaborations and highlight the expertise that already exists within the NYU community.

Libraries can also take a less formal approach to pointing their users to data sets by creating curated lists of data resources. Many libraries are making such lists available on their websites or through pages on the popular LibGuides platform. Indeed, a search for "data sets" on the LibGuides Community page, which searches across over half a million public guides, returns over 44,000 results as of this writing (Springshare 2017). Other resources like the Registry of Research Data Repositories (re3data) exist to help users navigate the complex world of freely available data (re3data.org Team 2016).

CONCLUSION

The policies and practices discussed here represent a variety of possible approaches to collecting data in health sciences library settings. Libraries should consider how best to meet the needs of their particular user groups within their technological, budgetary, and staffing constraints. Even in libraries for which a large-scale data collection is out of reach, opportunities exist to help connect users with the data they need to support their research, teaching, and clinical needs.

REFERENCES

Alpaydin, Ethem. 2014. *Introduction to Machine Learning*. 3rd ed. Cambridge, MA: MIT Press.
Ashinsky, Beth G., Christopher E. Coletta, Mustapha Bouhrara, Vanessa A. Lukas, Julianne M. Boyle, David A. Reiter, Corey P. Neu, Ilya G. Goldberg, and Richard G. Spencer. 2015. "Machine Learning Classification of OARSI-Scored Human Articular Cartilage Using Magnetic Resonance Imaging." *Osteoarthritis Cartilage* 23 (10): 1704–12.
bioCADDIE. 2016. "bioCADDIE: biomedical and healthCAre Data Discovery Index Ecosystem." University of California, San Diego, bioCADDIE. Accessed September 28. https://biocaddie.org/about.
BMIC (Trans-NIH BioMedical Informatics Coordinating Committee). 2014. "NIH Data Sharing Policies." National Library of Medicine, National Institutes of Health. Accessed March 18. https://www.nlm.nih.gov/NIHbmic/nih_data_sharing_policies.html.
———. 2017. "NIH Data Sharing Repositories." National Library of Medicine, National Institutes of Health. Accessed March 18. https://www.nlm.nih.gov/NIHbmic/nih_data_sharing_repositories.html.

Brown University Library. 2010. "Social Sciences Data Collection Development Policy." Brown University Library. https://library.brown.edu/about/datacenter/DataCollDevPoli cy_08-20-10.docx.

Carlson, Jake R., Michael Forsmire, Chris Miller, and Megan R. Sapp Nelson. 2011. "Determining Data Information Literacy Needs: A Study of Students and Research Faculty." *Libraries Faculty and Staff Scholarship and Research* (Paper 23):11–34.

Columbia University Libraries. 2016. "Electronic Data Service." Columbia University Libraries. Accessed September 28. http://library.columbia.edu/about/policies/collection-develop ment/format/electronic_data_service.html.

Cornell University Library. 2014. "Obsolescence: File Formats and Software." Cornell University Library. http://www.dpworkshop.org/dpm-eng/oldmedia/obsolescence1.html.

Georgetown University Library. 2016. "Numeric Data and Data Sets: Data Services Policy." Georgetown University Library. Updated July. http://guides.library.georgetown.edu/numer icdata/datapolicy.

Goodwin, Sara, John D. McPherson, and W. Richard McCombie. 2016. "Coming of Age: Ten Years of Next-Generation Sequencing Technologies." *Nature Reviews. Genetics* 17 (6): 333–51. doi:10.1038/nrg.2016.49.

Grisham, William, Barbara Lom, Linda Lanyon, and Raddy L. Ramos. 2016. "Proposed Training to Meet Challenges of Large-Scale Data in Neuroscience." *Frontiers in Neuroinformatics* 10: 28. doi:10.3389/fninf.2016.00028.

Heather, James M., and Benjamin Chain. 2016. "The Sequence of Sequencers: The History of Sequencing DNA." *Genomics* 107 (1): 1–8. doi:10.1016/j.ygeno.2015.11.003.

Hu, Xia, Peter D. Reaven, Aramesh Saremi, Ninghao Liu, Mohammad Ali Abbasi, Huan Liu, and Raymond Q. Migrino. 2016. "Machine Learning to Predict Rapid Progression of Carotid Atherosclerosis in Patients with Impaired Glucose Tolerance." *EURASIP Journal on Bioinformatics & Systems Biology* 2016 (1): 14. doi:10.1186/s13637-016-0049-6.

IBM Support. 2016. "Compatibility of SPSS Files (.sav, .sps, .spv, .spo) between Different Versions." IBM. Accessed September 28. https://www-304.ibm.com/support/doc view.wss?uid=swg21480797.

ICPSR. 2016. "ICPSR." Institute for Social Research, University of Michigan. Accessed September 28. https://www.icpsr.umich.edu/icpsrweb/index.jsp.

James Madison University Libraries and Educational Technologies. 2011. "Data Set Collection Development Policy." James Madison University Libraries and Educational Technologies. https://www.lib.jmu.edu/faculty/datasetcdpolicy.aspx.

Kung, Janice Yu Chen, and Sandy Campbell. 2016. "What Not to Keep: Not All Data Has Future Research Value." *Journal of the Canadian Health Libraries Association / Journal de l'Association des Bibliothèques de la Santé du Canada* 37 (2). doi:10.5596/c16-013.

Laurence McKinley Gould Library. 2015. "Data Collection Policy." Laurence McKinley Gould Library, Carleton College. Updated July. https://apps.carleton.edu/campus/library/assets/ DataCollectionDevelopmentPolicy_2015.pdf.

Leonelli, Sabina. 2015. "What Counts as Scientific Data? A Relational Framework." *Philosophy of Science* 82 (5): 810–21.

McCallum, Q. Ethan. 2012. *Bad Data Handbook: Mapping the World of Data Problems.* Sebastopol, CA: O'Reilly Media, Inc.

Michigan State University Libraries. 2014. "Collection Development Policy Statement: Data Services (Numeric Data)." Michigan State University Libraries. http://libguides.lib.msu.edu/ dataservicescollectiondevpolicy.

Mike Wirth Art. 2016. "The Lifespan of Digital Media." Mike Wirth Art. Accessed September 28, 2016. http://www.mikewirthart.com/projects/the-lifespan-of-storage-media/.

Molineris, Ivan, Ugo Ala, Paolo Provero, and Fernando Di Cunto. 2013. "Strategies and Models for Data Collection Development." International Association for Social Science Information Services and Technology Annual Conference, Cologne, Germany.

NCBI (National Center for Biotechnology Information). 2016. "All Resources." National Center for Biotechnology Information, National Library of Medicine, National Institutes of Health. Accessed September 28. https://www.ncbi.nlm.nih.gov/guide/all/.

Northern Illinois University Libraries. 2017. "Collection Development Policy." Northern Illinois University Libraries. https://library.niu.edu/ulib/content/aboutus/policies/collection-devpolicy.shtml.

NYU Health Sciences Library. 2016. "About the Data Catalog." NYU Health Sciences Library. Accessed September 28. https://datacatalog.med.nyu.edu/about.

Penn State University Libraries. 2005. "Social Science Statistical and Numerical Data Collection Development Statement." Penn State University Libraries. https://libraries.psu.edu/social-science-statistical-and-numerical-data-collection-development-statement.

PLOS. 2016. "Data Availability." PLOS. Accessed September 28. http://journals.plos.org/plosone/s/data-availability.

Purawat, Shweta, Charles Cowart, Rommie E. Amaro, and Ilkay Altintas. 2016. "Biomedical Big Data Training Collaborative (BBDTC): An Effort to Bridge the Talent Gap in Biomedical Science and Research." *Procedia Computer Science* 80: 1791–1800. doi:10.1016/j.procs.2016.05.454.

re3data.org Team. 2016. "re3data.org: Registry of Research Data Repositories." re3data.org. Accessed September 28. http://www.re3data.org/.

Schield, Milo. 2004. "Information Literacy, Statistical Literacy and Data Literacy." *IASSIST Quarterly* 28 (2–3): 6–11.

Sirota, Marina, Joel T. Dudley, Jeewon Kim, Annie P. Chiang, Alex A. Morgan, Alejandro Sweet-Cordero, Julien Sage, and Atul J. Butte. 2011. "Discovery and Preclinical Validation of Drug Indications Using Compendia of Public Gene Expression Data." *Science Translational Medicine* 3 (96): 96ra77. doi:10.1126/scitranslmed.3001318.

Snow, Richard. 1996. "Wasted Words: The Written Collection Development Policy and the Academic Library." *The Journal of Academic Librarianship* 22 (3): 191–94. doi:10.1016/S0099-1333(96)90057-9.

SpringerNature. 2017. "Authors and Referees: Policies—Availability of Data, Material and Methods." Macmillan Publishers, SpringerNature. Accessed May 23. http://www.nature.com/authors/policies/availability.html.

Springshare. 2017. "LibGuides Community." Springshare. Accessed May 23. http://community.libguides.com/.

Surkis, Alisa, and Kevin Read. 2016. "Building Data Management Services at an Academic Medical Center: An Entrepreneurial Approach." In *The Medical Library Association Guide to Data Management for Librarians*, edited by Lisa Federer. Lanham, MD: Rowman & Littlefield.

Tenopir, Carol, Suzie Allard, Kimberly Douglass, Arsev Umur Aydinoglu, Lei Wu, Eleanor Read, Maribeth Manoff, and Mike Frame. 2011. "Data Sharing by Scientists: Practices and Perceptions." *PLoS ONE* 6 (6): e21101. doi:10.1371/journal.pone.0021101.

Tenopir, Carol, Elizabeth D. Dalton, Suzie Allard, Mike Frame, Ivanka Pjesivac, Ben Birch, Danielle Pollock, and Kristina Dorsett. 2015. "Changes in Data Sharing and Data Reuse Practices and Perceptions among Scientists Worldwide." *PLoS ONE* 10 (8): e0134826. doi:10.1371/journal.pone.0134826.

University of California, Santa Barbara, Library. 2015. "Collection Development Policy for Social Science Data." University of California, Santa Barbara, Library. http://www.library.ucsb.edu/collection-development/collection-development-policy-social-science-data.

University of Ontario Institute of Technology Library. 2016. "Data Collection Development Guidelines." University of Ontario Institute of Technology Library. Accessed September 28. http://www.uoit.ca/sites/library/about_the_library/uoit-library-policy-and-related-documents/data-collection-development-guidelines.php.

Westra, Bonnie L., Thomas R. Clancy, Joyce Sensmeier, Judith J. Warren, Charlotte Weaver, and Connie W. Delaney. 2015. "Nursing Knowledge: Big Data Science—Implications for Nurse Leaders." *Nursing Adminstration Quarterly* 39 (4): 304–10. doi:10.1097/NAQ.0000000000000130.

Wilkinson, Mark D., Michel Dumontier, IJsbrand Jan Aalbersberg, Gabrielle Appleton, Myles Axton, Arie Baak, Niklas Blomberg, et al. 2016. "The FAIR Guiding Principles for Scientific Data Management and Stewardship." *Scientific Data* 3: 160018. doi:10.1038/sda ta.2016.18.

Xie, Iris, and Krystyna Matusiak. 2016. *Discover Digital Libraries: Theory and Practice.* Cambridge, MA: Elsevier.

Yale University Library. 2014. "Collection Development Statements: Science and Social Science Data." Yale University Library. http://web.library.yale.edu/collection-development/science-and-social-science-data.

Chapter Nine

The Hunt of the Unicorn

Collection Development for Special Collections in Health Sciences Libraries

Stephen J. Greenberg

If it were only so simple! Building a collection of exquisite rare texts in fine leather bindings and putting these treasures in front of a rapt audience of scholars and connoisseurs of the book arts. Reading rooms would have dark wood and comfortable leather chairs reminiscent of an exclusive private club, and donors would be lining up at the doors to donate their own collections or to write checks to buy what is wanted to fill up library shelves and vaults. At 2 p.m. (promptly), everyone would stop for sherry and biscuits.

In the real world, that's about as common these days as unicorns. Instead, special collections librarians are faced with demanding, multifaceted jobs requiring extensive cross-disciplinary training and skills, as they try to create and extend collections in a landscape where everything librarians knew (or thought they knew) has changed. Perhaps these changes are for the better; perhaps not. Most of the time, librarians and archivists are too busy to tell.

There is, at its core, a fundamental duality in the roles of health sciences librarians tasked with the creation and continuance of a special collection in the history of medicine and/or other health sciences. On the one hand, they act as rare book librarians, expected to be skilled in descriptive bibliography and the history of books as physical objects. They care about binding leathers and type fonts, chain lines and collations, mezzotints and wood engravings. The actual subject matter of the items in their charge is (almost!) irrelevant. On the other hand, they are expected to be subject specialists in the history of medicine; more properly, the history of the health sciences writ large: nursing, pharmacology, toxicology, dentistry, botany, veterinary medicine, or

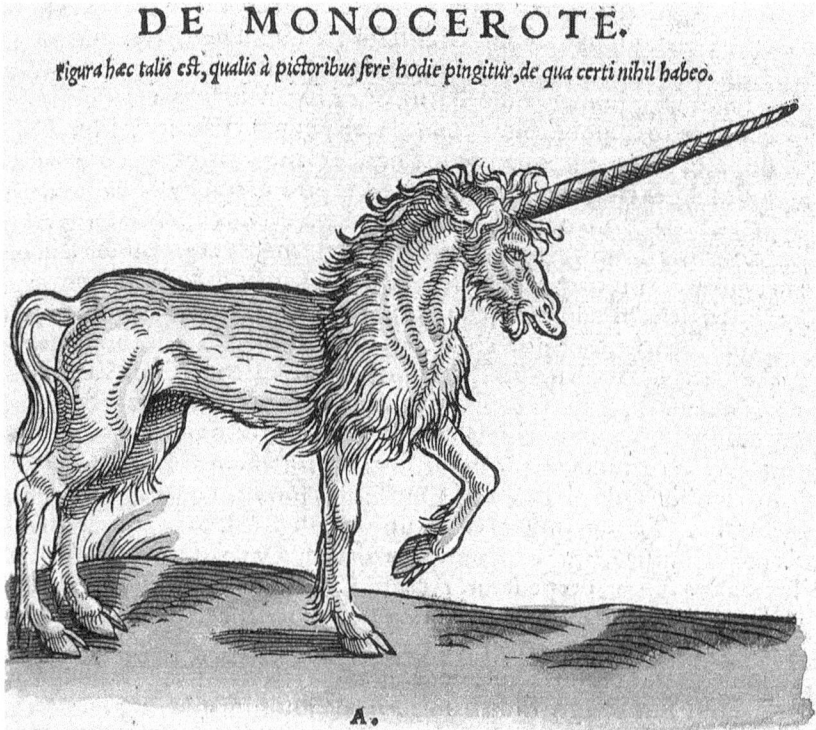

DE MONOCEROTE.

Figura hæc talis est, qualis à pictoribus ferè hodie pingitur, de qua certi nihil habeo.

A.

Figure 9.1.   Unicorn from Conrad Gesner, ***Medici Tigurini Historiae Animalium,*** **1:781 (1551). Photograph by Stephen Greenberg, courtesy National Library of Medicine**

zoology. The further back the collections go, the lower the boundaries are between the life sciences, and the more librarians must be aware of their roles regarding the books (i.e., the physical objects) and the text (the intellectual content they contain). In the first iteration, they are hardly medical librarians at all; in the second, they care chiefly about the message and are asked to subjugate the medium in which it was conveyed. It is the central contradiction in what special collections librarians do.

When one begins to consider collection development for special health sciences library collections (which in this chapter will be taken to mean rare and/or historical materials as print, as audio-visual materials, as images, and as archival collections), a whole new range of issues and considerations arise. In addition to all the usual concerns of collection scope, content, and access, librarians (and archivists) must deal with a heightened awareness of all the issues inherent in building and maintaining collections of fragile, hard-to-describe, often impossible-to-replace items whose sheer market value blots out normal considerations of whether an item belongs in a given collection and how access should be handled even for qualified researchers from among the library's core users. It is difficult to maintain a business-as-usual attitude while handing across a circulation counter a book with a documented value of thousands or even tens of thousands of dollars. On the other hand, these are libraries, not museums; it's impossible to read a book locked up in a vitrine. In the now-classic instructional film *How to Operate a Book*, narrator and cowriter Gary Frost notes how implausible it would be to expect a museum to allow hands-on examination of, say, its collection of seventeenth century silver, while special collections libraries routinely page items of similar age and greater fragility for patrons (Frost and Belanger 1986). If the institutional commitment does not exist to make its materials available for appropriate patrons, it is probably better not to build a special collection at all.

These considerations soon branch out into two separate but parallel lines of inquiry and concern. If one is dealing with an established collection, perhaps containing early editions of recognized classics of both great historical interest and significant market value, does one simply maintain the collection, acting as the good steward in balancing the demands of preservation and access, or does one attempt to "grow" the collection by adding additional materials, both primary and secondary, to burnish the luster of the primary item? A single copy of a great book is a curiosity, but adding supporting materials transforms it into a source for research. This should be why these items are in collections to begin with, but is there deeply rooted institutional support (intellectual, moral, and financial) to follow such a path?

THE NATURE OF SPECIAL HEALTH SCIENCES COLLECTIONS MATERIALS

If librarians are tasked with creating a new special collection, the choices that they are called upon to make are different but no less challenging. While the impetus to form a new special collection may come from a single (perhaps spectacular) gift from a donor seeking to honor his or her alma mater, or a long-time and presumably fruitful institutional affiliation, the question soon becomes a resounding "Now what?" The gift of a Vesalius or a Harvey may be inspiring, but, even with unlimited funding at one's disposal (a not-very-likely scenario to say the least), it would be no more possible to build from scratch a grand new collection of the world's accepted medical classics from Hippocrates to HIV than it would be build a new art museum stuffed with Rembrandts, Picassos, and Renoirs. This material is in finite supply, and most of it is already taken by institutions with deep pockets. This is not to say that the occasional papyrus or a subject collection of materials on eighteenth-century cookery might not show up on the rare book market (cookery is in scope for some history of medicine collections, but some institutions change their scope through time), but that market is hardly robust enough to supply a slew of purchases of Old Masters.

At this juncture, it is necessary to note in some detail the inherent differences in dealing with collections that are primarily print-based (which may be rare enough, but unlikely to be unique) as opposed to archival and manuscript collections, which by definition *are* unique. Here the rules (and the stakes) are different. The papers of a Nobel Prize– or Lasker Prize–winning researcher might well be offered to a variety of hosts. The professional responsibility of the would-be curator, in close consultation with the institutional administration and (of course!) the donor, is to determine what makes the most sense for the collection: What future home can provide the appropriate mix of preservation and access for future researchers? Does the potential host institution possess the expertise to properly curate the collection, including staff who arrange and describe the material, write a useful finding aid, make the collection "findable" with modern search tools, while all the time protecting the physical safety and integrity of the actual items that make up the collection? Moreover, there is the vexing question of context. The gift of the papers of a Nobel winner may be tempting indeed, but, if the recipient institution has no other related or supporting collections, while some other institution at an inconvenient commuting distance away already has a recognized mass of such holdings, the decision can become fraught. There is a point where the accretion of mutually supportive collections reaches a critical mass, and what was once an accumulation of interesting stuff becomes a major center for research. Of course, the sharing of digital files (of which there will be a great deal to say later) has gone a long way in addressing such issues, but some concerns remain. Sentimentality cannot be the sole criterion in such a decision, but neither can it be ignored. No one has ever said that donor relations were simple.

All of this leads to several related points that command attention. The first is that medicine, like art and literature, will continue to produce masterpieces that will need to be collected and documented for future generations of scholars and researchers. But many of these masterpieces are already in research library collections, albeit fragmented and as-yet unrecognized. Vesalius, Harvey, Darwin, and their ilk wrote books, but books are no longer the primary medium of medical communication. The peer-reviewed periodical medical literature will become the raw material, to be mined somewhat after the fact. At one level, health sciences librarians and archivists are more fortunate than their colleagues in the liberal arts; they have reasonably comprehensive indexes of the peer-reviewed medical literature going back to 1879 with the *Index Medicus*, and at least some subject-arranged coverage before that in the *Index Catalogue* (Gallagher and Greenberg 2009). They are also fortunate that a certain level of "greatness" is recognized somewhat earlier in the sciences than in the arts. Using the Nobel Prize as a crude, if convenient, measure, the mean age of laureates in literature between 1901 and 2015 is sixty-five; in medicine and physiology, the age is fifty-eight (Nobelprize.org 2016). Many of the winners in medicine and physiology were considerably younger: Joshua Lederberg was thirty-three; Marshall Nirenberg was forty-one; Harold Varmus, fifty. To document these advances, librarians and archivists need an awareness that relatively recent materials, both published and unpublished, need to be recognized and preserved when they are still "new." It is also vital that the institutional culture be attuned to and supportive of these efforts.

But collecting the original journal articles of the great scientists, while necessary, is not sufficient in itself. A wider context is required. What was the state of the scientific art when the great breakthroughs were made? For generations, librarians, acting in accordance with the best practices of their times, rebound their journals for convenience and shelving efficiency. Forgetting for the moment the conservation horrors inflicted by over-sewing and acidic library buckram, how much contextual information was lost by discarding covers and advertisements? Some years ago, the author dealt with a reference question about ads on the covers of *Index Medicus* volumes from the early twentieth century, when it was not a government publication but was privately printed with citations provided by the Army Medical Library (the precursor to the National Library of Medicine [NLM]). Months of research revealed a startling fact: no library in the United States, not even NLM, had copies of *Index Medicus* with original covers and advertisements for that period. And this concern is likely to become more acute. While covers and advertisements were often removed from journals in the past before binding, many bound library journals do still retain some of that content. As health sciences and research libraries discard bound printed journals in favor of electronic archives, however, this "less important" content is even more likely to be lost. Very few journal publishers have bothered to digitize covers, front and back material, and advertisements from their journals.

Another striking example of the importance of preserving context can be found by examining the issue of the journal *Nature* containing the brief but momentous announcement by James Watson and Francis Crick of their discoveries concerning the structure of DNA (Watson and Crick 1953). The same issue has two other articles on the subject; one coauthored by Rosalind Franklin, who did not yet know that Watson and Crick had been given access to her X-ray diffraction photographs without her knowledge, and a second by Maurice Wilkins, who is alleged to have leaked the photographs to Watson and Crick. Forgetting the drama for just a moment, a scholar with access only to a digital copy of the Watson and Crick article would lose the context of a

trio of simultaneous publications and its implication of prepublishing circulation and discussion.

To some extent, therefore, special collections librarians are expected to be
prescient, and that is not a subject covered in the professional training of
librarians, archivists, or historians. Moreover, they are expected to be all-
inclusive, and that is especially hard when the significance of what is kept, as
opposed to what is discarded immediately or weeded out later, will not be
demonstrated for years or even decades to come. Archivists have always
been attuned to this. Over twenty-five years ago, this author's instructor in
archives, who had decades of experience dealing with very large collections,
told his class that a working archivist needed two pieces of furniture to
approach a new collection: a big table to spread things out, and a big trash
can whose use should be obvious. He was being neither flippant nor unpro-
fessional. He was merely bowing to the reality that no one can keep everything. The Watson and Crick article is in no danger of disappearing (or at
least, not its text in digital form), but the physical volume is already an
endangered species. Textbooks and other less glamorous items are forever at
risk. Of course, only the very largest medical libraries have ever committed
to keep masses of print or manuscript material that may yet prove to be
historically important down the line; in theory, that is what national libraries
are for.

DEVELOPING A COLLECTION PLAN

Not surprisingly, the rules and standards for special collections development
have changed over time, although some basic benchmarks remain. In 1965,
the Association of College and Research Libraries issued a monograph as an
overall guide to the care and feeding of special collections. In the chapter on
acquisitions, Howard H. Peckham, director of the William L. Clements Library, University of Michigan at Ann Arbor, could already write,

> It is virtually impossible today for a library to begin a rare book collection
> from scratch, from absolute zero. . . . Rare books are naturally few in number,
> they are eagerly sought after, and patience is as necessary as willingness to
> pay. Fewer private collections come on the market today to offer the newcom-
> er an opportunity to collect in the process of redistribution. (Peckham 1965,
> 26)

Peckham then goes on to discuss the traditional options for acquisition: seeking local rarities, contacting specialist book dealers already vetted by the
Antiquarian Booksellers' Association of America, and perhaps attending
book fairs and auctions. None of this, of course, should be attempted before a
careful collection development statement is worked out by all parties con-

cerned at the home institution. A decade later, Roderick Cave, writing from the United Kingdom but for an American audience, could give remarkably similar advice (Cave 1976, 34–66). Again, he stresses the need to focus on a comprehensive collection development plan and to establish good relations with reputable dealers and potential donors. More gingerly, auctions are suggested, but only after much care and preparation.

Clearly, this part of the world has changed. The last significant auction of a private collection in the history of medicine was nearly two decades ago, when Christie's New York handled the sale of the Haskell F. Norman Library of Science and Medicine. The actual sale lasted four days spread over a seven-month period, and the three-volume sales catalog is still considered to be a valuable reference work in its own right. There is unlikely to be the equal of that sale again, as no collection of its size and specialization still exists in private hands. Auctions do take place, but they are far more likely to be held on eBay than in a setting out of Hitchcock's *North by Northwest.* Moreover, printed catalogs, while they still exist, have been largely displaced by websites, with all the pluses and minuses to be expected. But nothing of lasting value can be attempted without a collection development plan. There are three main factors in developing such a plan:

1. What is the perceived scope of the collection?
2. What clientele will be served?
3. What formats can the collection effectively both preserve and make available to its patrons?

Internally, there are other factors to be considered:

1. Is there a long-term institutional commitment to a special collection?
2. Is there an appropriate space and facility to house a special collection?
3. Is there a reasonable integration of the special collection with the larger library and the institution as a whole?

Steven K. Galbraith and Geoffrey D. Smith, drawing upon guidelines proposed by the International Federation of Library Associations, have condensed these ideas into four bullet points: selection, planning, public relations, and context (Galbraith and Smith 2012, 104). Each of these points must be approached with caution and seriousness. It is all too easy for a special collection to be seen as an indulgence or a novelty with little scholarly relevance, and the rare-book reading room becomes little more than an attractive venue for cocktail parties. In the academic medical world, the stakes can get higher very quickly. Can the institution justify the purchase of a rare text when the same money might be used to modernize a laboratory or fund a clinical trial? In an article published in *RBM,* the journal of the Rare

Books and Manuscripts Section of the Association of College and Research Libraries, devoted to assessing the role and relevance of special collections in today's (and tomorrow's) academic libraries, Sarah M. Pritchard wrote,

> The key challenge in special collections—in fact, in any part of the academic library—is getting the broader institution to care. How does one ensure that the university and its stakeholders will be willing to underwrite the support of special collections, arguably the most expensive component of a library as far as acquisitions, skilled professional staff, customized space, preservation, and security? Expecting an appreciation of the intrinsic goodness of special collections won't carry the day even in well-off, prestigious institutions, because— well, because at the top level "it's all about them." Our assessment program has to demonstrate the value of special collections to advancing the mission of the entire library, and in turn the value of the library in contributing to the accomplishment of the university's goals. (Pritchard 2012)

These are not easy questions to answer, especially when the librarian's role is reduced to being an onlooker at a board of trustees meeting. The donation of a valuable (intellectually, that is) archival collection makes a fine item in an annual report, but it takes time, money, and expertise to fetch the boxes from a damp garage, rehouse, arrange, possibly weed, and describe the material to the point where it becomes a resource for scholars.

Another point that could be raised here concerns the ongoing relations between the special collections staff and the staff in the general library. This often comes to a head over acquisitions (the dividing up of scarce resources) and can lead to open hostilities that reach far beyond the scope of this chapter. The cure lies in common sense and the clear and consistent application of a carefully worded and mutually accepted collection development policy. If there are two acquisition units working in parallel, they should respect each other's expertise and issues. One will never be required to chase down missing journal issues; the other will never wrestle with the niceties of converting U.S. dollars to Bulgaria levs to buy a unique item from a bookseller in Sofia. But both will know what frustration means.

Collecting Archival and Manuscript Materials

Assuming that these hurdles are past and there is money, space, staff, and commitment, it becomes necessary to distinguish again between archival and manuscript collections on the one hand, and rare book collections on the other. To obtain a desirable archival collection for one's collection is primarily an exercise in establishing and maintaining good donor relations with both the principal and the heirs. In the best case scenario, the principal is contacted long in advance of any donation date, and a proper deed of gift is written and signed. The Society of American Archivists (SAA) website (www2.archivists.org) is the first stop in identifying best practices and making sure that they are followed. Archival collections are sometimes offered for outright sale, and perhaps more often there is some competition between institutions for a particularly desirable collection. In such situations, there is no substitute for properly trained professional staff or at least good guidance. The most delicate point in the process is ensuring that the donors understand what they are gaining, and what they are relinquishing, on the day that the deed of gift is signed.

The acquisition of archival collections is not without its share of whimsy and/or the slightly macabre. Archivists read obituaries (it comes with the territory) and may need to contact grieving families quickly if no groundwork has been laid down in advance. SAA provides ethical guidelines, and good professionals follow them, but sometimes the race *is* to the swift. The whimsical part comes when unexpected things show up in the as-yet unexamined corners of a new collection. Any archivist who has been in the field for more than a few years has anecdotes: did the subject of the collection really save *that*? This is the time when the written collection development policy (sorry, we don't collect that; it's not our policy) and permission to weed come to the fore. Organizational archives are likely to have less drama, but, again, it is still vital that the deed of gift is detailed and specific. Once donated, the papers become part of the collection where they are housed. Proper access must be agreed upon at the outset, but legal ownership has passed hands.

If the collection development policy is to include a significant amount of archival material, the services of a professionally trained archivist are essential. Archivists and librarians do not always think alike; their training is different, as are their responsibilities. It is possible, in the short term, to hire archivists on a contract basis for a specific project, but a robust program of archival acquisitions requires the skills of a full-time, permanent professional.

Collecting Books

Returning to the subject of print materials, establishing ongoing and professional relations with specialist booksellers is a vital step. In many ways, this step is easier now than it has been in the past, with so many websites offering so much material. It is important, however, to know the sources. The gold standard for a rare books dealer is membership in the Antiquarian Booksellers' Association of America (www.abaa.org). Here one is assured of a standard of professional ethics (and a relatively uniform vocabulary of terminology for bibliographic description and condition). It is possible to pick up a few interesting items on eBay to bolster a collection, especially if the seller has a high approval rating, offers a return policy, and the librarian, as the buyer, is very knowledgeable about what he or she is looking at. But, in the long run, it is far safer to deal with a professional. Moreover, a bookdealer who is familiar with a library's wish list will be able to help obtain items and perhaps suggest other items of which the librarian was previously unaware.

Such caveats may seem appropriate when acquiring seventeenth-century texts but might be overkill with more recent materials. In fact, eBay can be a legitimate source; more than a few ABAA members sell items there. This raises issues about items that have been facetiously (but usefully) described as "medium rare." Such items may be hard to find, of growing historical interest, but not likely to show up yet in a Sotheby's sale. As long ago as their 1998 annual meeting, the Rare Books and Manuscripts Section of the Association of College and Research Libraries (RBMS/ACRL) discussed the impact of time: what was once commonplace, ephemera, and easily discarded was becoming historical (RBMS 1998). Many libraries, health sciences or otherwise, have defined "historical" by simply drawing a line in the sand. The National Library of Medicine draws its line at 1914 for monographs and 1870 for serials. Archives and manuscripts are exempted. Such lines move only with difficulty. Many larger and older collections, recognizing that history never sleeps, routinely scan their current collections for items fit to be transferred to special collections. This may be occurring more with recent shifts of many legacy health sciences library collections to storage. However, this is difficult to do systematically, and, as mentioned earlier, requires more prescience and a certain amount of luck. If a collection development policy runs to ephemera such as posters and pamphlets, new sources will need to be explored.

Collecting Audio-Visual Materials

Occupying a sort of middle ground are the issues raised when collecting audio-visual and other non-print formats. A remarkable amount of historical information is preserved in photographic prints and negatives, transparencies, microfilm, and its cousins (fiche and opaque microcards), filmstrips (with or with an accompanying recorded commentary), motion pictures in a dizzying array of formats, and sound recordings from wax cylinder, to compact disc, to streamed podcasts. This material is rarely costly to acquire and often a hugely valuable adjunct to print and archival collections, but keeping the information accessible to researchers will be a daunting task. Often, it is a challenge to simply identify the format. As time goes by, fewer and fewer people will have had firsthand experience with 16mm optical sound films or video formats like U-matic video tapes, which were once industry standards, not to mention a myriad of continuous-loop teaching tapes and non-standard audio cassettes that never quite became commercially viable.

If the institutional collection development policy includes collecting such materials, the decision to acquire will be tempered by two distinct but over-lapping concerns. The first is a question of information accessibility; simply put, what is required to access what's there? Photographic prints are simple, as are glass-plate or film-based negatives, microfilm formats, and most trans-parencies. An inexpensive scanner can enlarge, convert negative images to positives, and save images to (current) digital formats or even hard copy. Mysterious audio or video formats present a thornier problem. If the format can be identified, but hardware is not locally available, the next step can be problematic. Scrounging through the Internet and buying legacy hardware through eBay can be a temporary solution, but, sooner or later, a serious collecting commitment will require a systematic program of reformatting, knowing full well that the process will likely need to be repeated in years to come as technology changes. There are commercial sources that can reformat virtually anything, but such services are expensive, and the results will still be subject to additional issues of obsolescence in the future.

The second question is a matter of preservation. The complex chemical nature of such materials means that what conservators quaintly refer to as "inherent vice" is guaranteed to be rampant. "Archival" photographic prints and microfilm reels may have been created to last, but anyone who has ever seen a poorly washed print fading away or smelled vinegar emanating from a drawer of microfilm masters knows that permanence is a hard-fought battle that never quite ends. If the decision is made to collect such material and then to provide access to originals, the first responsible step must be to gather information from such sources as the Image Permanence Institute (www.imagepermanenceinstitute.org) and Wilhelm Imaging Research (www.wilhelm-research.com).

DIGITAL SURROGATES

In many ways, the proceeding discussion has been circling the proverbial elephant in the room: the increasingly complex relationship between original collection material and the constantly improving quality of digital surrogates. There are many iterations of the questions one might ask, but they all come back to this question: at what point, if ever, will access to a digital copy fully replace the need to see an original, possibly fragile, probably extremely valuable book? The image in figure 9.2, created by the author and provided courtesy of the National Library of Medicine, was created to demonstrate a point. The book is William Hunter's *Anatomia uteri humani gravidi tabulis illustrata* (The anatomy of the human gravid uterus exhibited in figures), published in Birmingham, England, by the master printer John Baskerville in 1774. It is a very big book; page size is 67 by 49 centimeters (26.4 by 19.3

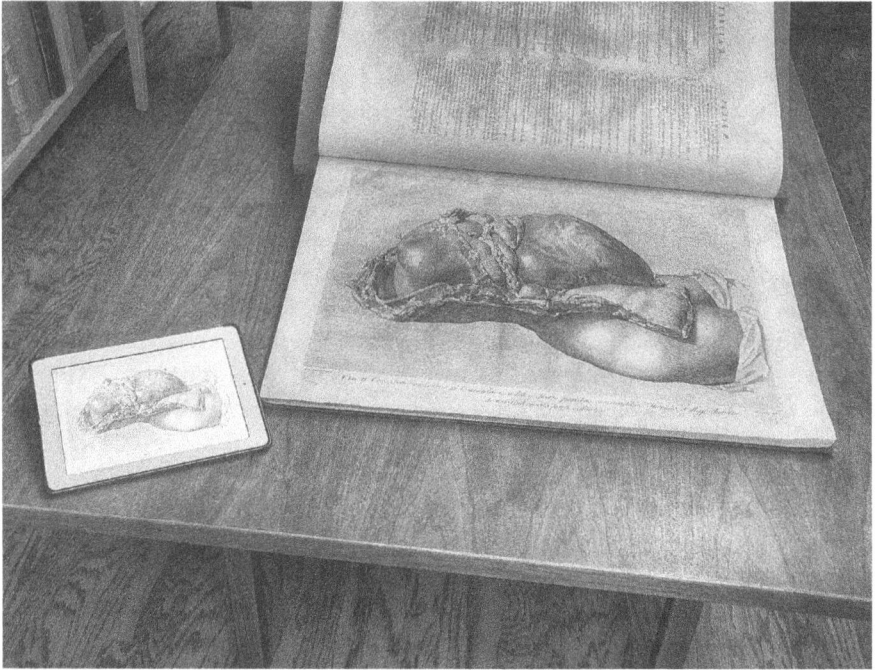

Figure 9.2.   Actual and Digital: William Hunter, *Anatomia Uteri Humani Gravidi Tabulis Illustrata* ["The anatomy of the human gravid uterus exhibited in figures"] , Table 2 (1774). Photograph by Stephen Greenberg, courtesy National Library of Medicine

inches). For scale, the device in the lower left showing a high-resolution digital copy of the illustration is not a cell phone, it is a 9.7-inch diagonal tablet. It is fair, and particularly germane, to ask two sets of questions here: why is the original so big, and is the high-resolution image, easily and freely available, a proper substitute?

To answer the first question, one must take a small detour through the history of childbirth, midwifery, and obstetrics. Hunter published his atlas at the point in medical history when physicians were seizing control of childbirth from the traditionally trained midwives, who had held a monopoly in the field since the Middle Ages. Hunter, along with such colleagues as William Smellie in England and William Shippen in America, sought to medicalize childbirth, making it a surgical procedure. These academically trained *accoucheurs*, as they were called, used their books and tools (such as forceps) as weapons. They could do dissections (midwives could not), and books with stunning, full-sized illustrations were an effective way to overawe the public and demean the midwives. The transfer of childbirth to hospitals (at least in urban settings) over the next seventy-five years had its own costs in the rise of deaths due to puerperal fever, but the obstetricians carried the day. To see Hunter in the original is to literally feel the weight of his arguments (Porter 1997, 129–30, 273–74, 369–70; Duffin 2010, 287).

Then what is the use of the scanned version? It may well be, if properly presented, quite considerable. Certainly, the details of the engraving can be more clearly seen in the digital version, given the ability to enlarge at will. The digital version can be shared more widely, and the original will be spared the inevitable wear and tear of patron use. After all, it is a flimsy sheet of paper that's almost 250 years old. Finally, NLM has posted (as would any responsible repository) excellent metadata that reveals evidence that might be concealed behind the shiny glass display, including its physical size. With such splendid free access, why should a library spend thousands of dollars to buy a Hunter for its own collections, and, moreover, how does a library justify such an expense to those who must raise the funds and sign the checks?

The lure of creating a virtual-only collection is compelling, and its charms will only increase. In the field we are seeing the continued rise of large digital collections of rare print materials, most notably the Medical Heritage Library consortium.

> The Medical Heritage Library (MHL), a digital curation collaborative among some of the world's leading medical libraries, promotes free and open access to quality historical resources in medicine. Our goal is to provide the means by which readers and scholars across a multitude of disciplines can examine the interrelated nature of medicine and society, both to inform contemporary medicine and strengthen understanding of the world in which we live. The MHL's growing collection of digitized medical rare books, pamphlets, journals, and films number in the tens of thousands, with representative works from each of the past six centuries, all of which are available here through the Internet Archive. (Medical Heritage Library 2017)

Currently, MHL has nine principal contributors, and over thirty content contributors in the United States, Canada, and the United Kingdom. These numbers can only be expected to grow.

The possibilities inherent in such a collection are staggering and must give pause to any institution still interested in developing and maintaining a paper collection. But digital collections will, in the real world of scholarship, continue to have their limitations. Michael F. Suarez, S.J, director of the Rare Book School at the University of Virginia but also, since 2010, editor in chief of Oxford Scholarly Editions Online, is quick to embrace the possibilities of the digital world, but is equally vociferous in pointing out the limitations to scholarship based solely upon the virtual, which he refers to as an "impoverishment"(Suarez 2012).

To develop a working collection in this new digital environment requires a level of cooperative vision previously unimagined. Who will hold the original, who will scan and upload, and who will settle for access to a digital copy only? Fortunately, such cooperation is made feasible by the same digital situation that makes it so essential. As Jeffrey S. Reznick, chief of the History of Medicine Division at NLM, has written,

> For historical medical libraries and archives to survive and thrive in the future, their unique stewardship of medical-cultural heritage—collecting it, cataloging it, preserving it, curating it, making it accessible, as well as refining collection development and retention policies related to it—must become future-oriented in terms of thinking, planning, and action. . . . How precisely historical medical libraries and archives will survive and thrive depends not upon technology, but upon informed and proactive leadership at all levels that can effectively navigate the digital world and corresponding factors of culture, economy, society, and politics. (Reznick 2014)

If the future of special collections lies in digital consortia and the creation of a scholarly equilibrium of traditional and digital repositories, then Reznick's emphasis on forward-thinking leadership becomes paramount. The task of collection development takes on a new role in the digital workplace, as collection equals cooperation.

THE FUTURE OF HEALTH SCIENCES SPECIAL COLLECTIONS

It may well be, as has been suggested by Simon Chaplin, director of Culture and Society at the Wellcome Trust and for ten years head of its library, that medical libraries, at least in their traditional form, are dying:

> Or at least some specific sorts of medical libraries—independent institutional libraries, owned by historic organizations, in historic buildings, with large historic collections—are under serious threat of themselves becoming part of the past. To mitigate this threat, there is a need to rethink the nature of the "historic" medical library. . . . Digitization has a role to play in this rethinking, but it is neither a panacea nor, in most cases, does it address fundamental questions about the sustainability and utility of legacy print collections and the spaces used to house them. (Chaplin 2014)

Chaplin reviews the many (mostly unappetizing, at least to traditionalists) options that face such collections: selling off, becoming "museums" (the Wellcome collection does in fact include artifacts), and so on. But he does close his article with some encouragement. New ideas, new technologies, new partnerships still have a place within for books and paper, although that place has and will continue to change in ways unimaginable a few decades ago. Certainly, if trends in health sciences libraries can be gleaned from recent articles and stories written in this book, many of the large print health sciences library collections are not necessarily being sold off but are in the process of being moved to off-site storage. Librarians are collaborating on print repositories to keep only one copy of items that were previously held in multiple institutions. Much of the material published today is only being collected in electronic format. New appreciation for special collections, however, may be gained when there is very little print material left in these libraries.

Few librarians entered the field of special collections librarianship and took up the responsibilities of collection development with the intention of overseeing the dispersal of their collections. And indeed, not all special collections librarians face the same challenges. Archival collections, by their very size and heterogeneity of format, are often not good candidates for total digitization. Perhaps the collection includes documents on five-inch floppy disks, written with some obscure software program that only works under DOS 3.1.

Now, too, archivists are faced with the problems of archiving born-digital content. Not the least of the difficulties in that endeavor is recognizing ephemeral web content quickly and finding ways of granting it permanence. NLM has made some effort to create formats and protocols for capturing born-digital content for future generations of historians, starting with the documentation of the 2014 Ebola pandemic (National Library of Medicine History of Medicine Division 2016).

For those whose holdings are still primarily print-based, the traditional ways of building collections can seem increasingly obsolete. There is some small comfort in pointing to such instances as William Hunter's atlas or the many other cases where only the original item can answer the needs of a researcher. Then, too, the medical field moves so quickly that many items become historical virtually as one watches. Textbooks come and go, and, while few libraries have the interest and the means to preserve every edition, and even fewer are purchasing new editions of these textbooks in print, it is important that someone does collect these. Due to copyright restrictions, such works are not easy to digitize, and online texts can update overnight, leaving no trace of their earlier content. They will all be historical someday, and, fifty or seventy-five years from now, historians will need to know what all the fuss was about concerning the Zika virus. The pace of journal publication shows no signs of abating. How will the historians of the future access the content of electronic-only journals that were only available on that quaint thing they used to call the Internet?

As the old proverb goes, librarians are cursed to live in interesting times, and those charged with building and managing special and historical collections feel it perhaps more acutely than others. The bricks and mortar of the grand buildings seem suddenly insecure. Librarians want to move forward, but the path is unclear. They are called upon to embrace the digital, without a guarantee of its permanence, at the same time as they struggle to make paper collections both accessible and relevant. On either front, there are increasing demands and uncertain resources. It won't be easy, but it really never has been. Pooling resources and expertise, creating new alliances with a forward-looking but flexible plan, is the only realistic approach to fulfilling our promises to the collections, the patrons, and successor librarians on either side of the actual (or virtual!) circulation desk.

This work was supported by the Intramural Research Program of the National Institutes of Health, National Library of Medicine.

REFERENCES

Cave, Roderick. 1976. *Rare Book Librarianship.* Hamden, CT: Linnet Books.

Chaplin, Simon. 2014. "The Medical Library Is History." *RBM: A Journal of Rare Books, Manuscripts, and Cultural Heritage* 15 (2): 146–56.

Duffin, Jacalyn. 2010. *History of Medicine: A Scandalously Short Introduction.* 2nd ed. Toronto: University of Toronto Press.

Frost, Gary, and Terry Belanger. 1986. "How to Operate a Book." In *How to Operate a Book from Punch to Printing Type*, directed by Peter Herdrich. Charlottesville, VA: Book Arts Press. Digitally remastered for DVD, 2004, 29 minutes.

Galbraith, Steven K., and Geoffrey D. Smith. 2012. *Rare Book Librarianship: An Introduction and Guide.* Santa Barbara, CA: ABC-CLIO.

Gallagher, Patricia E., and Stephen J. Greenberg. 2009. "The Great Contribution: Index Medicus, Index-Catalogue, and IndexCat." *Journal of the Medical Library Association* 97 (2): 108–13. doi:10.3163/1536-5050.97.2.007.

Medical Heritage Library. 2017. "About: The Medical Heritage Library." Medical Heritage Library. Accessed May 8. http://www.medicalheritage.org/about/.

National Library of Medicine History of Medicine Division 2016. "Future Historical Collections: Archiving the 2014 Ebola Outbreak." *Circulating Now* (blog), March 10. National Library of Medicine, National Institutes of Health. https://circulatingnow.nlm.nih.gov/2016/03/10/future-historical-collections-archiving-the-2014-ebola-outbreak-2/.

Nobelprize.org. 2016. "Average Age for the Nobel Laureates." Nobel Media AB. Accessed November 10. https://www.nobelprize.org/nobel_prizes/lists/laureates_ages/index.html.

Peckham, Howard H. 1965. "Acquisitions." In *Rare Book Collections*, edited by H. Richard Archer. ACRL Monograph Number 27. Chicago: American Library Association.

Porter, Roy. 1997. *The Greatest Benefit to Mankind: A Medical History of Humanity.* New York: W. W. Norton.

Pritchard, Sarah M. 2012. "Afterword: Special Collections and Assessing the Value of Academic Libraries." *RBM: A Journal of Rare Books, Manuscripts, and Cultural Heritage* 13 (2): 191–94.

RBMS (Rare Books and Manuscripts Section). 1998. "Getting Ready for the Nineteenth Century: Strategies and Solutions for Rare Book and Special Collections Librarians." The Thirty-Ninth Rare Books and Manuscripts Preconference. Association of College and Research Libraries. http://web.archive.org/web/19990429070318/www.princeton.edu/%7Eferguson/98precon.html

Reznick, Jeffrey S. 2014. "Embracing the Future as Stewards of the Past: Charting a Course Forward for Historical Medical Libraries and Archives." *RBM: A Journal of Rare Books, Manuscripts, and Cultural Heritage* 15 (2): 111–23.

Suarez, Michael. 2012. "The Future for Books in a Digital Age." Lecture, National Library of Medicine, Bethesda, MD, April 19, 2012. The lecture has not been published, but unedited video recordings are available through the National Library of Medicine.

Watson, James D., and Francis H. C. Crick. 1953. "Molecular Structure of Nucleic Acids." *Nature* 171 (4356): 737–38. doi:10.1038/171737a0.

Chapter Ten

The Future of Health Sciences Collection Management

Susan K. Kendall

It's risky to try to predict the future. Invariably, one gets some things right, some things wrong, and completely misses out on foreseeing some of the most important innovations. Why do it then? There are several reasons. Collection management librarians make decisions every day. These decisions will have ramifications not just for today, but also for the future, and sound decision making takes into account both current and future needs. Another reason for librarians to be thoughtful about the future is to tread that fine line of staying relevant without clinging to outmoded practices or wasting time on short-lived infatuations. A third reason is to create the future. Librarians don't just have to watch what happens from the sidelines; they can help shape what kind of future they want to see, because there is not just one preordained future. In his article "Librarian as Futurist," Brian Mathews says, "Futurists do not attempt to figure out *what will transpire* but instead focus on understanding *how things could turn out*" (Mathews 2014). He stresses that the point is not to forecast accurately what will happen but to develop diverse models of the future, predicting and strategically planning for different scenarios. In fact, he says, one common pitfall is choosing one scenario over another too early and then not being prepared when things go a different way.

Most predictions focus on the near future, extending present trends out into time just a few decades. A children's book, published in 1981 at the very beginning of the home computer revolution, presents an amusing picture of life filled with vacations to the "Space Islands," where computers can immediately translate your speech into other languages, and visits to the "Hovies," holographic, interactive, totally immersive videos. It also suggests some other innovations that will make life "great" in the future: electronic mail, learning via video computer (instead of at schools), and computer shopping of warehouse-style stores that deliver the goods directly to your home. One illustration shows medical experts testing a new operation using robot surgeons while an "editor" (really, a medical librarian!) in a *Star Trek*–inspired unitard inputs data into the electronic library as she watches. "In theory," the book states, "one huge electronic library could serve the whole world!" (Ardley 1981).

Glimpses like this into what people in the past envisioned can help put into perspective current predictions about the future, and they confirm Brian Mathews's advice to think broadly. The fact is that some mid-twentieth-century "world of tomorrow" predictions look very much like the present, but some of them, like holographic movies, are *still* being predicted for the future. Other predictions from the past, like ubiquitous space travel, are not even on the radar of today's futurists, except for science fiction writers. Many futures are possible, given current technology and trends. Before discussing the future of health sciences library collections, it might be helpful to look at what librarians in the past have predicted about the future for libraries and collections to see how far libraries have and have not come.

PAST PREDICTIONS AND CHALLENGES

The 1964 book *The Future of the Research Library* didn't so much predict the future as present goals for the future and problems to be solved. In it, Verner Clapp, then president of the Council on Library Resources, identified four gaps between what research library users require ("prompt, assured, and convenient access") and what research libraries can supply, as areas ripe for problem solving (Clapp 1964). Many of these can translate to health sciences libraries and their collections. First, he said, there was a gap between production and acquisition of library materials, with ever-increasing quantities of publications of which libraries can afford only a fraction. Second, there were obstacles to sharing resources. Third, there were bibliographic deficiencies— that is, a lot of information was hard to find due to insufficient indexing and cataloging. And finally, there were inadequate techniques in place for aspects of library management, namely, physical maintenance of collections, library record keeping, and library administration, including recruitment and training. Although this list of challenges refers, obviously, to print collections in the middle of the twentieth century, it is interesting that identical challenges face twenty-first-century health sciences libraries for electronic collections. Many of these have been mentioned in the chapters of this book. Chapter 1's discussion of the health sciences publishing landscape points out that the amount of publishing has only continued to rise. Budgeting to be able to afford what users need is even more of a challenge for today's libraries than those in the past. The obstacles to sharing resources in the past were physical. Now they rest in publisher licenses, digital rights management, and the technical limitations of some types of resources like e-books. Information remains hard to find even in the age of Google search and discovery tools, because the wide variety of vendor platforms and insufficient metadata make interoperability difficult. Finally, as will be discussed further below, aspects of library management are also still challenging, including the maintenance and preservation of electronic collections, technical support of diverse electronic resources, and recruitment and training of collection management librarians.

At the end of the twentieth century, librarians were publishing books and articles about the "twenty-first-century library." The focus was, naturally, on the transition from print collections to digital collections and the ramifications of that shift. In 1994, the same year that *Time* published a cover story on the "Strange New World of the Internet" (Elmer-Dewitt and Jackson 1994), F. W. Lancaster surveyed various thinkers of the day to write about "Collection Development in the Year 2025" (Lancaster 1994). Perhaps he was unable to see far enough into the future because he sounds like he's talking about today. He predicted that catalogs would be "gateways to resources beyond the walls of individual libraries," electronic resources would move from simple text to a full exploitation of the possibilities of incorporating hypertext and multimedia, that the nature of scholarship would change with the possibilities of manipulating text by computer and of research institutions taking a larger role in dissemination, and that librarians would be mediating access for users to information upon request while downloading for permanent acquisition only a subset of the materials available. Then he raised the same concerns Clapp did thirty years earlier: increased costs, inadequate bibliographic control, difficulty of sharing, and difficulty of preservation of electronic resources.

Richards and Eakin also talk about the future in their 1997 book *Collection Development and Assessment in Health Sciences Libraries* (Richards and Eakin 1997). They suggested that, in the "virtual" library, journals would fade and articles would be the unit of interest. There would be large-scale conversion of print collections to electronic. Librarians would be playing larger roles in the structure and design of systems for electronic information. They also pointed out the challenges of electronic publishing: concerns of quality control, intellectual property rights, distribution, retrievability, and preservation. Finally, the economics of information were a major concern, and the struggle for libraries to afford to build collections was forecasted to lead to an emphasis on acquiring materials at the time of need rather than in anticipation of need. More than twenty years later, the challenges and concerns raised by both of these books from the late 1990s still sound very familiar to librarians, despite the fact that the electronic resources known to those writers were on CD-ROM and floppy disc.

In 2005, Donald Lindberg and Betsy Humphreys from the National Library of Medicine looked ten years ahead and envisioned the medical library of 2015. In their version of the future, health care professionals, patients, educators, and researchers would have easy access to electronic information from anywhere from a variety of desktop, portable, and wearable devices. The electronic health record would be ubiquitous with linking that connected different types of information sources, making it easy to move from research data, to clinical data, to public health data, to published literature. All information retrieved would be customized to the individual needs of the patient or health care provider. They were conservative about some prognostications, suggesting that journals would remain important means of research dissemination and that a lot of scientific information would still require paid licenses.

Should one be disheartened that librarians are still grappling with many of the same challenges that were identified more than fifty years ago, or comforted that the concerns and values of librarians remain the same despite radical changes in the formats of information resources? Is it surprising that it is taking longer than predicted for information resources to be linked together? If these past predictions tell us anything, it is that the central concerns of librarianship are not simplistic, that librarian goals remain consistent over time, and that perhaps some of these problems may not ever be totally solved.

CURRENT PREDICTIONS OF THE FUTURE

Future of Collecting

What predictions have librarians made more recently about the future of health sciences collections or library collections in general? A 2014 special issue of the journal *Collection Management*, "We're Moving, Please Pardon Our Dust: Transformative Changes in Collection Management," explored changes for academic libraries, not specifically health sciences, but the article in that issue reporting the most radical change was a health sciences library that withdrew 90 percent of its print collection and transitioned to collection management based solely on usage statistics (Jarvis, Gregory, and Shipman 2014). The editors of that issue, Susanne Clement and Karen Fischer, concluded that transformative changes were taking place in collection-building practices, many in response to the economic downturn that had started around 2008, with a common theme being a user-centered rather than collection-centered focus. They found that collection building and management were becoming "nearly inseparable from access and discovery" (Clement and Fischer 2014). The editors concluded, however, that "it is in our opinion that although we may be observing several transformative changes in academic libraries, we are not yet at a paradigmatic shift in collection management. . . . Perhaps paradigmatic shifts must encompass more theoretical changes."

Other thinkers in the library field seem to be suggesting that libraries (at least academic libraries) are in the middle of a paradigm shift regarding their collections and will be experiencing the effects of this shift in the near future. They vary in how radically they believe the future will differ from the present. In 2002, Peggy Johnson's preface to the first edition of her textbook on collection management stated that "[c]ollection development and management are the meat and potatoes of libraries. If you don't have a collection, you don't have a library" (Johnson 2009, ix). In contrast, by 2011 Harvard's Dan Hazen was writing that "[c]ollections no longer lie at the center of research library operations and goals" (Hazen 2011). In 2016–2017, some library leaders like Lorcan Dempsey and Doug Way, started talking about the model of "collections as a service," which does seem to be a theoretical change, at least for research libraries (Way 2017; Dempsey 2016). The course for librarians going forward into the future, according to this model, is similar to the pragmatic approach that Clement and Fischer found some libraries had already adopted: librarians put users in contact with content (the "facilitated collection") regardless of format or location, and they maximize that access and their budgets by working together cooperatively to minimize duplication in their collections. While Dempsey and Way both suggest that owned collections will diminish even more than they have, the owned collections of research libraries, at least, are still part of the spectrum of collections in their visions for the future. Others take the idea of facilitated collections even further. In an *Against the Grain* interview (available for listening on podcast), Anja Smit, library director at Utrecht University, talks about the future "library without a collection" (Smit 2016). Like the other thinkers mentioned here, her point of view is as a research librarian. Her concept of no collection is based on predictions (and plans by such initiatives as OA2020) that most research materials (at least journal articles) in the future will be available for free, as open-access materials (Max Planck Digital Library 2016a). Furthermore, she suggests that librarians need to give up the idea of libraries being gateways to content, forget about the catalog, and leave discovery to Google. Librarians in her future will function as consultants for accessing and assessing information and helping to preserve information of many types, including data, for the future.

Most librarians writing about the future mention open access as one influence on the direction of future collecting, but they also recognize that most library collections contain other types of materials that are not part of any open-access plans. There are a couple of different proposals for how collecting might be different in the future. One is that collecting will become even more cooperative, beyond consortial licensing. Thinking about the "collective collection" was the theme of the 2017 Librarian Initiatives Conference of the Big Ten Academic Alliance, a consortium of large, mostly public, research universities predominantly located in the Midwest region of the United States, many of which have medical schools (Big Ten Academic Alliance 2017). A break-out session of that conference challenged collection management librarians to react to the vision statement that, by 2027, all collection management for these university libraries would take place on the consortial level. Others are thinking in a different direction, suggesting that librarians encourage all publishers to move toward a patron-driven model of acquisitions for *everything* in the future. In a panel session of the 2016 Charleston Conference (available for listening on podcast), Rick Anderson suggested that that is where the future lies, for both monographs and journal articles, and that the prices paid for materials under these models could and should be completely negotiable by each institution according to its own needs and usage (Anderson 2016).

Lorcan Dempsey, of OCLC, has spoken and written about "outside-in" and "inside-out" resources (Dempsey, Malpas, and Lavoie 2014). The first are the materials librarians purchase or license from external providers, and the second are resources created by the library or its larger institution that librarians can make available to the world. Although there are diverse opinions about what the future of collecting looks like, most of the thinkers named above and others (of academic libraries, mostly) agree with Dempsey that librarians will shift focus to "inside-out" resources, contributing more and more to the creation and curation of local content and adding value to that content by making it discoverable.

So much discussion of the future of libraries and collections is focused on academic libraries. Of course, many of these ideas about future collections are already reality in some kinds of health sciences libraries, and this may simply demonstrate that, as usual, health sciences libraries tend to point toward the future for other kinds of libraries. Health sciences libraries, particularly those serving health professionals for patient care, more than researchers, have always been focused on present access to the most current information. The idea of collections as a service, and even the idea of not building a collection at all but simply facilitating access to information resources through a combination of aggregators, subscription databases, and on-demand requests, will not be new to many librarians at smaller special libraries, hospital libraries, and libraries supporting medical schools established in the twenty-first century. What is new is that other types of libraries serving the health sciences, such as smaller and community colleges and even research libraries, look like they might go in this direction, too. Because the small libraries look to the larger ones to preserve the scholarly record, these changes will have an impact on them as well.

Future of Information Resources

But perhaps it is putting the cart before the horse to talk about the future of collections without talking about the future of the information resources themselves and how they will be used by library patrons in the functions that health sciences libraries serve: research, patient care, and education. Librarian David Lewis has studied the concept of "disruption," developed by business theorist Clayton Christensen, and applied it to library concerns in his book *Reimagining the Academic Library* (Lewis 2016a). Disruptive innovations, according to Christensen's theory, are technological changes that also come with a completely new business model. It is the new business model that causes trouble for the traditional institution, not necessarily the new technology. For libraries and scholarly publishers, subscription e-journals and purchased e-books are not disruptive. They merely continue the library role as provider of published content by many of the same publishers from the past.

What is disruptive is all of the free material now available on the web to anyone: crowdsourced and distributed content like Wikipedia, open data sets, YouTube videos, SlideShare, and podcasts. Through these types of resources, people share information with each other for free without the intervention of publishers or libraries. Information is no longer a scarcity to be managed and supplied to users by libraries. Librarians and professors shudder at medical students using Wikipedia and YouTube to gather information, and they would be right to be worried. Nevertheless, these sources, coupled with more traditional resources that are also now available on the web for free, such as Google Books, open-access journal articles, and bootlegged medical textbooks, are competing with library resources, and it is worth considering what aspects make them popular besides being free.

Lewis suggests that maybe we are going back to becoming more of an oral than a written culture (Lewis 2016b, 24). The rise in popularity of YouTube and podcasts and the decline of blogs seems to point that way. The popularity and usability of many of the free web resources stands in stark contrast to some of the electronic resources for which libraries are paying good money. Librarian and former provost James O'Donnell quipped in a panel presentation at the 2016 Charleston Library Conference (available for listening on podcast) that "the challenge of the things we now call e-books is that they aren't books, and they're only moderately 'e,' and they just plain don't work very well" (O'Donnell 2016). He went on to say that publishers might want to take note that the bootlegged PDF versions of textbooks seem to be a lot easier to use and access than the legitimate versions, so it is not just price that drives users to the bootlegged version. At that same conference, plenary speaker and university librarian emeritus James Neal predicted that by 2026 there would be no information industry targeting the library marketplace. Self-publishing would dominate, many resources would be open access and open source, and other content would be sold directly to consumers.

Lewis points out other changes in information resources that should cause both librarians and publishers to reconsider the future for traditional resources (Lewis 2016b, 15–18). Digital scholarly documents can have multiple versions, can be commented on by users, and can incorporate many types of media, data sets, and visualizations. The fluid nature of these materials will likely grow in the future and presents a challenge for libraries to control or preserve in traditional ways.

Customization of products and experiences is a very current trend in all of society, and it even extends to health care and discussions of the future for "personalized" or "precision" medicine. Artificial intelligence is a technology that is part of this trend, and many believe it will transform information resources as it is transforming many other sectors of society. Artificial intelligence (AI) involves computer programs functioning in such a way that they display what looks like human intelligence. The machine adjusts to the human, rather than the human adjusting to the machine.

This might mean that a point-of-care resource could become more capable of helping with diagnosis over time as health care professionals input data and refine the questions that they ask of it. Research literature databases could learn from an individual researcher's queries over time to adjust to that person's specific needs to identify (much better than they can today) exactly which newly published articles are of interest. An artificial intelligence expert and futurist, Jerry Kaplan says that "the essence of AI—indeed, the essence of intelligence—is the ability to make appropriate generalizations in a timely fashion based on limited data" (Kaplan 2016, 5).

In a way, it seems ludicrous to talk about some of the databases health sciences libraries subscribe to being able to learn and do intelligent searches for users when their search engines now are barely able to do basic keyword searches and return relevant results; that is where it is important to remember Brian Mathews's concept of considering diverse futures and the librarian's role in influencing what will come about. One interesting aspect that remains to be seen is how limited the data can be for AI to work. Medical subject headings (MeSH), created by humans at the National Library of Medicine and available freely to use, are currently an important part of the success of many of the "smart" search engines created by various companies for the medical literature. How much will expert librarian input (old-fashioned "bibliographic control") count versus non-expert user input for the development of the "smart" search engines of the future?

Constraints on Change

The above predictions represent different views and ideas about the future, some bolder than others. A realistic view of the future is perhaps that there will be major changes in format and distribution of information resources and that technology will very likely bring exciting new products that people today are unable to even dream of. What will be the successor to smart phones and tablets? It is impossible to tell. But, it is important to remember that technology is rarely as seamless, trouble-free, and "smart" as predicted.

Because technology exists in a world of humans, human concerns like money, power, politics, and prestige have to be taken into account. Companies are competing against each other and must focus on profitability and what's new, not necessarily on perfecting what already exists. Scholarly societies have to compete for their share of money to stay alive, and this affects their decisions about the publications they sell. Researchers and scholars, who create the health sciences information resources, are concerned with keeping their jobs, getting tenure, and progressing in their careers, which involves impressing colleagues and granting institutions with numerous prestigious publications. Students would like not to spend money on books. Health care institutions and universities are also very much concerned with their bottom lines, which can be affected by governments and the political concerns and values of those in power. And, finally, everyone in the industries involved (authors, graphic designers, managing editors, copyeditors, information technologists, programmers, educators, scientists, health care professionals, and librarians) would like a reasonable paycheck in exchange for their work. These are many of the day-to-day reasons why some recent envisioned transformative projects like the Google Book Project, Massive Open Online Courses (MOOCs), and open textbooks have fallen short of the "disruption" they were supposed to wreak on these industries (Gose 2017; Somers 2017; Hill 2016). In light of this, while it is interesting to entertain predictions that self-publishing, open-access, crowdsourced, and open educational resources will make health sciences collections obsolete, it seems highly unlikely that, in the future, large amounts of valuable health information will simply become free.

CONTINUING TRENDS AND CHALLENGES

So what about the future for health sciences collections in particular? In the spirit of Brian Mathews, multiple options for the future can be considered based on the trends discussed in this book: first, about the nature of information resources; second, about the nature of collections; and, finally, about how collection managers and other librarians will be interacting with the collections.

Nature of Health Sciences Information Resources

Scholarly journal publishing is still very much in flux, and it is difficult to predict where it will end up and how libraries will be affected. Will there be the large-scale transition of all scholarly journals to open access (OA) by 2020 as the international OA2020 initiative calls for and as envisioned by those who think libraries will no longer need to have collections (Max Planck Digital Library 2016a)? It is certainly one possibility that most scholarly publishing, particularly in the sciences and health sciences, will be open access in the future. But it seems equally, if not more, likely that this will not be the case.

The roadmap is fairly vague and assumes that libraries (at research institutions) will be the leaders (Max Planck Digital Library 2016b). But the system of research grants, publication, tenure, and university faculty reward is deeply conservative (especially in the life and medical sciences) and does not change quickly. Yes, the amount of open-access material has grown enormously, and that is a major change from the past. However, research is driven by grant money, and the power for change rests with grantors. While some grantors are requiring open-access publication, governments in many countries have compromised with publishers to allow embargoes, and this will likely continue.

Preprint servers like BioRxiv will grow in popularity, as younger scientists find them useful for fast dissemination of work (Cold Spring Harbor Laboratory 2017), but they are supplemental to formal publication and do not take its place. This doesn't mean that the concerns about the sustainability for library budgets of ever-rising journal prices for libraries will go away, but it has already been predicted that, for the sciences, 100 percent OA would not cost research libraries less. In fact, as discussed in chapter 3, it would likely cost more, and it is not any more sustainable than the present situation (University of California Libraries 2016).

Second, the gap between health sciences library budgets and the costs of library resources will probably continue to widen, and collection managers will be called upon to prioritize more than ever. For health sciences libraries, this is not just about research journals. The large-scale omnibus resources discussed in this book, the specialty databases for point-of-care or drug information, and the packages of medical e-books are challenging libraries just as much, if not even more, than journal subscriptions. Health sciences libraries are already starting to say "no" to some of these e-book packages and omnibus resources. At present, some publishers have found offering only package models for e-books to be lucrative. But that policy may backfire in the future. If enough libraries choose not to purchase an entire package in order to get access to one classic book, the readership of that book may start to diminish, and possibly its reputation in the field.

Medical and other health professional textbooks and educational resources are an area of publishing that is definitely being affected by the disruptive elements of the web that Lewis talks about. Furthermore, there has been a shift at many universities and medical schools away from requiring students to purchase textbooks and toward the expectation that libraries will provide the informational resources that students need. This has been an unprecedented opportunity for collaboration between librarians and faculty for guiding professional health sciences education into the future. However, publishers should take note that their pricing models may have an effect on which books, if any, get chosen for the next generations of students. Medical and nursing faculty have created some of their own curricular resources and open-source textbooks and, while there are concerns with the sustainability of the open textbook movement (Gose 2017), the movement toward open educational resources is one optional future. Students are choosing free, whether it is the web or library resources, and they are less and less likely to make individual purchases. No matter what happens with the medical and other clinical textbook market, it does seem clear that the vast array of clinical monographic material published every year by traditional publishers is not sustainable.

Of course publishers, too, are looking toward the future and trying to figure out how they can thrive in a new information environment and compete with free. At a 2006 symposium on the Research Library in the Twenty-First Century, Karen Hunter, a librarian and senior vice president at Elsevier at the time, said that the largest challenge facing scholarly publishers is to show return on investment in improving, adding features, and adding functionality to electronic products (Hunter, Waters, and Wilson 2010).

This is no doubt why electronic resources remain so disappointingly unusable, and James O'Donnell's criticisms of e-books resonate with most health sciences librarians. They are difficult to navigate, and they don't reflect how anyone (students, health care professionals, professors) would intuitively think they *should* be able to use them. The different designs, different file formats, and different terms of use are challenging, and the limitations placed on these books, presumably to keep users from posting them illegally, make them at times so unusable as to cause collection managers to wonder why they are spending money on them at all. Also, now that health college curricula are online, faculty want to integrate library e-book content into that curricula, but they are stymied by archaic licensing and terms of use. Databases, too, fall short of the goal of simple usability principles, not to mention accessibility for all library patrons. Most health sciences collection managers have the experience of learning about a new database, reading the promotional literature, and trialing it only to find it doesn't work very well to answer real-world information questions.

Librarians can sympathize with publishers that electronic resources present many challenges for sustainability, but it seems that there are two alternatives for the future. One is that vendors and publishers figure out how to invest in the improvement of their electronic products, develop standards among themselves, ease up on restrictions, and develop policies that truly open up these resources to support education. The other is that these resources become more irrelevant, as faculty members and students turn to other sources of information. The success of products with simple, but *effective*, interfaces (not to be confused with simple merely in appearance) will have to be a model for publishers to compete.

Following on this, in contrast to research publication and dissemination, which, as noted above, tends to follow time-honored traditions and is slow to change, publication of information resources to support patient care is showing rapid evolution. The wildly successful point-of-care tool UpToDate, among practicing health care professionals and their institutions, took many in the library and publishing worlds by surprise. Traditional publishers have responded by trying to capitalize on their existing classic textbook and/or journal content to create competing products, but one cannot put a search engine on traditional content and call it a point-of-care tool. UpToDate's success happened because its content was created specifically for its own purpose, and it provides an easy means for clinicians to access the exact information needed. Leaving aside questions of whether UpToDate is the best information resource, whether its pricing model is sustainable for institutions, or whether it is evidence-based, it seems clear that the future of clinical information looks more like UpToDate than like textbooks. What does this mean for health sciences libraries and publishers? Both may need to give up the idea of creating and collecting so many textbooks in all of the clinical subject areas. There is room for competition in this new market, but the competition will have to think outside the box of traditional publication.

Nature of Health Sciences Collections

As the nature of health sciences information resources changes, so will the nature of health sciences collections. Much has been written about the transformations that have taken place in the physical footprints of many health sciences library spaces (Lynn, FitzSimmons, and Robinson 2011). Health sciences libraries have been some of the first to give up the idea of ownership, although academic health sciences libraries still hold out for that ideal with e-journals and some e-books. But so much material is merely licensed, and health sciences libraries have already started substituting on-demand article purchasing for some journal subscriptions. Health sciences collections will likely be much smaller and more focused, especially when it comes to clinical material, much of which can be redundant.

Some of the proposals mentioned above for collection building in the face of budgetary pressures are possible options for health sciences libraries of all types. Anderson's suggestion that patron-driven models for journal article acquisition may be even more cost-effective than on-demand purchasing will be very attractive to some kinds of libraries. Certainly many librarians would welcome the opportunity to purchase clinical textbooks on demand rather than maintain pricey subscriptions. This may never become an option, however, unless there are larger changes to the books themselves or economic pressures on the publishers.

Collaboration and resource sharing are already deeply entrenched values for libraries, and that will not change in the future. But, as has been pointed out in various chapters of this book, inattention to restrictions imposed by licensing has hampered sharing of electronic resources among libraries. This is another area where librarians have the opportunity to shape their future. Many librarians have insisted on licenses that allow for interlibrary loan of e-journal articles and e-book chapters. If e-books evolve and become more usable (instead of more irrelevant), librarians should insist on being able to loan and borrow whole e-books just as they did printed books.

For libraries that are still interested in ownership and collection building, consortial licensing could be joined by consortial collaborative collection management. This is already taking place for legacy print collections, and the trend for libraries to cooperate to preserve and provide access to their print materials, while downsizing their individual collections, will continue in the near future. The development of shared print repositories means that fewer copies of the older materials will exist in the world, but libraries will be assured that enough copies are being preserved for future research.

With a few exceptions, the transformation of most health sciences libraries (academic and hospital/special) to electronic collections with only small physical collections on site will likely be complete within the next ten years. The approximately 126 libraries supporting medical schools that are members of the Association of Academic Health Sciences Libraries (AAHSL) have been reporting around 95–97 percent of their collection expenditure going toward electronic resources for the last five years (Squires 2015, 2016, 2017).

This may have hit a plateau. As noted in other chapters of this book, there has been pushback on electronic books, from people of all ages, and even some "born-digital" libraries like Western Michigan's (described in the story following chapter 1 in this book) have ended up purchasing small print collections at the request of users. Print will not likely go away completely for some kinds of books. But many of those same AAHSL libraries are also, as a group, in the middle of a mass deaccessioning of print materials (especially journal volumes now online) and movement of their older print collections to storage. The combined total number of volumes owned by all

AAHSL libraries has decreased from a high of over 33 million in 2006 to 22 million in 2016, and that number will probably continue to decline. The total number of volumes these libraries have stored remotely has steadily increased during that same ten-year period from 3 million to almost 6 million. Around 650,000 volumes went into storage between 2015 and 2016 alone.

The story in this book from Texas (see chapter 5) about building a shared print repository is potentially a look into the future for more health sciences libraries. In 2016, despite the trends above, less than half of the AAHSL libraries had any volumes stored remotely at all, and not all libraries have a remote facility available to them. As group efforts like MedPrint increase, it is likely that more libraries, and more different types of health sciences libraries, will be able to share remote collections. The next several years will be a unique period of time in which, ironically, collection managers and library staff spend more time with their print collections than they may have spent in years.

The logical next step from shared print repositories would be for these same cooperating libraries to coordinate print purchasing and collection development in the future. If some printed copies of classic texts are wanted, for use or preservation, perhaps only a few copies are needed per consortium. As mentioned above, collaborative collection management is being proposed at the consortial level. It remains to be seen whether librarians have the will to pursue this vision.

Future Collection Management Librarian Activities

One question that has not been addressed is who will manage the health sciences collection of the future. New generations of health sciences librarians are graduating without much training or experience in collection management or collections issues (Kendall and Monosoff-Richards 2015). One hope is that this book can serve as a resource for learning about the basics as well as the current issues that affect collections work. Perhaps it can spur interest in this fascinating aspect of librarianship. There has been a trend downward in the amount of professional FTE that even large academic health sciences libraries are devoting toward collection development responsibilities. Even though the mean number (around twelve to thirteen) of professional staff that work in the health sciences libraries that are members of AAHSL did not change from 2006 to 2016, the mean number of professionals dedicated to collection development activities decreased during that time period from 0.85 (median 0.70) to 0.60 (median 0.5) (AAHSL 2017).

While aspects of the job are quite complicated, other aspects are being automated and some are being cut entirely. Perhaps some of the duties of collection managers are being farmed out to librarians with other titles: assessment librarians, electronic resource managers, liaison librarians, usability specialists, and scholarly communication librarians. Certainly this book has pointed out that many of those functions are important parts of collection management today. Nevertheless, with less time to spend on collections, collection managers will have to be even more strategic and intelligent about their activities to keep up the quality of collections that institutions will require.

What activities will the collection management librarians of the future be focused on? Collection assessment is one. There will be many decisions on bringing sustainability to library budgets, and institutional administrators will increasingly require data that shows the library providing value. Demonstrating value is a larger societal trend for all the sectors that health sciences libraries serve: health care, higher education, and research. Toward that end, librarians have been questioning the kinds of statistics that they gather for some years now.

For example, to measure collections-related elements, the AAHSL statistics report yearly volume counts, title counts, circulation, expenditures, and occasionally staffing (by library activity) and lists of key subscribed resources. Having consistent data over time is helpful for showing trends, and several of the authors of chapters in this book have used AAHSL data to demonstrate the radical changes that have occurred with health sciences libraries' collections. But many complain that none of this data demonstrates impact. Impact is extremely hard to measure, though, and is individual to each institution.

One proposed, seemingly "easy" way of showing the value of the library is high usage of library resources. However, this author was a member of the AAHSL Committee on Assessment and Statistics during a time when electronic resource usage was proposed and trialed as a measured data point. It was not successful. It turns out that electronic usage statistics across multiple institutions, even of the same resource, are not very meaningful and are very time-consuming to compile. Furthermore, David Lewis cautions against libraries trying to provide numbers that demonstrate "value of return on investment" (Lewis 2016b, 90). He says that libraries are a "commons infrastructure," like parks or bridges, for which that type of analysis is usually impossible.

It is true that the outcomes librarians hope to assess, like student learning, better patient care, and successfully funded grants, are removed from the kinds of statistics that are possible to collect. If the future is indeed about showing impact, librarians will have to find means other than statistics of demonstrating that at their institutions. Perhaps storytelling will be the answer instead of hard data: showing the money saved by students and residents, for example, when the library provides medical textbooks; having a faculty member report how much a data set provided by the library has raised the quality of her grant proposal, or publicizing how a subscription resource has helped a clinician make a diagnosis.

A focus on discovery will continue to be important for health sciences collection managers of the future. This is contrary to both Anja Smit and Lorcan Dempsey, cited above, who have both told librarians to forget about discovery. (Dempsey says to focus on discoverability of one's locally created collections instead.) But health sciences resources, particularly those for patient care, are more varied than the journals and monographs that make up the majority of resources for other subject areas, and they are not necessarily found through a Google search. A Google search also won't point a library user to the version of a medical textbook that is licensed by the library. Librarians and vendors have been working on increasing discovery of electronic collections for quite a while, but there still is no seamless way to bring all of the information resources together into one place that users can learn to access on their own. Perhaps more standards for interoperability will help solve this problem in the future. The future will involve meeting users where they are (physically and mentally) rather than expecting them to make a special effort to seek out the electronic library and adjust to its demands, and artificial intelligence will help make the resources more personalized. The integration of information resources into electronic health records is a start in this direction, but the usability of both the resources and the electronic health records themselves needs work. Lindbergh and Humphrey's vision of the seamless health sciences library for 2015 will need to be extended some more years. Collection managers in the future will be collaborating closely with discovery and metadata librarians, liaison librarians, and programming and web design librarians to help create and customize these systems.

Another key aspect of collection management will be preservation for the future of collections in all kinds of formats: print, digital, audio-visual, and data sets. Since this chapter is looking toward the future, it is worth considering what primary source materials about such topics as the state of the art of health care from the twenty-first century will be available to historians in, say, the twenty-second century, when such resources as ClinicalKey, UpToDate, and AccessMedicine are long gone. Collection managers at academic health sciences libraries, along with their counterparts for the other disciplines, are currently spending a lot of time on preserving printed content from the nineteenth and twentieth centuries in collaborative repositories. This paper material, representing the not-so-distant past, seems to have the most secure future out of all the formats listed above even if, as pointed out in chapter 9, it is not always very organized.

The ephemeral nature of electronic resources, whether owned physical formats such as DVD or CD-ROM, websites, or electronic internet resources housed on a publisher's server, presents a large problem that librarians are only just beginning to tackle. A few libraries (such as the National Library of

Medicine) are preserving some data and information from websites. But it is still very little. Preserving local data through data management programs will also be part of that challenge. And, for materials that reside on publisher sites, librarians are only able to encourage publishers to use such services as Portico and LOCKSS (discussed in chapter 1) for preservation of materials. Collection managers will not have to think about preservation alone. Many academic research libraries are hiring digital preservation specialists and data management librarians, as these are young and growing fields. These are also fields that consortia are talking about for collaboration.

CONCLUSION

Mathews has said that "as a profession, librarians are obsessed with talking about our future" (Mathews 2014). He thinks it is more important to focus on factors driving change in society and in the communities libraries serve and with which they partner. The goal of this chapter and of this entire book has been to point out these factors in the areas of education, health care, and scholarship, and to highlight what effects current changes are having on collections. There are common threads running through all of the predictions and continuing trends discussed above. These are sustainability (for budgets, collection size, scholarly publishing, and staff time), the wisdom of collaboration and sharing at all levels, a need to demonstrate the value and relevance of library collections for the intended user communities, and the expectation by users that the resources libraries present to them will be easy to use and personalized for their needs. Furthermore, while the technologies being discussed change radically, it has been noted that the challenges identified for the future for health sciences librarians remain quite consistent over time because they are based on values rather than the specifics of one place and time. In 2014, the American Library Association established the Center for the Future of Libraries (http://ala.org/libraryofthefuture/). Miguel Figueroa, its director, has said that

> [o]ne of the biggest lessons my colleagues and I have learned while developing the Center for the Future of Libraries is that studying change is useless without considering values. As we bring together our observations of change with the constancy of our values, we can begin to exert influence. We can learn which trends advance our work and which might challenge our work. (Figueroa 2017)

This has been the second goal of the discussion in this chapter and this book. Health sciences librarians can specifically look to the Medical Library Association Code of Ethics for Health Sciences Librarianship (MLA 2010) for a list of librarian values as they apply to the health sciences field. Each trend and change to health sciences collections that has been discussed here must be evaluated and debated in light of whether it helps promote informed decision making in health care, research, and education; promotes access to health information for all; maintains conditions of freedom of inquiry, thought, and expression; and protects the privacy and confidentiality of clients. Collection management librarians and other librarians working with various aspects of the collections will see a great deal of change during their careers, much of which is impossible to predict, but, with these values and goals in mind, they will be able to nudge and guide the decisions of the publishing world, their libraries, and their larger institutions toward a fuller realization of a future in line with those goals.

REFERENCES

AAHSL (Association of Academic Health Sciences Libraries). 2017. *Annual Statistics of Medical School Libraries in the United States and Canada: Descriptive Library Surveys (2006–2016)*. Association of Academic Health Sciences Libraries, accessed May 12. http://aahsl.ccr.buffalo.edu/.

Anderson, Rick. 2016. "The Road Ahead? Patron-Driven Acquisition Might Become . . ." (Panel Presentation at the 2016 Charleston Conference). *ATGThePodcast* (podcast). Against the Grain. http://atgthepodcast.libsyn.com/podcast/atgtp-005-patron-driven-acquisition.

Ardley, Neil. 1981. *School, Work, and Play*. New York: Franklin Watts.

Big Ten Academic Alliance. 2017. "Library Initiatives." Big Ten Academic Alliance, accessed May 19. https://www.btaa.org/projects/library/home.

Clapp, Verner W. 1964. *The Future of the Research Library*. Urbana, IL: University of Illinois Press.

Clement, Susanne K., and Karen S. Fischer. 2014. "Introduction to the Special Issue 'We're Moving, Please Pardon Our Dust': Transformative Changes in Collection Management." *Collection Management* 39 (2/3): 53–59. doi:10.1080/01462679.2014.914418.

Cold Spring Harbor Laboratory. 2017. "About bioRxiv." Cold Spring Harbor Laboratory, accessed May 11. http://biorxiv.org/about-biorxiv.

Dempsey, Lorcan. 2016. "The Facilitated Collection." *Lorcan Dempsey's Weblog* (blog), January 31. http://orweblog.oclc.org/towards-the-facilitated-collection/.

Dempsey, Lorcan, Constance Malpas, and Brian Lavoie. 2014. "Collection Directions: The Evolution of Library Collections and Collecting." *portal: Libraries and the Academy* 14 (3): 393–423.

Elmer-Dewitt, Philip, and David S. Jackson. 1994. "Battle for the Soul of the Internet [cover story]." *Time*, July 25, 50–56.

Figueroa, Miguel. 2017. "Our Futures in Times of Change." *American Libraries* 48 (3/4): 32–37.

Gose, Ben. 2017. "Growing Pains Begin to Emerge in Open-Textbook Movement." *The Chronicle of Higher Education*, April 14, B12–B13.

Hazen, Dan. 2011. "Lost in the Cloud: Research Library Collections and Community in the Digital Age." *Library Resources & Technical Services* 55 (4): 195–204. doi:10.5860/lrts.55n4.195.

Hill, Phil. 2016. "MOOCs Are Dead: Long Live Online Higher Education." *The Chronicle of Higher Education*. http://www.chronicle.com/article/MOOCs-Are-Dead-Long-Live/237569.

Hunter, Karen, Donald Waters, and Lizabeth Wilson. 2010. "Panel 3: Into the Glass Darkly: Future Directions in the 21st Century." In *The Research Library in the 21st Century* (Proceedings of The Research Library in the 21st Century Symposium, Sept. 11–12, 2006), edited by Douglas Barnett and Fred M. Heath, 66–86. New York: Routledge.

Jarvis, Christy, Joan M. Gregory, and Jean P. Shipman. 2014. "Books to Bytes at the Speed of Light: A Rapid Health Sciences Collection Transformation." *Collection Management* 39 (2/3): 60–76. doi:10.1080/01462679.2014.910150.

Johnson, Peggy. 2009. *Fundamentals of Collection Development and Management.* 2nd ed. Chicago: American Library Association.

Kaplan, Jerry. 2016. *Artificial Intelligence What Everyone Needs to Know.* New York: Oxford University Press.

Kendall, Susan K., and Mari Monosoff-Richards. 2015. "Training a New Librarian in the What, How, Where, and Why of Health Sciences Collection Management." *Proceedings of the Charleston Library Conference*: 147–54. doi:10.5703/1288284316246.

Lancaster, F. W. 1994. "Collection Development in the Year 2025." In *Recruiting, Educating, and Training Librarians for Collection Development*, edited by Peggy Johnson and Sheila S. Intner, 215–29. Westport, CT: Greenwood Press.

Lewis, David W. 2016a. "Force One: Disruption." In *Reimagining the Academic Library*, 3–12. Lanham, MD: Rowman & Littlefield.

———. 2016b. *Reimagining the Academic Library.* Lanham, MD: Rowman & Littlefield.

Lynn, Valerie A., Marie FitzSimmons, and Cynthia K. Robinson. 2011. "Special Report: Symposium on Transformational Change in Health Sciences Libraries: Space, Collections, and Roles." *Journal of the Medical Library Association* 99 (1): 82–87. doi:10.3163/1536-5050.99.1.014.

Mathews, Brian. 2014. "Librarian as Futurist: Changing the Way Libraries Think about the Future." *portal: Libraries and the Academy* 14 (3): 453–62. doi:10.1353/pla.2014.0019.

Max Planck Digital Library. 2016a. "Open Access 2020." Max Planck Digital Library. https://oa2020.org.

———. 2016b. "OA2020 Roadmap." Max Planck Digital Library, last modified October 26. https://oa2020.org/roadmap/.

MLA (Medical Library Association). 2010. "Code of Ethics for Health Sciences Librarianship." Medical Library Association. http://www.mlanet.org/page/code-of-ethics.

O'Donnell, James. 2016. "The Evolution of E-Books" (Panel Presentation at the 2016 Charleston Conference). *ATGthePodcast* (podcast). Against the Grain. http://atgthepodcast.libsyn.com/podcast/against-the-grain-the-podcast-008-the-evolution-of-e-books.

Richards, Daniel T., and Dottie Eakin. 1997. "Research Questions and Future Issues in Collection Development." In *Collection Development and Assessment in Health Sciences Libraries*, 225–36. Lanham, MD: Scarecrow Press.

Smit, Anja. 2016. "Views from the Penthouse Suite, Interview by Erin Gallagher and Matthew Ismail, November 16." *ATGthePodcast* (podcast). Against the Grain.

Somers, James. 2017. "Torching the Modern-Day Library of Alexandria." *The Atlantic.* https://www.theatlantic.com/technology/archive/2017/04/the-tragedy-of-google-books/523320/.

Squires, Steven J., ed. 2015. *Annual Statistics of Medical School Libraries in the United States and Canada, 2013–2014.* 37th ed. Seattle, WA: Association of Academic Health Sciences Libraries.

———, ed. 2016. *Annual Statistics of Medical School Libraries in the United States and Canada, 2014–2015.* 38th ed. Seattle, WA: Association of Academic Health Sciences Libraries.

———, ed. 2017. *Annual Statistics of Medical School Libraries in the United States and Canada, 2015–2016.* 39th ed. Seattle, WA: Association of Academic Health Sciences Libraries.

University of California Libraries. 2016. "Pay It Forward: Investigating a Sustainable Model of Open Access Article Processing Charges for Large North American Research Institutions." Mellon Foundation. http://icis.ucdavis.edu/wp-content/uploads/2016/07/UC-Pay-It-Forward-Final-Report.rev_.7.18.16.pdf.

Way, Doug. 2017. "Transforming Monograph Collections with a Model of Collections as a Service." *portal: Libraries and the Academy* 17 (2): 283–94. doi:10.1353/pla.2017.0017.

Index

Contributors

Bruce Abbott, MLS, is a medical librarian at the Blaisdell Medical Library, which serves the University of California Davis Health System in Sacramento, California. There he is liaison to the School of Nursing and the UC Davis Hospital's Patient Care Services Department; his expertise is in online searching, collection development, and electronic resource management. He received his MLS from Louisiana State University.

Nancy G. Burford is the veterinary collections curator at Texas A&M University Medical Sciences Library. She is an associate professor within the Texas A&M University Libraries faculty and has worked at the Medical Sciences Library for over thirty years. Her primary responsibilities from 2001 through 2011 were with the current collections and included collection development, acquisitions, cataloging, and collection evaluation. Burford actively participated in a regional collection development group for a number of years. Most recently she provided leadership for decisions and operations in moving half of the current collections to remote storage. Since 2012 her focus has been on the development of the historical veterinary research collection, a unique collection dating from the sixteenth through the early twentieth century, and consisting of over six thousand print and manuscript items and over three thousand artifacts.

Esther E. Carrigan, MLS, is the associate dean and director of the Texas A&M University Medical Sciences Library. Carrigan holds the rank of professor, is currently the Mary and James Crawley '47 Endowed Professor, and is a distinguished member of the Academy of Health Information Professionals of the Medical Library Association. She has held numerous leadership positions in the Veterinary Medical Libraries Section of the Medical Library

Association. She is the recipient of the Texas A&M University Association of Former Students Distinguished Librarianship Award (2004) and the Louise Darling Medal for Distinguished Achievement in Collection Development in the Health Sciences, awarded by the Medical Library Association (2007). Carrigan was a member of the author team that was awarded the Daniel T. Richards Prize for Best Published Article on Collection Development in the Health Sciences by the Collection Development Section of the Medical Library Association (2011). She received her master's of library science degree from the State University of New York at Buffalo and is a frequent presenter at regional, national, and international conferences. She has authored numerous articles and book chapters, and has served as editor of two monographs. Her research interests include collection development, library assessment, and trends in veterinary libraries.

Joseph A. Costello, MSIS, is an informationist at Western Michigan University Homer Stryker M.D. School of Medicine in Kalamazoo, Michigan. His background includes combat veteran, poetry editor, library information services technician, and telecommunication infrastructure technician. He provides instruction and service in the fields of evidence-based medicine, health literacy, advanced searching, and critical analysis of scientific literature. Costello's research interest is at the intersection of narrative analysis, trauma, and motivation. He has a BBA in telecommunications and information management from Western Michigan University and an MS in information studies from the University of Texas, Austin.

Lisa Federer, MLIS, MA, currently serves as research data informationist at the National Institutes of Health Library, where she provides training and support in the management, organization, sharing, and reuse of biomedical research data. She is the author of several peer-reviewed articles and the editor of *The Medical Library Association Guide to Data Management for Librarians*. She also blogs about data science and data librarianship at www.librarianinthecity.com. She holds a master's of library and information science from the University of California, Los Angeles, and graduate certificates in data science (Georgetown University) and data visualization (New York University), and she is a doctoral student at the University of Maryland.

Stephen J. Greenberg, MSLS, PhD, received his doctorate in early modern history from Fordham University with a dissertation on early printing and publishing. After teaching for several years, he returned to school and earned his library degree from Columbia University, specializing in rare books and archival management. Since 1992, he has worked in the History of Medicine Division at the National Library of Medicine, where he is currently head of the Rare Books and Manuscripts Section. His research and publications span several fields, including the history of printing and publishing, the history of medical librarianship, and the history of medical photography. He is a past chair of the Medical Library Association (MLA) History of the Health Sciences Section and past president of Archivists and Librarians in the History of the Health Sciences (ALHHS). He has lectured and taught nationwide through such groups as the NIH Speaker's Bureau, the Medical Library Association's Continuing Education Program, and Rare Book School at the University of Virginia. Dr. Greenberg is the recipient of numerous awards, including the ALHHS Publication Award (2011) and National Institutes of Health Award of Merit in 2013. Dr. Greenberg is also an adjunct professor at both the Catholic University of America and the College of Library and Information Studies at the University of Maryland (College Park), where he lectures on the history of the book.

Joseph J. Harzbecker, Jr., MS(LS), MA, AHIP, is the head of Reference and Electronic Collections Management at the Boston University Medical Center, Alumni Medical Library, Boston, Massachusetts. He received his MA in history from the University of Massachusetts, Boston; MS(LS) in library science from Simmons College, Boston, Massachusetts; BA in history and political science from Drew University, Madison, New Jersey; and an academic fellowship in history from the Graduate Center, City University of New York (CUNY). He also holds a Certificate of Librarianship from the Commonwealth of Massachusetts, Board of Library Commissioners. He manages a reference department staff of six librarians who provide information services to the Boston University, Boston Medical Center, and Boston Library Consortium communities. He also participates in the libraries' educational activities with the schools of dentistry, medicine, graduate program, and public health. He has been managing collections for the health sciences for twenty years and collaborates with other librarians throughout the Boston University campuses regarding reference and electronic collections, specifically planning, development maintenance, and purchasing. He has held committee appointments in the Medical Library Association and has also been professionally active in the American Library Association, Association of College and Research Libraries, Massachusetts Health Sciences Library Network (MaHSLIN), North Atlantic Health Sciences Libraries, Inc. (NAHSL), and the Freedom to Read Foundation.

Emma Cryer Heet, MA, MSLS, is the associate director of Collections Services at the Duke University Medical Center Library and Archives, Durham, North Carolina. She received her MS in library science from the University of North Carolina at Chapel Hill. At the Duke Medical Center Library she leads the Departments of Technical Services, Access Services, ILL, and Collections. She has managed library collections for the biomedical sciences at Duke for eight years. She has held leadership positions in the Collection Development Section of the Medical Library Association and been active professionally in the American Library Association and the North American Serials Interest Group. She has published several articles on scholarly communication and collections topics.

Iris Kovar-Gough, MA, MLIS, is the liaison librarian to the College of Human Medicine at the Michigan State University Libraries, East Lansing, Michigan. She received both her MA in classical archaeology and her MLIS from the University of British Columbia, Vancouver, BC, Canada. She has worked as a health sciences librarian at Michigan State University since 2014 supporting medical school curriculum development, teaching, and research needs, and has done collection development for clinical medicine since 2016. Kovar-Gough is professionally active at the state and national levels in health sciences library organizations and is a member of the Association of Academic Health Sciences Libraries Task Force Evaluating Association of American Medical Colleges Core Entrustable Professional Activities. She has published articles with medical school faculty and has also published and presented on various topics in health sciences librarianship.

Elizabeth R. Lorbeer, EdM, MLS, AHIP, began her role as the founding library director at Western Michigan University Homer Stryker M.D. School of Medicine in 2013. Lorbeer's career spans over twenty years as a librarian and education administrator. She previously held positions at Boston University, Rush University Medical Center, the State University of New York at Buffalo, and the University of Alabama at Birmingham. She has held leadership positions in the Collection Development Section of the Medical Library Association, and she has been the principal investigator for three National Network of Libraries of Medicine Express Library Digitization Award grants and the recipient of the Association of Academic Health Sciences Libraries Leadership Scholarship. She speaks and publishes on topics such as digital scholarship, collection management, and publisher-vendor-library relationships. She regularly consults for publishers and vendors and is a distinguished member of the Academy of Health Information Professionals. She holds the rank of associate professor and is the chair of the Department of the Medical Library. Lorbeer attained her master's in library sciences from State University of New York at Buffalo. She then completed a master's of education in higher education administration at Boston University.

Sarah McClung, MIS, is the collection development librarian at the University of California, San Francisco (UCSF). She received her BA in English from the University of Mary Washington in Fredericksburg, Virginia, and her MS in information sciences from the University of Tennessee, Knoxville.

She has worked in academic health sciences libraries for nine years, and in her current role, she oversees the overall development and management of the UCSF Library's extensive collections. She has held leadership positions in the Northern California and Nevada Medical Library Group and the Librarians Association of the University of California. Additionally, she has presented nationally at numerous library conferences and volunteers for the Oakland Public Library.

Rikke Sarah Ogawa, MLIS, is the team leader for Research, Instruction, and Collection Services at the UCLA Louise M. Darling Biomedical Library. At UCLA Library, she leads a team of four librarians who provide instructional, consultation, and advanced research support services to UCLA's health and life sciences communities. She has been the liaison for medical school curriculum (at both UCLA and Stanford University) for seventeen years and has coordinated collections for the health and life sciences for five years. She has held various leadership positions in the Medical Library Association, including member of the board of directors, chair of the Educational Media and Technologies Section, and various task force memberships.

T. Scott Plutchak, MA(LS), is director of Digital Data Curation Strategies at the University of Alabama at Birmingham (UAB). In that capacity he works with units throughout the university to develop institutional policies and services for the management and curation of research data. From 1995 to 2014 he was the director of UAB's Lister Hill Library of the Health Sciences. He received his MA in library science from the University of Wisconsin, Oshkosh, in 1983, and was a postgraduate library associate fellow at the U.S. National Library of Medicine. From 1999 through 2005 he was the editor of the *Journal of the Medical Library Association (JMLA)*, and he serves on editorial boards for *The Journal of eScience Librarianship*, *JMLA*, and *The BMJ*. He is a founding member of the Chicago Collaborative, a group dedicated to finding common ground among the librarian, publisher, and editorial communities. In 2009 he was a member of the Scholarly Publishing Roundtable, which submitted a report to the U.S. Congress in January 2010 with recommendations on providing public access to federally funded research results. He is a frequent speaker to publisher and library groups on topics ranging from intellectual property to scholarly communication to the future of librarianship.

Heidi M. Schroeder, MLIS, is the accessibility coordinator and science collections coordinator at the Michigan State University Libraries in East Lansing, Michigan. She received her master's in library and information science from Wayne State University, concentrating in health sciences librarianship. At the Michigan State University Libraries, Schroeder currently coordinates and oversees all library accessibility initiatives and leads a team of six librarians who provide information services to the university's science colleges/departments. Previously, she served as the nursing librarian and managed the nursing collection at the MSU Libraries and has held leadership positions in the Nursing and Allied Health Resources Section of the Medical Library Association and the Michigan Health Sciences Libraries Association. She has presented numerous times on the accessibility of library e-resources and was instrumental in the creation and charge of the Big Ten Academic Alliance Library E-Resource Accessibility Group.

Jessica Shira Sender, MLS, MET, is a health sciences librarian and liaison for the College of Nursing and the Department of Communicative Sciences and Disorders at the Michigan State University Libraries in East Lansing, Michigan. She received her master's in library science from Indiana University and her master's in educational technology from Boise State University. Previously she held positions as instructional technology and information literacy librarian at the Michigan State University Libraries and instructional technology librarian at Guilford College in Greensboro, North Carolina. She has been active in the American Library Association, chairing the Committee on Literacy, and was an Emerging Leader in 2011. She has also held leadership positions with ALA's New Members Round Table and the Association of College and Research Libraries, and is an active member of the Nursing and Allied Health Resources Section of the Medical Library Association.

Steven W. Sowards, PhD, MLS, is the associate director for collections at the Michigan State University Libraries, East Lansing, Michigan. He received his PhD in history as well as his MLS from Indiana University, Bloomington. At the Michigan State University Libraries he is responsible for overall direction of collection development and management, including budgeting and license approval, and for the work performed by subject liaison librarians serving all parts of the campus. He has been in this role for twelve years, after previously serving as head of reference for the Michigan State University Libraries and as a reference librarian in liberal arts college libraries. He has been professionally active in the American Library Association and served on editorial boards for the journal *Library Hi Tech* and ALA's *Guide to Reference*. He has written a variety of articles and numerous book reviews.

Kathleen Strube, MLS, is the director of library services for Aurora Health Care, Inc., a not-for-profit integrated health care system in eastern Wisconsin and northern Illinois. She received her BA in history from the University of California, Los Angeles, and her MLS from the University of Missouri, Columbia. With Aurora Health Care for twenty-five years, she leads a team of ten librarians, four library assistants, and an intern who work in seven hospital libraries. Strube's start as a reference librarian and her interest in having great online information resources led her to start a consortium to leverage lower prices for online journals. The Aurora Libraries are known for their high-quality reference and embedded librarian work, and for "lots" of journals on their library website. They also manage subscriptions for the whole organization and have an institutional repository. Strube has published various articles over her career, mainly in *Medical Reference Services Quarterly* and *Journal of Hospital Librarianship*.

Susan E. Swogger, MLIS, is the librarian liaison for the College of Graduate Health Studies and the Missouri School of Dentistry and Oral Health at the A.T. Still University in Kirksville, Missouri. She received her MLIS and an Endorsement of Specialization in the Design and Structure of Digital Resources from the University of Texas at Austin in 2002. She was previously collections development librarian at the University of North Carolina at Chapel Hill's Health Sciences Library and has held leadership positions in the Collection Development Section of the Medical Library Association. She is an editor of the most recent edition of the widely used textbook *Introduction to Reference Sources in the Health Sciences*, is subject editor for the Health Sciences and Medicine section for ALA's *Resources for College Libraries*, and has published a number of book chapters, articles, and reviews.

Ana G. Ugaz, MLIS, is the collection development and strategic initiatives coordinator at Texas A&M University Medical Sciences Library. She received her bachelor of science in nutrition and dietetics from the University of Texas at Austin and her master of library and information science from Dominican University. Ugaz has been working in resources management since 2004, researching and writing on topics related to her lead role in collection development, assessment, and management of health sciences and veterinary medicine collections at the Medical Sciences Library. She is an associate professor within the Texas A&M University Libraries and is a senior member in the Medical Library Association's Academy of Health Information Professionals.

Linda A. Van Keuren, MLS, AHIP, is the associate director for resources and access management at Dahlgren Memorial Library, Georgetown University Medical Center. She has a master's in library science from the University of Pittsburgh and an undergraduate degree from Carnegie Mellon University. In her position, she acquires and manages the resources that comprise the Dahlgren Memorial Library collections. She also supervises the library's access and delivery services to ensure that high-quality resources are readily available in support of academic, clinical, and research missions of the Georgetown University Medical Center. Prior to her appointment at Georgetown, she was the systems manager at Grace Library, Carlow University in Pittsburgh, Pennsylvania, as well as adjunct faculty, Department of Management, and was awarded the Adjunct Excellence in Undergraduate Teaching Award. She is an active member of the Medical Library Association and the Academy of Health Information Professionals.

About the Editor

Susan K. Kendall, PhD, MS(LIS), is the coordinator for health sciences at the Michigan State University Libraries, East Lansing, Michigan. She received her PhD in cell and molecular biology from the University of Michigan, Ann Arbor, and her MS in library and information science from the University of Illinois, Urbana-Champaign. At the Michigan State University Libraries, she leads a team of five librarians who provide information services to the university's health colleges. She has managed collections for the biological sciences for fifteen years and coordinated collections for the health sciences for eleven years. She has held leadership positions in the Collection Development Section of the Medical Library Association and been active professionally in the Special Libraries Association and the Association of Academic Health Sciences Libraries. She has served on the editorial board of the journals *Collection Management*, *Journal of the Medical Library Association*, and *Biomedical Digital Libraries* and has published several book chapters, articles, and reviews.

Lightning Source UK Ltd.
Milton Keynes UK
UKHW012333050619
343834UK00006B/226/P

9 781442 274211